Choices in
RECOVERY

27 Non-drug Approaches for
Adult Mental Health

An Evidence-Based Guide

Choices in
RECOVERY

27 Non-drug Approaches for Adult Mental Health

An Evidence-Based Guide

For those with mental health issues
and their loved-ones

CRAIG WAGNER

Onward Mental Health

Onward Mental Health Press
South Lyon, Michigan USA
www.OnwardMentalHealth.com
Printed in the United States of America
Library of Congress Cataloging-in-Publication Data
Choices in Recovery, Non-drug Approaches to Adult Mental Health, an Evidence-Based Guide 1st ed. 1.7.2019
Includes bibliographical references and index.
ISBN: 978-0-9966080-0-8
eISBN: 978-0-9966080-1-5
   1. Psychiatry, 2. Mental Illness – Alternative Treatments
Wagner, Craig 1954-

Cover Design by Marty Somberg - www.SombergDesign.com

Pay it forward. To make this information available to those who need it, we provide free or steeply discounted books to those in financial hardship and to nonprofits who will use the book for education. To gain access to and support this effort, see www.OnwardMentalHealth.com.

Author. Contact Craig@OnwardMentalHealth.com.

For Batchawana
Only love, fully love, always love

Contents

Preface

My large extended family has witnessed mental health issues up close and personal. Frankly, too close and too personal.

We have experienced the dramatic mood swings of bipolar, the disembodied voices and delusions of schizophrenia, the black dog of depression, the spiral of alcoholism, the gripping fear of phobias, and the last resort of suicide attempts. We have faced the difficulties of withdrawal from antidepressants and the indignities of being forced into psychiatric care against our will. We have seen dramatic turnarounds to recovery. And we have seen relapses.

We have many stories. Each is owned by a single person who experienced these difficulties and who courageously fought to overcome them. Each story is very personal and will be told or kept private by the person at its center. I honor that ownership and decision to maintain privacy.

But I also have a story. I entered the world of mental health out of necessity. It wasn't a career choice, but a survival instinct when a loved one experienced a mental health crisis. For our entire family, the experience was painful, confusing, frightening, and disempowering.

To make sense of what we were going through, I connected with the local affiliate of the National Alliance on Mental Illness (NAMI). I enrolled in their education class taught by volunteers who faced similar difficulties. Our class learned the basics of mental health and were given a good dose of pragmatic advice and warm, supportive companionship. What especially caught my attention was the wide-ranging presentation on non-drug approaches. They seemed to hold great promise. A seed of interest had been planted. It drove me to systematically research this new world of alternative treatments.

I decided to start at a trusted place: medical journals. Although at first a bit daunted, I picked up their vocabulary and research methods quickly enough, reading everything I could find about non-drug options. All the while, I jotted notes and ideas. I realized that a vast range of non-drug options was available and the extent of research supporting them was staggering. Soon my notes coalesced into a paper that I shared with interested NAMI volunteers, and later in public conferences.

But something was gnawing at me. If these medical journals were accurate, why wasn't I hearing about non-drug options from psychiatrists?

In the space of thirty minutes, I posed that question to two psychiatrists who worked at one of America's leading hospitals. I was interested in calibrating my new-found knowledge about mental health issues with people extensively trained and actively practicing in the field.

First, I spoke with a smart and engaging psychiatrist who had recently finished his medical internship. I was interested in how the positive research on nutrient therapy was being used to improve clinical care. The newly minted psychiatrist made his position clear: taking supplements posed possible drug-interaction issues. He said it was important to stop the vitamins and other supplements unless there was a clear medical reason for taking them. He obviously viewed vitamins and nutrients as having little benefit. In fact, he viewed them as potentially detrimental to the true solution: drugs.

I walked away feeling embarrassed. Maybe I hadn't understood those medical journals all that well. But then I recalled the many studies documenting the benefits of nutrients both alone and with drugs. Regaining a bit of confidence, I set off for my next conversation.

The head of the psychiatric department was waiting for me, a man with decades of clinical experience and front-line mental health management. He smiled and invited me into a meeting room. After introductions, I asked him about recent studies that had received notoriety in the medical press, including a prominent blog by the Director of the National Institute of Mental Health.

The studies' findings were startling: antipsychotics (drugs taken for schizophrenia and other disorders) appeared to do more harm than good in the long run. People who used them had *more* hallucinations than those who didn't. Plus, their brains physically shrank in proportion to the amount of antipsychotics consumed. These findings seemed to shake the very core of recommended care for psychosis. I wanted to know what to make of these conclusions. Trying not to be intimidated by his degrees and expertise, I posed my question.

The answer I received stunned me.

He was unfamiliar with the studies. The head of a world-renowned psychiatric department was unfamiliar with the studies.

For a moment, I sat speechless. When I regained my composure, I forced out a few more questions, to which he gave insightful responses. But my mind was elsewhere. We soon exchanged pleasantries and I departed, feeling stunned.

And I continued to feel stunned. Yes, I could forgive anyone for missing one study in thousands that stream through their inbox. But this wasn't just one insignificant study. It was a bright yellow caution sign held aloft by the head of the American agency coordinating all mental health research.

As I stood rooted to the floor, a familiar feeling started to come over me. After spending years in business, I knew the sensation: inertia. It seems to infiltrate all large organizations. Even when individuals know better, the machine they are a part of often doesn't. The status quo changes slowly, even when compelling, peer-reviewed, scientifically-calibrated and well publicized studies point in a better direction.

In that moment, this book was born.

I had searched long enough to know that a comprehensive layman's guide to the full breadth of non-drug treatments didn't exist. So, I decided I had better write one.

My goal was to answer one question: What are my best options? But before I started, I wanted to check to see if others believed that was the correct question.

I turned to leaders and lay people in the mental health field for wisdom.

United Nations Secretary-General Ban Ki-moon, in speaking about the global health crisis of depression, urges:

[We need] an international effort to increase access to a wide variety of effective and affordable treatments.[1]

Dr. Barbara Van Dahlen, a psychologist who founded Give an Hour, a non-profit group that pairs volunteer mental-health professionals with recently returned U.S. war veterans, says:

We want suffering veterans to understand that feeling better is possible.... We need options for mental health care, traditional and alternative approaches that are readily available and easily accessible.[2]

Monica Cassani, a mental health activist who has seen the system from both sides, as a social worker and a person with a mental health diagnosis, writes:

The idea behind all of my advocacy around mental health [is that] we need [to make] a smorgasbord of options available.[3]

Finally, a man I will call Andrew G offered the perspective of someone who has seen more than a dozen mental health specialists in an attempt to recover from his issues:

We learn from listening to consumers... Consumers should be presented with many options from which to choose. Options provide hope, and hope—in many cases—is the only force that has the ability to sustain someone struggling with mental health issues.[4]

These sentiments echo a recurring theme, an urgent plea, and a critical need in the field of mental health: **people need options**.

This plea arises from the fact that the most prevalent conventional option involves psychiatric drugs (also known as psychotropics), which rarely offer a completely acceptable answer. In some cases, they work very well. But often they only reduce the severity of some symptoms while leaving others untouched. And far too often they introduce a dizzying and distressing array of side effects.

Fortunately, many non-drug approaches can be used with psychotropics—or in place of them. In some cases, these approaches target underlying causes of mental health symptoms and can legitimately be called cures. In others, non-drug approaches can provide substantial and prolonged symptom relief as good as, or better than, what psychotropics offer, and with minimal or no side effects. Still other approaches can reduce symptoms so that lower doses of psychotropics are needed. The message is loud and clear: *substantial scientific findings support using non-drug options.*

We are drowning in a sea of information about mental health, thanks to the internet. But often it raises more questions than it answers. So many competing claims from so many sources espouse so many perspectives with so many agendas. It's hard to make sense of the masses of sometimes conflicting advice.

I bring two primary skills to this roiling sea: information management and communication. My academic background and career have required unearthing, evaluating, synthesizing, distilling, and communicating information—separating the wheat from the chaff, differentiating the hyperbole from the truth, making the complex understandable, and making the important compelling.

I applied these skills to the work of brilliant psychiatrists and researchers who have already navigated and charted portions of this sea. I am significantly indebted to them for their many valuable maps. My goal was to stitch together and harmonize these maps for people with mental health issues and their loved ones. This job required overlaying maps from opposite sides of the world regarding illness and wellness, science and humanity, pragmatism and hope. In the process, I've discarded medical jargon when it wasn't necessary and translated critical information I believe can help you or your loved one recover.

My priority is to present non-drug approaches with sound scientific evidence. In fact, the summary of *Most Promising Therapies* found in Chapter 8 offers approaches in an order based on the strength of evidence regarding their effectiveness.

I strove to make this information balanced, easy to understand, and prudent. I have tried to avoid overstating the benefits or risks of any approach. I tried to create a logical structure and context for the enormous quantity of information. Most importantly, this book attempts to make information comprehensible, actionable, and useful.

Believing that we all need options, this information is more complete than brief. People with mental health issues need a great deal of information about their treatment options.[5] This book isn't *the* answer to the question *What should I do?* as much as it is a menu and roadmap to help you create your answer to the question "What *will* I do?"

The field is constantly evolving. What I offer isn't bullet-proof because few easy answers exist. I'm not offering shocking new discoveries. But I am offering the first book I've seen that attempts to present the full breadth of proven non-drug approaches to mental health, extracted from the bowels of clinical research and translated into a usable and empowering tool for those who need a path to recovery.

And in writing this book, I found more than scientific methods to recovery. I also found tremendous hope.

I want to be clear on an important point: what I offer isn't an invitation to self-diagnosis or self-treatment. Nor is it an invitation to quickly abandon psychotropics. Instead, *Choices in Recovery* presents the broad array of non-drug options so that psychotropics can be correctly viewed as one potential piece of a much larger puzzle.

This book is intended to inspire hope from the experiences of many people who live in recovery. I invite you to explore non-drug modalities and identify any that can help you. And I urge you to trust yourself enough to lead your own recovery, within the context of a team. Ultimately, accepting this personal responsibility becomes an "Ah-ha!" moment, both a turning point and a burst of energy that helps propel you on your journey to wellness.

This book is a place to start and a potential light on your path of recovery.

I have a simple premise.

Mental health recovery can be achieved through a courageous individual process of prudent experimentation. The likelihood of success skyrockets when the process is grounded in self-determination, fueled by hope, assisted by talented practitioners and caring supporters, and enabled by non-drug options validated by science–where the golden nuggets, warts, and any unknowns are clearly stated.

This book is based in respect for all who engage in the mental health struggle: those with mental health issues, their families, mental health professionals, researchers, teachers, and communities.

In writing this book, I sought to make available a resource that would have helped and encouraged me and my family members many years ago. I hope that it will help and encourage you right now.

Onward,

Craig Wagner

Introduction

This book is for those with mental health issues and their loved-ones. It can help you understand, select, and use non-drug options as part of your individualized mental health recovery plan.

Structure

Chapter 1 introduces the significant paradigm shift in psychiatry that is underway. It explores the motivations and forces behind this shift, which is ushering in an expansive new set of solutions for mental wellness.

Chapter 2 focuses on the concept of mental health recovery. It outlines the stages of recovery; reviews the attitudes, knowledge, and skills needed to create recovery; and emphasizes the importance of self-determination and experimentation, which are at the root of recovery. It also introduces the overarching framework for the many non-drug options of recovery.

Chapters 3-7 contain an overview of each of the 27 broad non-drug approaches, offering a quick understanding of the options. These include therapies from conventional Western psychiatry and from a variety of traditional medicine systems. Each approach is then subdivided into individual therapies, along with summaries of the most compelling medical evidence supporting them. Endnotes provide internet links.

Information on each non-drug approach is consistent, providing:

- *Essence* – an overview of the approach
- *Evidence* – key studies that show that the approach is effective
- *Considerations* – things to keep in mind if you choose to use the approach
- *Real World Experience* – case studies and practitioner stories of success
- *Resources* – links to additional information and tools

Chapter 8 distills and prioritizes the non-drug options down to a short-list of those most promising for seven different mental health diagnoses: ***depression, schizophrenia, bipolar, anxiety, dementia, substance abuse,*** and ***insomnia.*** These lists are laid out simply; each is only about five pages long, enough to give a quick view of the full breadth of non-drug options. They are organized by the stage of recovery in which each is most beneficial. *All are linked to earlier parts of the book, where the options are presented in more detail.*

Chapter 9 takes readers beyond the elimination of mental illness to the creation of mental well-being. Personal growth and mental health recovery fit into a broader framework of wellness.

Appendices cover biomedical lab testing protocols; directories of practitioners and resources; and much more.

To make this book easier to use, references to parts of the mental health framework are italicized and capitalized (for example, *Wellness Basics*). Detailed discussions are placed in starred endnotes (for example, "PTSD[*36*]"), in an effort to streamline the themes. I tried to minimize use of medical jargon, to improve readability. Hundreds of links lead to the original studies.

Grounding

This book is evidence-based, grounded in approaches that have been validated in well-designed studies that have withstood the scrutiny of peer review. Although black-and-white definitions clarify whether something is evidence-based or not,[*6*] to be realistic, we must consider evidence on a sliding scale – a spectrum ranging from very strong to very weak. Randomized Controlled Trials (RCT, see *Glossary*, p. 337) are often the best place to start, since they offer strong validity. My information is grounded overwhelmingly in RCTs. At the same time, we need to consider less robust evidence, since many people recover using approaches that are not strongly evidence-based.[7]

I've added case studies, to give a dose of humanity to the clinical data. Stories and quotes are paraphrased to convey the essence of the message.

Source material

Thousands of clinical trials form the basis of my primary research; most are Randomized Controlled Trials. Other trial designs are used in cases where more rigorous trials are unethical, impractical, or unavailable.

Secondary research summarizes and analyzes the work of primary researchers. I focused on meta-analyses that reveal meaningful statistical patterns across similar studies. Secondary research includes:

Cochrane Collaboration,[8] arguably the leading and most rigorous source of medical research summaries.

Psychosocial Research Summaries. I carefully considered recommendations from psychological associations in the United States,[9] Canada,[10] the United Kingdom,[11] and Australia.[12]

Guidelines, texts, practice recommendations, and therapy summaries. The World Health Organization,[13] American Psychiatric Association,[14] Brown,[15] Fredrick,[778] Lake,[16, 17, 18] Walsh,[19] Stradford,[20] Sarris,[21] Zessin,[22, 23] Mental Health America[24] are my sources. I also include summaries for schizophrenia,[25] bipolar,[26] and post-traumatic stress disorder.[27]

Integrated Web Resources

www.OnwardMentalHealth.com is a companion to *Choices in Recovery*. It features many web-based tools including infographics, monographs, self-help tools and more. Web updates occur quarterly. This includes online updates to many of the appendices in this book. We encourage you to use and share the wealth of information available at the site.

Acknowledgments

It takes a village. Many friends and colleagues have provided tremendous help to improve this book and make it available to those in need.

First, I am greatly indebted to two friends who believed in the book and who tirelessly labored with me in its boiler room. My ever-optimistic editor Cindy Furlong Reynolds wielded a keen understanding of the English language and a sharp machete in the face of my tendency for completeness over brevity. Researcher and author Dion Zessin poured over the clinical detail and provided scores of references, case studies, personal observations and ideas that significantly strengthened the book's evidence-base.

Many thanks to Emma Bragdon, PhD, founder and Executive Director of Integrative Mental Health for You (www.IMHU.org) for her detailed guidance on improving this book; to Bob Nassauer, mental health advocate, educator and National Alliance on Mental Illness (NAMI) volunteer for his early review of the material and his pragmatic mental health efforts in Michigan; to Kurt Scholler, instructor and mental health advocate for his initial introduction to non-drug treatments; and to Penney Acosta, NAMI education coordinator for inviting me to deliver the non-drug message as an adjunct to local NAMI training programs.

Also, thanks to alternative mental health organizations that have helped me bring the message to a broader audience: the American Psychiatric Association's Caucus on Complementary, Alternative and Integrative Medicine and its leader Dr. Lila Massoumi, for the opportunity to help share the non-drug message with U.S. psychiatrics; Safe Harbor (www.AlternativeMentalHealth.com), and its president and founder Dan Stradford, for giving me the chance to participate as Executive Director; the Mad in America community of contrarians (www.MadInAmerica.com) and its fearless leader Robert Whitaker, for inviting me onto their blogging team; and the Washtenaw County Michigan NAMI affiliate (www.NAMIWC.org) and its many dedicated volunteers for helping me in my time of need and for allowing me to include the essence of this book in their public conferences.

Additionally, thanks to Dr. William Shaw, PhD, Director of Great Plains Laboratory (www.GreatPlainsLaboratory.com) for his extensive mental health test panels; and to Dr. Ray Pataracchia, an Orthomolecular medical professional of the Naturopathic Medical Research Clinic (www.nmrc.ca), for his detail on his testing protocol and content contribution.

From a creative perspective, many thanks to Marty Somberg for his graphic design expertise and keen sense of color that resulted in the cover design. Also, thanks for select infographic templates designed by Freepik.

Finally love and thanks to my dear wife, Kristin, for her support and partnership, infectious optimism and continuous outpouring of kindness; and to our wonderful children, Lance and Tess, who continue to sustain me.

1 – Mental Health Care in Transition

This book introduces scores of non-drug options for adult mental health.

It describes them, categorizes them, provides evidence that they work, suggests when they might be helpful, and assists in identifying practitioners who can skillfully administer them. It also provides many resources to help you use them, and an important caution you should read now (See *Disclaimer,* p. iv).

If you want to immediately jump into the detail of the therapies, skip this preamble, turn to Chapter 8, and find the section on your particular diagnosis. You will find a summary of the most promising therapies you should consider, distilled from the many options this book discusses. But, at some point, come back here for context to help you navigate today's world of psychiatry, which can be overwhelming.

The crux of the situation is this:

Mental health care is undergoing a critical paradigm shift driven by the serious risks and limitations of today's psychiatric drugs. The emerging paradigm – *Integrative Mental Health* **– accepts drug therapy when needed but asserts that non-drug options strongly supported by scientific evidence are vital. The shift holds tremendous promise for those with mental health issues.**

Figure 1 (p. 20) offers a birds-eye view of this paradigm shift, comparing conventional psychiatry to the emerging field of *Integrative Mental Health.*

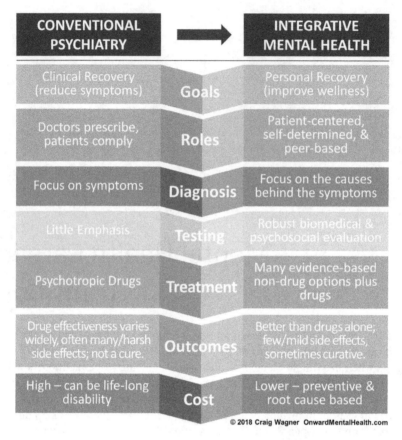

CONVENTIONAL PSYCHIATRY	➡	INTEGRATIVE MENTAL HEALTH
Clinical Recovery (reduce symptoms)	**Goals**	Personal Recovery (improve wellness)
Doctors prescribe, patients comply	**Roles**	Patient-centered, self-determined, & peer-based
Focus on symptoms	**Diagnosis**	Focus on the causes behind the symptoms
Little Emphasis	**Testing**	Robust biomedical & psychosocial evaluation
Psychotropic Drugs	**Treatment**	Many evidence-based non-drug options plus drugs
Drug effectiveness varies widely, often many/harsh side effects; not a cure.	**Outcomes**	Better than drugs alone; few/mild side effects, sometimes curative.
High – can be life-long disability	**Cost**	Lower – preventive & root cause based

© 2018 Craig Wagner OnwardMentalHealth.com

Figure 1- Psychiatry in Transition

The need for this paradigm shift is evident worldwide. A United Nations report calls for "urgent" change and advises us to "abandon the predominant medical model" of conventional psychiatry.[28] Thankfully, change is being driven by groups within and outside of the mental health profession.

Within the profession, clinicians and researchers are proving the value of expanded treatment options. Some approaches strike at the core of known causes of mental health issues with therapeutic programs customized to a person's individual blood chemistry and circumstances. Others are borrowed from non-Western medicine and psychology. Many practitioners are championing the expansion of therapeutic options, seeing the mounting evidence of the limited effectiveness and significant risks and limitations of psychiatric drugs.

The growing movement outside the profession includes people who have experienced recovery first-hand. They value the clinical science, but add a strong dose of humanity, emphasizing the dignity, empathy, and self-determination needed for mental healing. Understanding the sometimes debilitating side effects of psychotropics and stigmas, they believe that recovery is much more than symptom relief; it must also involve personal growth and change. They seek a broad range of therapeutic options to facilitate this change. This group's perspective is often called the *Recovery Model*.

Together, these groups are revolutionizing mental health practice.[29]

Changes in Grounding

There is an extraordinarily important difference between conventional psychiatry and *Integrative Mental Health*. This difference influences how their respective practitioners spend their consultation time; how they test, diagnose and treat; and ultimately, how much positive impact they help create. In many ways, this difference is the reason behind the limited effectiveness of conventional psychiatry and the significant momentum behind the paradigm shift to *Integrative Mental Health*. The difference is this:

Unlike nearly every other branch of medicine, conventional psychiatry is grounded in providing *uniform* solutions (very similar treatment for everyone) based on *symptoms*. Other medical disciplines, including *Integrative Mental Health*, are grounded in providing *unique* solutions (customized for each individual) based on *causes*.

An example is helpful. Consider people who come to the doctor with abdominal pain. There can be any number of causes: a broken rib, food poisoning, a urinary tract infection, appendicitis, and many more. Each possible cause requires a radically different treatment. Although we can expect to see broad symptom improvement if all of these people are given pain-killers, we cannot expect healing if pain-killers are the only form of care.

Conventional psychiatry is much akin to dispensing pain-killers for abdominal pain. It gives a uniform set of treatments to people with similar symptoms with little search for underlying causes. Although conventional psychiatry can sometimes provide great value in symptom reduction, it is generally incapable of healing. As a counterpoint, forward-looking psychiatrists are using *Integrative Mental Health* to test, analyze, and probe the body, mind, and emotions of each person individually, looking for causes, knowing that if healing is to occur, it must be grounded in the best possible understanding of exactly what is wrong.

This shift to cause-based care is an incredibly promising evolution in psychiatry, made possible by extensive gold-standard research that has uncovered many treatable causes and influencers of mental health symptoms.

Changes in Diagnosis

The causes of mental health issues are varied and can be difficult to detect. As a result, most conventional psychiatrists focus on understanding, categorizing, and relieving symptoms. The drugs they prescribe aren't considered a cure, but a means to manage symptoms.

Integrative Mental Health practitioners readily admit there is much we *don't* understand about the causes of mental health issues, but they focus on the many causes and influencers we *do* know. Figure 2 identifies some of the major factors directly associated with mental health issues. Sometimes their combined weight can "break the camel's back" and lead to psychiatric crisis.

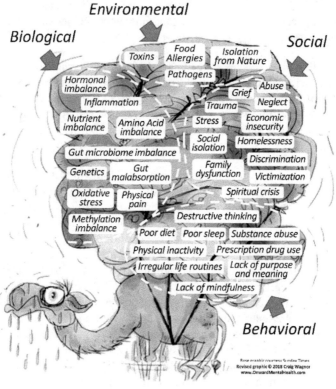

Figure 2 – Factors in the "web of causation" of mental distress

Integrative Mental Health practitioners use a common-sense approach: they systematically check for these many causes and influencers and treat those found. They know that everyone's constellation of factors is different, and these factors constantly interact in a dynamic web of causation where the line between cause and effect becomes blurred. Their appreciation of this complexity leads them to use individualized combinations of therapies to target each person's unique situation. It also leads them away from the simplistic model of conventional psychiatry that often discounts multi-factor causation and usually offers only a single one-size-fits-all solution: drugs.

This more exhaustive and insightful paradigm opens new doors to recovery. In some cases, it fully eliminates symptoms—to the point where drugs become unnecessary. In most other cases, symptoms are reduced, often significantly, so that smaller drug doses (with fewer associated side effects) can be used.

To understand how this plays out, consider the differential diagnosis process – the detective work practitioners use to determine an individual's specific disorder or disease. The DSM-5 (see Glossary, p. 337) is the "diagnostic bible" of psychiatry in the United States. Although psychiatrists and other practitioners passionately debate the DSM-5's validity and usefulness,[1556] it does provide a clear six-step process for differential diagnosis.[30]

Unfortunately, having a clear process doesn't mean it is used properly. Dr. Michael First, the DSM-5 editor, notes that diagnostic shortcuts are often taken:

> *There is a tendency to come up with a diagnosis in 30 seconds based on the gestalt [of the situation]...We call that 'premature closure,' and the problem is that you close your mind off to other possibilities....*[31]

Premature closure is much like a detective charging a suspect without collecting proper evidence. In conventional psychiatry, the problem is often an inadequate search for evidence in step three of the diagnostic process, when medical conditions and psychosocial stressors[32] are evaluated. It is in this critical step that First indicates, "the treatment implications are potentially profound".[33] Many *Integrative Mental Health* practitioners avoid premature conclusions by shifting into overdrive during step three. They use comprehensive *Biomedical Test Panels* (p. 323), full psychosocial assessments, and other methods to identify potential underlying issues.

The American Psychiatric Association (APA) shares this passion for detailed diagnostics and strongly encourages psychiatrists to use them. Its "Choosing Wisely" campaign emphasizes the critical importance of a "thorough assessment of possible underlying causes of target symptoms, including general medical, psychiatric, environmental, or psychosocial problems."[1454]

In the past, lab testing played only a peripheral role in the diagnosis and treatment of mental health concerns,[34] due to many factors: crushing demands on overworked practitioners; concern over the cost of diagnostic testing; the failure of medical schools to teach alternative therapies; and many market forces.

But increasingly, *Integrative Mental Health* practitioners are conducting rigorous testing to seek the root causes of symptoms, so they can better help people toward sustainable wellness. It is important to choose practitioners willing to undertake this more thorough approach. (See *Integrative Biomedical Practitioner Finder*, p. 320.) Your recovery may well depend on it.

Changes in Treatment

Conventional psychiatry relies almost exclusively on psychotropic drugs to relieve symptoms and increase a patient's ability to function. *Integrative Mental Health* practitioners, however, use a broad set of evidence-based options including drugs. Many of these non-drug options are considered ***Complementary and Alternative Medicine*** (CAM) since they can be used with (complementary), or instead of (alternative), conventional Western psychiatry.

Nutrition is beginning to take center stage in this new paradigm. The International Society for Nutritional Psychiatry Research notes, "Nutrition and nutraceuticals should now be considered as mainstream elements of psychiatric practice, with research (and)…policy reflecting this new paradigm." [35]

Increasingly, psychiatrists are aligning with *Integrative Mental Health* and are joining the APA caucus on Complementary, Integrative, and Alternative Medicine to share best practices.[36, 37] *Integrative Mental Health Organizations* (see p. 341) are also expanding the breadth of recovery approaches.

But, before we go into detail on non-drug options, **we need to discuss the benefits and downsides of psychotropics.** First, the **benefits**.

- **Psychotropics can save lives.** Especially in cases of violent behavior, potential suicide, and extreme breaks with reality, they can stabilize crises.
- **Psychotropics provide symptom relief.** Many studies conclude that psychotropics relieve symptoms of mental distress. Although, relief is very often only partial, it can sometimes be substantial.
- **Psychotropics are widely available.**[38] They are commonly prescribed and widely available. Although some are very expensive without insurance, they are covered under most medical insurance prescription plans.
- **Psychotropics require little effort.** It is as easy as swallowing a pill. Time-release injections are also available when consistently taking pills is an issue.
- **Psychotropics can help people cope.** Some people consider them indispensable,[39] providing normalcy and relief. They activate the placebo effect and may provide additional symptom relief. This can create a receptive state to consider non-drug options that often help create sustainable wellness.

But **psychiatric drugs come with serious risks and limitations.**
- **Psychotropic drugs do not cure**[40] **and rarely fully relieve symptoms.** Drugs are rarely a complete answer. Half of people with depression have unresolved symptoms even after taking antidepressants.[41] More troubling, antidepressants work only slightly better than placebo (sugar pills), with the benefit so small that it may not be noticeable.[42, 43] An FDA executive flatly observes, "we all agree… the difference between [antidepressants] and placebo is rather small".[44] For schizophrenia, antipsychotics "have substantial limitations in their effectiveness;"[45] most people continue to experience persistent functional impairment while on antipsychotics.[46, 127]

- **The short-term side effects of psychotropic drugs can be substantial**. These drugs are powerful and often have adverse effects so pronounced that many people stop taking their medications.[47] Psychotropics can cause negative neurological, cognitive, metabolic, sexual, endocrine, sedative, and cardiovascular side effects.[127] Antidepressants have startlingly frequent side effects[48] and some significantly increase the risk of birth defects.[49] These serious side effects prompted the FDA to issue a black box warning – the most serious type of warning for prescription drugs – on all antidepressants as well as all 1st and 2nd generation antipsychotics.[50, 51]

- **The long-term use of some psychotropic drugs can be debilitating**. Yet long-term use is common. For schizophrenia, the past Director of the National Institute of Mental Health indicates[52] that antipsychotics appear to *worsen* the chance of long-term recovery[53] and may impede wellness.[54] A twenty-year study found that unmedicated schizophrenia patients had significantly *less* psychosis than those taking antipsychotics.[55] The long-term use of antipsychotics is linked to brain shrinkage–the larger the dosages, the greater the shrinkage.[56]

- **Psychotropics can *cause* mental health symptoms.** In fact, they can cause the very symptoms they attempt to relieve: hallucinations, panic, delusions, suicidal thoughts/behavior, mania, psychosis, anxiety, hysteria, depression, and violent behavior.[57] One-third of people using the antipsychotic clozapine develop or worsen obsessive-compulsive disorder (OCD) symptoms.[58] Taking anti-anxiety benzodiazepines for six months almost doubles the risk of developing Alzheimer's.[59] Veterans taking psychotropics for PTSD are at significantly increased risk of later developing dementia.[1555] Taking antidepressants triples the likelihood of later developing mania.[60]

- **Psychotropics do not address underlying medical issues that often cause mental health issues.** Over one-quarter of people with mental health issues have an underlying physical issue that causes or exacerbates their mental disorder.[61, 62] For lower socioeconomic status individuals, the figure approaches one-half.[63] Psychotropics aren't designed to address these underlying physical issues, so relying exclusively on them impedes recovery.

- **Psychotropics do not address underlying trauma, stress and unhelpful thinking that often cause mental health issues.** The ravages of war and sexual abuse, the experiences of trauma, the cumulative impact of stress, and the knots of destructive thinking are at the core of many mental health issues. Drugs may be able to take the edge off, but they don't resolve these issues.

- **Psychotropics are often not rigorously tested for the diagnoses for which they are prescribed.** [64] Increasingly[65] they are prescribed "off-label" in ways not evaluated by the FDA. Although legal, this prescribing practice is poorly supported by evidence. See *Off-Label* & *Polypharmacy* Risk (p. 263).

- **Withdrawal from psychotropic drugs can be very difficult.** Stopping use often results in withdrawal symptoms..[66] In fact, Allen Frances, the DSM-4 committee chair, says, "Often the withdrawal problems are worse than the original condition."[67] Typically, the longer you take meds, the more difficult the withdrawal.[68] Benzodiazepine withdrawal is life-threatening and is so common it is labeled a "syndrome".[69] Regrettably, psychiatrists have little literature[68, 70] and training[71] in drug withdrawal, even though most psychotropics have withdrawal symptoms.[72]

- **Psychotropics rarely deliver recovery.**[73] Most people find a combination of therapies that include non-drug approaches works best for recovery.[74]

Putting drug limitations in a visual context helps us understand the size and extent of the challenges in their use. First, consider antidepressants (Figure 3).

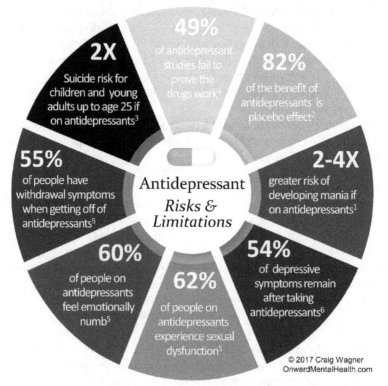

Figure 3 - Limitations of antidepressants
(See supporting studies[75])

Significant limitations are also found with antipsychotics (Figure 4, p. 27), the most common drug for schizophrenia, and benzodiazepines (Figure 5, p. 28), often used for anxiety.

These limitations are well-supported with evidence. They also represent a significant wake-up call to exercise great caution when considering psychiatric drugs and a strong incentive to search for a more complete solution.

Non-drug approaches paint a very different picture.

- **Non-drug approaches are helping deliver mental health recovery today.** Integrative Mental Health practitioners are helping many people dramatically improve their lives. Open-label trials show that over 70% of people who receive *Nutrient Therapy* (p. 167) see substantial symptom improvement across a spectrum of diagnoses including schizophrenia, bipolar, depression, anxiety and autism.[19] Thousands of gold-standard trials support the use of non-drug options.

- **Psychological non-drug options often work better than drugs.** For depression, *Cognitive Behavioral Therapy* (p. 117) works better than antidepressants.[76] In addition, psychological approaches are as effective as, or superior to, psychotropics for anxiety; significantly better for obsessive-compulsive disorder; preferred for post-traumatic stress disorder; and helpful in avoiding bipolar relapse.[10] These therapies don't have the side effects of psychotropics. Despite this compelling evidence, people rarely receive psychological therapy.[77]

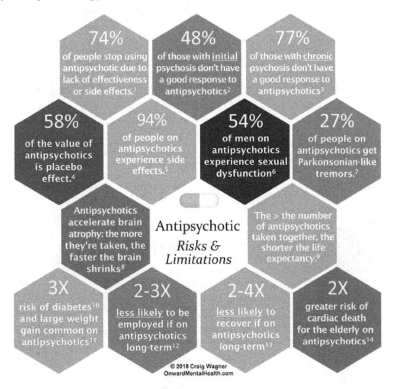

Figure 4 - Limitations of antipsychotics
(see supporting studies[78])

- **Non-drug treatments have far fewer and milder side effects than drugs.** [16] Their safety should encourage us to prudently experiment with them under a practitioner's care.[15]
- **Many non-drug approaches precisely target potential causes of mental health issues.** Robust biomedical and psychological evaluation can help identify the most appropriate non-drug approaches. NAMI, indicates that psychotropics have "buckshot"[79] accuracy, whereas *Nutrient Therapy* has the potential for "rifle-shot precision."[19]
- **Mental health advocacy groups see value in non-drug therapies.** Looking at the evidence, NAMI's medical director says that psychotropics are rarely enough[80] and notes that many people report that a combination of treatments is most effective.[81] Both NAMI[82] and Mental Health America advocate select CAM treatments. "[I]n many cases, with a little experimentation, effective CAM treatments can be found."[24]

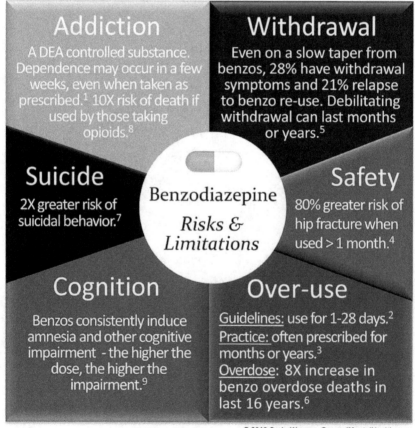

Addiction
A DEA controlled substance. Dependence may occur in a few weeks, even when taken as prescribed.[1] 10X risk of death if used by those taking opioids.[8]

Withdrawal
Even on a slow taper from benzos, 28% have withdrawal symptoms and 21% relapse to benzo re-use. Debilitating withdrawal can last months or years.[5]

Suicide
2X greater risk of suicidal behavior.[7]

Benzodiazepine
*Risks &
Limitations*

Safety
80% greater risk of hip fracture when used > 1 month.[4]

Cognition
Benzos consistently induce amnesia and other cognitive impairment - the higher the dose, the higher the impairment.[9]

Over-use
Guidelines: use for 1-28 days.[2]
Practice: often prescribed for months or years.[3]
Overdose: 8X increase in benzo overdose deaths in last 16 years.[6]

© 2018 Craig Wagner OnwardMentalHealth.com

Figure 5 - Limitations of benzodiazepines
(see supporting studies[83])

Psychiatric drugs remain an option and can provide significant symptom relief for some people. However, individual responses to drugs vary widely, and they have significant risks and limitations, while being only partially effective. This reality has spawned the formation of several organizations who seek to limit psychotropic drug use and help people withdraw from them (see p. 341).

Changes in Roles

Traditionally, psychiatrists evaluate the patient, offer a diagnosis, and recommend treatment (most often, psychotropics), expecting their patients to comply and take the prescribed drugs. Once treatment is underway, the most common psychiatric appointment is a fifteen-minute medication review.

But *Integrative Mental Health* shifts greater responsibility to the patient, emphasizing the importance of *self-determination* (p. 87) in recovery. Patients are expected to co-author and co-manage their recovery plans as much as possible. (See *Building your Recovery Plan*, p. 270.) With this greater control, patients are not only recipients of care, but co-creators of their own wellness.

In a coordinated effort with practitioners, *we must prudently experiment* with treatments in our recovery plan to see what works. There are no guarantees. Each individual situation is unique. When done with care and insight, *prudent* experimentation opens the doorway to recovery.

> **Failing to experiment with non-drug approaches is perhaps the largest single impediment to mental health recovery. Without investigating these proven techniques, we often accept a sizable and sometimes life-altering downside: resigning ourselves to limited symptom relief and possible significant drug side effects.**

There are many reasons why we should not only *participate* in non-drug therapy experimentation, but *lead* it.

- **Recovery requires experimentation. Experimentation is a cornerstone of psychiatry.** Significant research[98] shows recovery to be an active, individual process of experimentation.[16] In fact, the World Health Organization emphasizes that experimentation is *the* fundamental medical process.[84]
- **Conventional psychiatrists seldom experiment with non-drug treatments, so you must lead the effort.** Their biggest concern is malpractice liability[15,16] since non-drug treatments are not yet standard practice.[1465] Financials also play an important role. Psychiatrists often earn $150 for three fifteen-minute medication reviews and only $90 for forty-five-minute talk therapy sessions.[85] Additionally, psychiatrists often find new treatments are not easily integrated into their practice.[86]
- **Experimentation isn't a shot in the dark. Sound scientific research can guide experimentation.** Comprehensive lab tests and in-depth psychological assessments help target the best choices of non-drug treatments.

- **People who lead experimentation and make their own decisions have better outcomes.** Choosing your own therapies is an act of self-determination, a cornerstone of recovery. One study concluded that the ability to make therapy choices was the leading factor in good mental health outcomes.[87] The British Psychological Society underscores the importance of choice: "We need to stop telling people what to do and start supporting them to choose…Professionals need to acknowledge that the only way someone can find out for sure what helps them personally, is to try."[104]

- **You are not a statistic, so you must experiment to know what works for you.** Personal experimentation offers personal solutions. Proof that an approach worked for some people doesn't mean it will work for all. Likewise, an approach that shows statistically modest benefits for the general population may provide substantial benefits for an individual. The only way to know for sure is to experiment.

- **America's mental health system has proven unreliable in coordinating therapy experimentation, so you should lead it.** To evaluate recovery options, patients need to coordinate their recovery plan with psychiatrists, therapists, primary care physicians, and possibly specialists, since it is uncommon for practitioners to do this adequately.[1462]

- **New breakthrough drugs aren't expected, so non-drug experimentation is the best path to recovery.** Psychotropic drug research funding has been dramatically cut[88] while research in non-drug options is growing.

- **Limiting options is rarely a good idea.** A guiding concept in *Integrative Psychiatry* is to "leave no stone unturned."[15] According to one psychiatrist, "If the goal is to increase the quality of life…it doesn't make sense to limit one's self to either conventional or non-conventional treatment."[1465]

REAL-WORLD EXPERIENCE

Case Study 1 – Access to therapy information

Keris Jän Myrick is President of the National Alliance on Mental Illness, the largest mental health advocacy group in the U.S. She is also diagnosed with schizoaffective disorder.

"We are now finding that there are many things that contribute to one's recovery," she tells audiences. "I am a person who values what works for each individual in their recovery…We are all different!

"I believe each person should have as much information as possible, so they can make the decisions with their treatment team, families, and other supporters who will help them realize the meaningful lives of their dreams. I found the combination of interventions that allows me to lead the best possible life."[89]

Bottom Line*: Keris believes that self-determination and access to information on therapies is vital to help people create their own recovery plan. This book was written in that spirit.*

---

2 – The Art & Science of Recovery

What is Recovery?

For decades, that question has been debated by clinicians, researchers, and people with mental health issues. Although they have different perspectives,[90] their conclusions are finding common ground.

Not surprisingly, most medical professionals focus on *clinical recovery,* which emphasizes the relief of specific mental health symptoms. If their prescribed treatment significantly reduces or eliminates these symptoms, they decide their job is done: they have corrected what was wrong.

People suffering from mental health issues agree that *clinical recovery* is certainly important, but they often take a larger view.[91] They don't consider themselves passive recipients of treatment; they consider themselves active partners who help build, lead, and maintain their own recovery plan.[92] They are not just looking for outward intervention; they need something inward, something very personal. To them, recovery isn't just clinical. They want to launch a broader definition of wellness. Their recovery is *personal recovery.*

> [Personal recovery is] a process of change through which individuals improve their health and wellness, live a self-directed and fulfilling life,[1461] work toward a meaningful purpose, and create loving and supportive relationships,[91] even if some limitations persist.[93]

Why is this expanded definition of personal recovery important?

Because serious mental illness can do harm far beyond the mental health symptoms. It threatens our personhood and our sense of self, and therefore it can affect every facet of our lives[94] and the lives of those around us. Because the impact is that expansive, we need an expansive definition of recovery.

This book makes the following recommendations about recovery.

- **Seek personal recovery**. For enduring wellness, create meaning and positive relationships in addition to seeking clinical symptom relief.
- **Expect personal recovery**. A positive expectation can become a self-fulfilling prophecy, motivating us to do the hard work of recovery. People in mental distress who feel positive about their mental health, are much more likely to recover than those who don't, *even when they receive no treatment.*[95]
- **Look beyond drugs**. Psychiatric drugs alone can't deliver personal recovery because they only target symptoms. Non-drug approaches are necessary.
- **Own it**. Personal recovery only happens with a strong sense of self-determination. No one can recover for us. We must accept personal responsibility for our own wellness and make the many choices to create it.
- **Accept help**. Although self-determination is key, we shouldn't isolate ourselves. Involve practitioners who seek personal recovery and who have a demonstrated history of helping people realize it. Involve family and friends who will be positive and helpful.
- **Take it one step at a time**. Recovery is a process, not an event. Take steps toward recovery each day, no matter how small. Try new things. Experiment. Gain confidence in each step taken.

Even though we seek *personal recovery*, we must work within a mental health system that has predominantly been financed and structured to deliver *clinical recovery*. But, with creativity and perseverance, we can succeed.

Stages of Recovery

Personal recovery is a journey of growth and change. Signposts along the way help us stay oriented and offer a sense of accomplishment as we make progress. Be warned, though: this journey is seldom an overnight excursion. Instead, we proceed through five common stages,[96, *97*] often over months or years (Figure 6. p. 33).

Stage 1 - Distress.
Journeys often start with a sense of chaos and dependency. Sometimes a crisis triggers them, and we begin to feel a sense of denial, confusion, hopelessness, and withdrawal. We may feel that we've lost our self-identity.

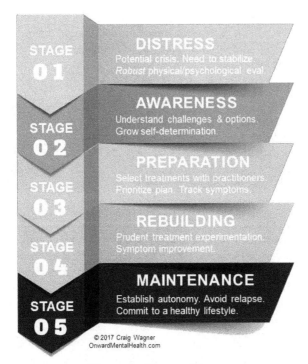

Figure 6 - Stages of Recovery

Stage 2 - Awareness.

We shift from distress to self-examination. We need to assess our personal strengths, weaknesses, needs, passions, and challenges. This is a time to rebuild our self-image. To move forward from this stage, it helps to adopt 3 perspectives:

- *A strong desire to change our situation.* This is often a desire to significantly improve or eliminate symptoms and rebuild our lives. It is a desire born in pain; a desire to alleviate that pain. This desire gives us incentive and motivation to do the hard work of recovery.
- *A belief that change is possible, even probable.* This isn't wishful thinking. It's pragmatic realism. We must acknowledge the fact that many people have already recovered, and there are many tools to help us do the same.
- *A commitment to the work needed for change.* This requires self-determination. We aren't "going it alone," although we do need confident self-leadership. We need to trust ourselves enough to step into uncharted territory. We also need the strength and humility to accept help.

When we accept the facts that we need to change, and that change requires work, we reach a turning point, from hopelessness to hopefulness. We are no longer dependent; we can navigate our route to recovery—with qualified help. We can now face the hard work ahead.

Stage 3 - Preparation.
We need to set goals, learn about recovery options and treatments, and be willing to experiment with different recovery techniques. We also need to connect with people who can help.

Stage 4 - Rebuilding.
Once we've prepared ourselves, the action begins. The rebuilding stage involves *doing*—working toward goals and actively managing the process of recovery. Although we'll be experimenting with approaches that have proven track records, we may face setbacks as we seek the best treatments for our own situation. Along the way, we need to work hard to solidify our relationships— with caregivers, friends, and family members. This stage requires resilience and independence.

Stage 5 - Maintenance.
This is the final stage of recovery, when we've reached a state of well-being. We have accepted who we are, and we have established autonomy, positive relationships, and a new sense of purpose. We make a commitment to sustain this state. Even if some mental health symptoms still exist, we know that we can live rich and meaningful lives, that we can actively respond to setbacks, and we can maintain a positive attitude about our future.

Although we have defined the stages of recovery, everyone's experience progressing through them is unique.[98] There is no cookie-cutter approach. The path to recovery can be unpredictable. We may reach periods of stagnation or abrupt change. Sometimes the struggle might seem overwhelming and the setbacks might seem daunting—but there can also be breakthroughs and a liberating sense of renewal if we persevere.

Each recovery stage comes with its own set of challenges and choices. We'll experience growing pains, false starts, and confusion. We'll make mistakes.*[107]* But, we'll also develop the ability to adjust and move forward when we face difficulties.

This book will help in each stage of the journey. But, a word of advice: using a technique in the wrong stage may be unproductive. To help select what is best for your current situation, look at tables of the *Most Promising Therapies* for each major mental health diagnosis found in Chapter 8.

The recovery journey offers few shortcuts. We must prepare ourselves for a voyage, not a jaunt. But, there are clear maps (see *Roadmap of Recovery*, p. 49) that mark the way, written in the sweat of thousands who faced similar challenges and recovered.

People of Recovery

Figure 7 identifies key people who can help in our recovery. Although we need a strong sense of personal self-determination, we must resist the urge to run solo. Many people can help, either actively or by their encouragement.

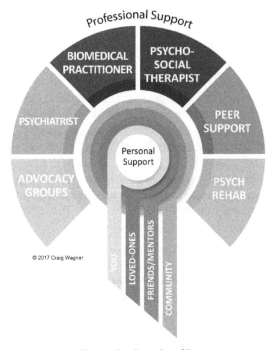

The inner portion of the diagram depicts personal support. It starts with "You" – the person with mental health issues. This person must always be the top priority. Your personal network then expands outward, from family, to friends, to your community. These people already know you and care about you and can be strong allies in recovery.

Figure 7 – People of Recovery

The outer portion of the diagram is professional support. It includes people with varied specialization, training and licensing. There is a tendency to regard the psychiatrist as the most important team member since they are doctors. However, it is best to consider them all to be peers—with each other and with you. Each brings a unique perspective, with some filling multiple roles. They have one job: to help you recover on your terms, and you should continually evaluate them on that basis. The major people involved in recovery are:

- *Biomedical Practitioners* focus on physical issues that may cause mental health symptoms. They run lab tests looking for things like thyroid disorders, nutrient imbalances, digestive issues, and much more. They also offer specific therapies to address whatever issues they find. Many different types of practitioners can fill this role. *See Integrative Biomedical Practitioner Finder* (p. 320) for more detail, and the directories to help you find one.

- *Psychosocial Therapists* focus on psychological development and how we relate to our world. They offer "talking therapy" and other ways to address past traumas, emotional difficulties, and unhelpful thinking. Psychologists and psychotherapists are examples. More broadly, a "therapist" specializes in any recovery approach including biofeedback, massage, acupuncture, etc.

- *Psychiatrists* are medical doctors that diagnosis and treat mental health issues. Conventional psychiatrists treat almost exclusively with drugs. Integrative psychiatrists can prescribe drugs but use a broader set of options.
- *Peer Support* (p. 131) is provided by people who have recovered from mental health issues. This "I've been there" support can be extremely valuable.
- *Psychiatric Rehabilitation* (PR) helps people function better in society, gain employment and housing, and improve their overall wellness. The Psychiatric Rehabilitation Association (www.uspra.org) is a major U.S. PR organization. PR workers have a variety of titles including case worker and social worker.
- *Advocacy Groups* offer information, training, and influence. Mad in America (www.MadinAmerica.com) is the largest online mental health forum. It seeks to rethink the drug-centered methods of psychiatry, fosters a variety of perspectives, and has excellent research analysis. Mental Health America (www.MentalHealthAmerica.net) and The National Alliance on Mental Illness (www.NAMI.org) are large U.S. advocacy groups predominantly aligned with conventional psychiatry.

In the U.S., *Community Mental Health* organizations bring a variety of these mental health professionals together. They typically offer psychotropics, case management, and psychosocial therapies. Access is limited, but people on Medicaid with severe mental health issues often can gain free services.

Finding the right professional support takes work.

Start with recommendations from people you trust. If you are out of crisis, look for an integrative biomedical practitioner and a psychotherapist. Both work to find and address underlying mental health issues. They can recommend a psychiatrist if drugs are needed. As you build your team, consider what set of *Wellness Continuum* therapies (Figure 9, p. 47) each is skilled in delivering.

But, do you really need three practitioners? Unfortunately, often the answer is "yes". Their perspectives and approaches differ; each has unique therapies to offer. Engaging all three helps expand the breadth of options to aid your recovery. The good news is that your private, Medicaid, or Medicare insurance often helps defray at least partial costs for all three.

Your insurance will play a large role in practitioner selection. Going "in-network" reduces your expenses but limits your choices. Going "out-of-network" gives you more options, at greater cost. Also, many doctors in private practice don't take insurance, which means you must pay up front and assume the risk of working with your insurance company for reimbursement. Perhaps the most painful reality is that there simply aren't enough mental health practitioners using non-drug treatments to satisfy demand.

Within these sizable constraints, be as selective as you can when choosing practitioners. Use *Questions To Ask Your Mental Health Practitioners* (p. 328) to help you decide if they are a good fit for you. Find people you trust, people with whom you can develop a rapport. Evidence indicates that a strong therapeutic alliance is especially critical for psychosocial therapies.[11]

Make sure the practitioners you choose expect you to recover. Research shows that people have better outcomes when they work with practitioners who share optimistic recovery expectations.[99] See Case Study 23 (p. 110) for a sense of the power of a positive therapeutic outlook.

You need to coordinate your practitioners, since they rarely do it for you. Keep a **documented recovery plan** giving a timeline of the therapies and drugs you have used, the changes in your symptoms resulting from their use, and a list of the therapies you would like to explore. Share it with all your practitioners.

Plan for mental health crisis so that you are prepared. Hospital rankings may not be a good indicator of patient-perceived quality, so contact local integrative mental health practitioners and people with diagnosis who have experienced the hospitals first hand. Also, research *Peer Respites* (p. 132). Too often psychiatric care in hospitals is impersonal; patients say they need the staff to treat them with more respect, talk to them, listen to them, and involve them in treatment decisions.[101] *Peer Respites*, though few in number, are an alternative designed to respond to these human needs in a less clinical setting. Also, learn about the assisted/involuntary treatment laws that may impose treatment on you.*.[100]*

Competencies of Recovery

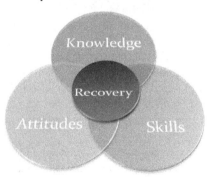

Figure 8 - Competencies of Recovery

The competencies of recovery (Figure 8) include *Attitudes*, *Knowledge*, and *Skills*. Our path to recovery will be much smoother when we develop these competencies.

Some apply more to those with mental health issues, others for their supporters, but all are valuable. Like muscles, the more we use them, the stronger they become.

Attitudes

Our attitudes, or core perspectives, color how we think and frame our decisions. They are the powerful lens through which we see the world, and they heavily influence our level of success in recovery.

Eight attitudes are essential for everyone—but particularly those of us facing mental health issues. If we adopt and develop these attitudes early in the recovery process, our path will become easier to navigate. (See notes on the *Awareness Stage*, p. 33.) Without them, recovery becomes much more difficult.

Respect the individual.

Perhaps the most important attitude is a profound sense of respect for those with mental health issues. People in distress desperately need their own and others' respect and compassion. Supporters must be able to look beyond the chaos and stress (see *Look Deeper*, p. 343) to value the humanity of the person in pain. Sometimes we can forget that the person we see in distress is the same person we love and appreciate.

In surveys and workshops, people with mental health issues repeatedly stress the importance of being treated with respect.[101] They are not problems to solve, but individuals to accept, encourage, and help. The stigma created by a lack of respect is a sizable barrier to recovery.[102]

Psychotherapist Michael Cromwell, who experienced psychosis first-hand, calls this respectful attitude *loving receptivity*.[103] He urges supporters to listen and spend quiet time with patients instead of peppering them with questions or imposing demands. Respect and love create an important *Emotional Sanctuary* (p. 101) for those with mental health issues, a place of calm and a refuge.

Honor the individual's experience.

We don't need to understand or agree with an experience, but we do need to honor it. We must acknowledge that someone we care about is undergoing a powerful and often frightening experience, and that person needs our time and attention. We must accept that this experience is a painful and difficult reality, regardless of how it compares to our reality. We can honor their experiences and earn their trust only if we support them without judgment. Being non-judgmental is important. So is ignoring the stigmas associated with specific illnesses.

Each person in mental distress regards the challenge differently. Some view it as a chemical imbalance in the brain; others regard it as a sickness, a spiritual crisis, a set of strong emotions out of control, or an opportunity for relief and growth. Supporters aren't helping in the recovery if they insist that their loved-one accepts one framework of understanding.[104]

The best way we can assist in mental health recovery is to understand the patients' perspective. *Their* recovery must be grounded in *their* perspectives and needs. To force another viewpoint is like standing far away and demanding, "Come here!" instead of going close and asking, "How can I help?" The first approach rarely succeeds. The second is one of the best ways to express respect.

Mental health crises often become difficult balancing acts. Those with mental health issues may not be able to make decisions to keep themselves and others safe. In this case, paternalism can be the best course, with actions and decisions aimed at protecting others and stabilizing the individual. However, too often paternalism means wrongfully judging someone as incapable, which interferes with that person's self-determination—and recovery. In fact, a person's right to self-determination is considered one of the fundamental measures of enlightened health care.[105]

Accept the situation.

Acceptance of the current situation is crucial. Accepting doesn't mean giving up, but calmly acknowledging what *is*. This offers an effective starting point for recovery. When we can respond thoughtfully and without undue emotion, we establish an atmosphere for productive change. (See the broader set of *Attitudes of Mindfulness* in Figure 15, p. 76.)

Courageously accept responsibility.

Accepting responsibility is the first major step in recovery. According to SAMHSA, "Individuals have a personal responsibility for their own self-care and journeys of recovery... Families and significant others have responsibilities to support their loved-ones."[1461]

It takes courage to accept this responsibility. We may not feel prepared for it. But in the end, we *must* accept this responsibility. (See *Attitudes of Effective Self-management*, Figure 17, p. 85.) Start small, with one step, and increase as you are able.

Trust yourself.

We all have strengths at our disposal, and when mental health issues arise, we need to use them—all of them, even if they are hidden or rusty. Research proves that better mental health outcomes occur when we focus on our strengths. So does our sense of satisfaction with life.[106] We must trust ourselves if we want to succeed at anything.

Be hopeful—there is good reason to be.

Hope is the essential catalyst for recovery.[1461] Hope provides a strong motivation to do the hard work necessary for success. Hope isn't a flimsy pipe dream, but a strong reasonable expectation. The many case studies in this book illustrate the power of hope. Hope doesn't gloss over challenges but helps us mount a powerful assault on them. Hope isn't a weak person's way of seeing the world through rose-colored glasses; it's a strong person's way of motivating oneself to get things done.

Hope, and the lack of hope, become self-fulfilling prophecies (see quote on p. 104). Without hope, we won't strive to recover. With hope, we concentrate on taking the many small steps to recovery. Hope can be helped by the broader set of *Attitudes of Belief, Hope & Self-transcendence* (Figure 22, p. 106).

Relax your expectations.

We all have expectations for ourselves and others. These expectations provide motivation, a sense of meaning, positive goals, and standards of behavior to guide us. On the flip side, we get frustrated when we fall short of our expectations. To avoid frustration, we need to relax expectations about things that aren't truly important. This doesn't mean abandoning our goals but prioritizing them. If we set aside expectations that are less important and relax the timetables on other goals, we can maximize and focus our energy on the major priority: recovery. As we make progress, we can gradually incorporate new goals and expectations.

Take the long-term perspective.

Achieving mental health takes time, so we need to adopt a long-term view, recognizing that we'll face ups and downs. Don't be discouraged if you don't see immediate results with a new approach. Most non-drug solutions require more time—but they can deliver impressive long-term results. For help in taking the long-term perspective, see *Attitudes of Purpose & Meaning* (Figure 21, p. 95).

While we work to develop and strengthen essential positive attitudes, we need to remember to forgive ourselves for the times we don't exhibit them. Changing and refining our attitudes take time. No one is perfect. *Everyone* makes mistakes.*.[107]* Mistakes are always part of the naturally messy process of recovery. But, fortunately, recovery is resilient. We can make progress despite our mistakes.

Knowledge

The second element of competency is knowledge. When we understand mental health fundamentals, we can greatly improve our prospects for recovery.

- **Know that there are many effective non-drug options.** Although conventional psychiatry rarely considers them, *Integrative Mental Health* uses them extensively. This book introduces the breadth of options available.

- **Know how to respond in an emergency.** A psychiatric emergency typically occurs when someone in mental distress becomes a danger to themselves or others. In an emergency, call 911. Hospital emergency psychiatric services usually focus on short-term stabilization with drugs. Although cooperative care is the aim, forced drug treatment or physical restraint is sometimes used when considered necessary. Such forced treatment is often frightening and sometimes traumatic. 58% of those forced to take psychiatric meds find it severely distressing.[108] Though few in number, *Peer Respites* (p. 132) offer a less distressing home-like alternative to hospitals with greater emphasis on "being with" and less emphasis on drugs. Prior to an emergency, consider a *Psychiatric Advance Directive,[109]* a legal document that outlines preferences for care should the patient become too unstable to communicate.

- **Know that your practitioners are trusted advisors, not your boss.** Your practitioners are your skilled advisors, allies, and partners. They have a single goal: to help you recover. Respect them, understand their guidance, but decide for yourself. Unless you are underage or under a court order, you are the ultimate decision maker. Periodically evaluate your practitioners on whether they are fulfilling their single goal; are they helping you recover? If you decide after a reasonable time that the therapies your practitioner recommended are not helping your recovery, consider respectfully changing practitioners. That is your right and, ultimately, your responsibility.

- **Know that access to services can be difficult.** The demand for mental health services is much greater than supply. *Integrative Mental Health* care is even harder to find, but with diligence many forms are available. Ask for help from family, friends, and public programs, if needed. Mental health phone apps (p.

328) and online psychosocial therapies, including computer-based *Cognitive Behavioral Therapy* (p. 117), can help. These tools are most effective when you have email and/or phone support from a therapist.

- **Know the nuance beyond the sound bites.** Mental health recovery is complex and often hampered by sound bites, or pithy tidbits of wisdom, that lack the broader perspective we need to make informed choices. Here are a few common sound bites that can be misleading.

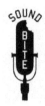

We don't understand the causes of mental ill-health, but they seem to be a combination of genetic, environmental, and stress issues. Since we don't understand the causes, we can only address symptoms.

A more complete perspective: This is one of the most powerfully misleading assertions in mental health. Mental health diagnoses are complex; interrelated causes vary among individuals. Many things can cause, influence, or exacerbate mental health symptoms: substance abuse, poor lifestyle choices,[110] allergies, heavy metal toxicity, electromagnetic fields, vitamin/nutrient deficiencies, microbial infections, digestive issues, low blood sugar, poor sleeping habits, thyroid disorders, methylation issues, inflammation, past trauma, social isolation, grief, lack of self-determination, excessive stress, and many more. Regrettably, we don't yet know all the causes.

To help someone showing mental health issues, a commonsense scientific approach is to test for the many known potential causes, and then treat any that are evident. In many cases, biomedical disorders can be diagnosed after simple lab tests, and they can be treated quickly and simply. For example, a thyroid test may uncover thyroid dysfunction, which can cause mental health issues. If a thyroid disorder is detected, thyroid therapy often fully eliminates the symptoms.

Conventional psychiatrists rarely perform robust biomedical tests. However, biomedical issues occur much more frequently in people with mental health issues.[61] Finding and treating these issues may avoid years of distress.

A major premise of this book is that thorough assessments for root causes of mental health symptoms should be mandatory. These tests include Biomedical Test Panels (p. 323) and a thorough psychosocial assessment.

They should be performed by practitioners who value the testing and regularly use it for diagnosis and treatment. Your mental health is too important to do anything less. Your primary care physician or psychiatrist will probably recommend common tests (among them thyroid, liver enzymes, and cholesterol), but you should also ask them to investigate all reasonable avenues, including allergies, broader endocrine issues, nutrient deficiencies, inflammation, and more. You may need to ask for referrals to endocrinologists, allergists, and other specialists appropriate for testing and evaluation in their areas of expertise.

Mental health issues are caused by an imbalance in neurotransmitter brain chemistry that we can address with the chemistry of psychotropics.

A more complete perspective: The neurotransmitter imbalance theory (a.k.a the *medical model*), has long been accepted as the explanation for mental health issues. Over the last decade, however, it has been widely discounted for lack of evidence. Some researchers call it a "dead end".[111] A United Nations report recommends abandoning it.[28] Both the British Psychological Society[104] and NAMI[81] advocate expanding beyond it. "We have hunted for simple neurochemical explanations... and have not found them."[112]

Other conceptual models are showing much more promise. The *bio-psycho-social* model suggests a much broader set of potential causes of mental health issues and underscores the effectiveness of psychosocial therapy.[12,113] The *biochemical individuality* model evaluates each person's unique body chemistry and recommends customized responses.[19] Many CAM approaches are grounded in a *stress model,[15]* aimed at reducing cellular, emotional, and physical stressors. The *Power Threat Meaning Framework* synthesizes evidence on the causal roles of power dynamics, meaning and narratives in mental health.[114]

Accepting the narrow view of the medical model leads to over-valuing its narrow set of solutions (psychotropics) and under-valuing the many proven non-drug approaches. Many people who have successfully recovered attribute their success to a winning combination of mental health approaches.

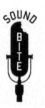

Psychotropics are the "Gold Standard" mental health therapy, since they are proven by "Gold Standard" clinical trial techniques.

A more complete perspective: Randomized Controlled Trials (RCTs, see *Glossary*) are an excellent method for scientific testing. Because they give unbiased and consistent results, they are sometimes called a "Gold Standard" technique. In practice, however, psychotropic RCTs only provide data for drugs' effectiveness over a short period of time. Psychotropic studies seldom provide quality data on the:

- Severity, frequency, and duration[115] of psychotropic side effects.
- Long-term impact of psychotropic use.
- Real-life psychotropic effectiveness when prescribed by doctors.
- Withdrawal difficulties.[116] Most psychotropics have withdrawal symptoms.[117]
- Results by diagnosis biotype. Results are nearly always given by an umbrella diagnosis (such as depression), ignoring biochemical differences in individuals. For instance, most people with depression have low serotonin and respond well to SSRIs. However, 30% of the people with depression have an elevated serotonin biotype. For them, SSRIs could be harmful.[19]

Even more troubling is the big picture. Pharmaceutical companies fund between 85 and 90% of all RCT drug trials. Those trials are four times as likely to produce results that support psychotropics than do independently run experiments.[118] Also, one-third of trials with negative psychotropic results go unreported[119]—especially those that find serious side effects from drugs.[120] In response to these troubling statistics, a U.S. House Investigations Subcommittee criticized the pharmaceutical industry for publishing only studies with positive outcomes,[121] and the World Health Organization unambiguously stated, "Registration of all trials is a scientific, ethical, and moral responsibility."[122]

Researchers know that RCTs have limitations.[123] They can be impractical, unethical, or impossible[124] at times, especially for psychological therapies.[125] The medical community must expand beyond RCTs to gain better real-world validity.[126] The true mental health "Gold Standard" is often a customized mix of therapeutic options[74] that may—or may not—include psychotropics.

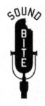

Mental illness is like diabetes. Both should be managed with a lifetime of drug therapy.

A more complete perspective: Comparing mental illness to diabetes is misleading. Many people become sustainably stable and can end psychotropic use. The psychiatric diagnostic bible is clear on potential exit ramps from drugs.[127] Further, you should adopt healthy skepticism regarding life-time drug use, since the long-term effectiveness of psychotropic drugs are not well proven.[128] Although some long-term drug trials are positive, others suggest that antipsychotics actually do more harm than good.[55]

Instead of expecting to be on a lifetime of drugs, expect to find answers in prudent experimentation with non-drug alternatives. As you experiment, accept the benefits and side effects of psychotropics as long as you need them.

Psychotropics are safe because they are FDA-approved.

A more complete perspective: Psychotropics are very powerful drugs, and their safety varies by individual. Psychotropics go through extensive clinical trials and gain Food and Drug Administration (FDA) approval when there is substantial proof that they reduce symptoms in the short-term. However, the side effects of these drugs are sometimes serious and often numerous. Studies on the long-term impact of psychotropics are troubling for both schizophrenia[52] and bipolar.[129] An extensive synthesis[130] of the FDA database on serious drug-adverse effects indicates that 19 of the 34 drugs that might cause violent behavior[131] are psychotropics. And, the FDA warns that antipsychotics increase the chance of death in the elderly.[132] In general, the risks of side effects and death are considerably greater for psychotropics than for non-drug therapies.

Despite these issues, FDA approval is valuable. We should therefore have healthy skepticism of common psychiatric practices that are <u>not</u> FDA-approved. (See *Off-Label & Polypharmacy Risk,* p. 263.)

Vitamins and supplements aren't safe because they aren't FDA-approved.

A more complete perspective: Most vitamins and supplements fall into a category called nutraceuticals.[133] Instead of clinical trials, the FDA requires that nutraceutical "recipes" contain only components already known to be safe.[134]

There are two grades of nutraceuticals.[778] *Pharmaceutical grade* products must meet 99% purity standards and must use manufacturing processes approved by the FDA. *Food grade* products, usually of good quality, are less pure and less costly, often have fillers and dyes, may have variable potency, and are available over the counter (OTC).

Nutrient and herbal therapy is generally safe, but, like drugs, nutrients and herbs can have side effects. If you do use nutrients, supplements, or herbs, discuss them first with trained practitioners familiar with current research, your medical history, and lab tests. (See *Biomedical Test Panels,* p. 323.) Your practitioners can advise on benefits, risks, and especially interactions.

Major retailers (including GNC, Walmart, Target, and Walgreens) have been accused of marketing fraudulent *food grade* herbal formulas.[135] Check the FDA website for alerts.

Skills

The third element of competency is skills—critical capabilities for those with mental health issues as well as their supporters.

Empathic communication. Empathy is the ability to see the world through

another person's eyes, to share and understand their feelings, needs, and concerns. Developing empathic communication skills is especially important for everyone dealing with mental health issues. Empathy provides emotional and practical support, helping us "be there" in times of distress.

To communicate well, choose moments for discussions when everyone involved will be most receptive—which means stopping everything else, eliminating all distractions, and listening with openness, respect, appreciation, and acceptance. This is a time for unconditional love, not judgment. Speak with warmth and let your concern show. Ask open-ended clarifying questions. Be clear and direct in your statements, honest and kind.

Empathic listening skills are equally important. Focus on your loved ones. Relax, smile, look into their eyes, and use welcoming body language. Nod, play back what you hear, and always maintain eye contact. Don't take everything at face value; look for the emotional content behind the words.

Problem-solving and change. Problem-solving skills and the ability to adapt to

change are critically important in reaching your recovery goals. Face and address issues as they appear; don't let them fester. Work collaboratively to identify problems, brainstorm ideas, evaluate alternative ideas, choose the optimal direction, plan steps, and act.

Advocacy. Advocacy skills help you collaborate with and influence practitioners, insurance companies, and other allies in your recovery, to get what you need. Strong, mutually beneficial relationships are especially important when mental health support resources are scarce. To effectively advocate:

- *Be respectful and friendly.* Express your needs clearly. Control your feelings. If you don't, you can become part of the problem, not the solution. Listen carefully to others' thoughts and recommendations. Ask questions until you understand. Give others the opportunity to help.
- *Be confident.* Don't be intimidated by professionals, even though they have the training and expertise that you don't have. Their job is to help you recover. Few things in mental health are black and white. You must live with the decisions, so feel comfortable asking questions and expressing concerns, without shyness or embarrassment. Make eye contact and speak clearly. You know your situation better than they do.
- *Be prepared.* Decide what you want to get out of a meeting before it starts. Come with questions (See *Questions for your Practitioners*, p. 328.) and any helpful or requested information. (See *Mental Health Tracking*, below.) Choose a meeting time when you are at your best, not tired or hungry.
- *Be clear.* Describe and express the situation, its impact, and what you would like to see happen. Use an appropriate level of urgency. Summarize the past concisely.
- *Be realistic.* Practitioners aren't miracle workers, and they often have limited resources. If you are not getting what you need, ask them to suggest the best way forward. Most are genuinely trying to help you.
- *Be assertive, not aggressive.* Push back on initial "no" answers if you need to—firmly and pleasantly. Ask for the pros and cons of suggested alternatives. Don't let practitioners brush off an interest you may have in alternative options.
- *Be grateful.* A well-timed "Thank you" and a letter of praise written to a supervisor do wonders for establishing and maintaining relationships.

Self-care. When we try to help loved ones with mental health issues, we sometimes shoulder huge responsibilities that can feel stifling and all-consuming. To be effective, we must maintain an identity apart from our role as caregiver—and if we do, we both will benefit. So will our friends and family members.

Self-care recognizes that we can't pour from an empty cup. It means we set boundaries, find others who can help, make our own physical health a priority, keep in touch with friends, exercise, find meaningful and relaxing activities that have nothing to do with our role as care-provider, and set aside time for our own pursuits. As caregivers or as patients, we should work on *Wellness Basics* (p. 55). BC Partners for Mental Health[136] and Rethink Mental Illness[90] offer suggestions and guidance. We all need to determine what will help us thrive during difficult circumstances and rely on those things while avoiding common traps: guilt, negativity, and helplessness.

Options of Recovery

This book reviews 27 non-drug approaches to mental health recovery. These approaches can be life-changing tools. *Integrative Mental Health* uses these treatments along with the drugs of conventional psychiatry to create a best-of-both-worlds model that accelerates mental health recovery.

One way to understand these 27 non-drug approaches is to place them into a *Wellness Continuum* of the U.S. Institute of Medicine and European Union of General Practitioners/Family Physicians.[137] (See Figure 9, p. 47)

This commonsense wellness framework has 4 categories of interventions:

- **Preventive** approaches are wellness basics for your body, mind, and spirit. They help minimize and avoid mental health issues—yet everyone can benefit from them. Exercise, nutritious eating, and social interaction are a few important basics. People often overlook the fact that what is healthy for the general population can have a profound effect on one person's mental health.

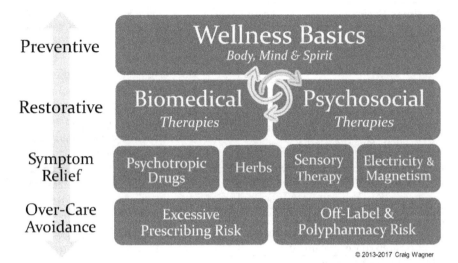

	Wellness Basics *Body, Mind & Spirit*	
Preventive		
Restorative	Biomedical *Therapies*	Psychosocial *Therapies*
Symptom Relief	Psychotropic Drugs / Herbs	Sensory Therapy / Electricity & Magnetism
Over-Care Avoidance	Excessive Prescribing Risk	Off-Label & Polypharmacy Risk

© 2013-2017 Craig Wagner

Figure 9 – Mental Health Wellness Continuum

- **Restorative** approaches address possible underlying influences and causes of mental health symptoms. They are either *biomedical* (related to the body) or *psychosocial* (related to the mind); both can have a tremendous impact on mental health, since our body and mind are so tightly entwined. Diagnostic procedures (including psychosocial evaluations as well as blood and urine tests) provide solid information to guide diagnosis and treatment. When targeted *Restorative Therapies* are used, they can often significantly reduce, and in some cases eliminate psychiatric symptoms. The cause-seeking perspective of *Restorative* approaches is shared with Functional Medicine.[138]
- **Symptom Relief** approaches don't aim to cure, but to minimize mental health symptoms, bringing someone to a more stable and receptive state so *Preventive* and *Restorative* approaches can be used. Psychotropics are by far the most common *Symptom Relief* therapy, but many more are available.
- **Over-Care Avoidance** means avoiding unnecessary and potentially harmful intervention. Psychotropics should be taken in minimum effective dosages for no longer than is needed—and in combinations proven to be effective and safe. This is vital since medical errors are the third leading cause of death in the U.S. behind only heart disease and cancer.[139] The American Psychiatric Association is working to curb two over-care practices: *Over-prescribing,* when drugs may not be warranted or necessary at high dosages (p. 259), and *polypharmacy,* prescribing too many drugs at once (p. 263).

The framework in Figure 9 provides context. It shows the big picture and how the pieces relate. It offers a visual reminder that the "higher" in this continuum you focus (toward *Preventive*), the better—though we often need to work in all four categories simultaneously.

Wellness Basics	# Techniques
1 Housing & Security	12
2 Diet & Digestion	4
3 Exercise & Sleep	6
4 Calm Awareness	10
5 Effective Self-management	10
6 Purpose & Meaning	4
7 Social & Outer Engagement	5
8 Belief, Hope, & Self-transcend.	5
9 Mind-Body Disciplines	3
Psychosocial Restorative Therapies	
10 Cognitive Behavioral Therapy	8
11 Individual Psychotherapy	8
12 Interpersonal, Family, & Peer	6
13 Cognitive Enhancement	1
14 Creative Engagement	9
15 Biofeedback	6
16 Dialogue & Exposure Therapy	12
17 Energy Therapy	7
Biomedical Restorative Therapies	
18 Nutrient Therapy	62
19 Endocrine Therapy	14
20 Food Allergy Therapy	3
21 Detoxification Therapy	4
22 Pathogen Therapy	12
Symptom Relief	
23 Herbal Therapy	56
24 Sensory Therapy	11
25 Electromagnetic stimulation	11
Over-care Avoidance	
26 Excessive Prescribing	3
27 Off-Label & Polypharmacy	2
Total	**294**

Figure 10 - The Non-drug Techniques for
Mental Health Recovery

It also clarifies the purpose and limitations of each approach. For instance, psychotropics are a form of *Symptom Relief.* They are not designed to address root causes and create core wellness, but they can relieve distress of certain symptoms. If you want more than *Symptom Relief,* you must look beyond meds.

And finally, this framework helps us avoid a myopic view of the importance of psychotropics. Figure 9 shows that psychotropics represent one of many options. They can be an important, but not exclusive, aspect of recovery.

These four categories of the *Wellness Continuum* are composed of 27 broad approaches, subdivided into 294 recovery techniques (Figure 10). These large numbers are good news, so don't feel overwhelmed. They represent many possible avenues to recovery. Chapter 8 helps you winnow down this large number of options quickly, to a much more manageable set of options that are most promising for your individual diagnosis and situation.

As you work toward recovery, realize that *Wellness Basics* and *Restorative Therapies* may not kick in as quickly as drugs. Many take days, perhaps weeks, and in some cases months, to deliver full results. But they often deliver significant and sustainable wellness gains. Patience and resolve are invaluable here.

Also realize that there is a strong bias toward psychotropics in our mental health system. Some conventional psychiatrists advise against using *Nutrient Therapy* and *Herbal Therapy,* citing the legitimate lack of robust research on their interactions with psychotropics. However, a growing number of Integrative

Mental Health practitioners consider this position much too restrictive, especially given the very favorable benefit/risk profile of nearly all non-drug approaches.

Taking a step back, know that there are thousands of well-designed studies that support the use of non-drug approaches. They work. Not all the time, and not for everyone, but they work. Some take time and effort—they aren't as easy as popping a pill. But, for many people, when we find the right combination of approaches that strike at the root causes of *our* symptoms, the payoff is enormous, sustainable, and life-altering.

Roadmap of Recovery

The world of mental health is complex, so consider a ten-step roadmap on your recovery journey (Figure 11, p. 50). Keep faith, hope, and confidence that you, like so many others, will reach your recovery destination and find the prospect so much better than you ever imagined.

If in crisis, quickly stabilize. Mental health crises can be dangerous. People in crisis often don't fully understand their situation and can't stabilize themselves. If you or your loved one appears to be in danger, call 911. Hospital emergency rooms are typically the front lines of defense. Although stabilization is often achieved with psychiatric drugs, increasingly, non-drug approaches are proving effective.

Although their numbers are small, *Peer respites* (p. 132) offer crisis intervention in less traumatic and lower-cost home-like settings, and often rely much less on drugs.

Create a calm haven of support. People with mental health issues often feel very vulnerable and need to be treated with calmness, kindness, and respect. Create a safe, quiet, reduced-stress, supportive environment—physical and emotional. Limit the demands placed on them while supporting their self-determination and social interaction.

Engage supporters and practitioners to bring vital expertise and humanity to your situation. *Integrative Mental Health* practitioners - those who value both conventional approaches as well as a variety of complementary and alternative approaches - offer the widest menu of recovery options. (See *The People of Recovery*, p. 35.) Family members, friends and peer support specialists are also often important to recovery.

Contact local *Community Mental Health* organizations (p. 36) to learn about their services and eligibility requirements. If you are a veteran, see *Veterans and Mental Health* (p. 335). Use the *Integrative Biomedical Practitioner Finder* (p. 320) to help build your team. Consider *Questions for Your Mental Health Practitioners* (p. 328) to help you find someone right for you. Practitioners have one role: to help you recover. The best practitioners fulfill their roles with skill, wisdom, creativity, and empathy.

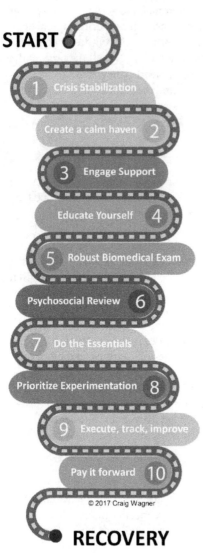

START

1 Crisis Stabilization

Create a calm haven 2

3 Engage Support

Educate Yourself 4

5 Robust Biomedical Exam

Psychosocial Review 6

7 Do the Essentials

Prioritize Experimentation 8

9 Execute, track, improve

Pay it forward 10

© 2017 Craig Wagner

RECOVERY

Figure 11 - Roadmap of Recovery

Educate yourself. There is much to learn in the world of mental health. Start with *Psychoeducation* (p. 126). Many people have found *Advocacy Groups* (p. 36) helpful for basic information, local emotional support, and personal connections, though they typically offer little assistance with non-drug approaches. Consider the wealth of information found in *Additional Resources* (p. 341) and study this book for the broad picture of the therapies available. Meanwhile, consider your *Attitudes* (p. 37), *Knowledge* (p. 40), and *Skills* (p. 44) needed during the *Preparation* stage (p. 34) of recovery.

Robust biomedical exam. Start by finding a skilled *Integrative Biomedical Practitioner* (p. 320) who can investigate possible physical disorders that might cause or influence your symptoms. They should use full *Biomedical Test Panels* (p. 323) to aid diagnosis. When underlying issues are found, they will recommend specific *Biomedical Restorative* therapies (p. 165) to address the issues, sometimes advising the engagement of other specialists (e.g. an endocrinologist).

Psycholosocial review.[140*] A licensed psychotherapist can assess past traumas, significant stressors, and destructive patterns of thoughts and emotions that directly influence mental health. If found, *Psychosocial Restorative Therapies* (p. 115) can target underlying issues. In many cases, these therapies are as effective as psychotropics and more sustainable in the long term. The quality of your relationship with a therapist can be as important as the therapy itself.

Do the essentials. Address *Wellness Basics* (p. 55) that are most out of balance.[141] *Housing & Security* (p. 57) are top priorities. Find a safe home, connect with people, eat well, reduce stress, sleep regularly,[142] and find creative, uplifting activities. Work to stop or reduce substance abuse. Don't try to take on too much at once, though, while you find the motivation to develop new daily habits that will help you make changes that you can sustain. Add new activities and therapies slowly.

Prioritize experimentation. With your practitioners' advice, consider the 27 broad non-drug approaches and the many techniques within them—as well as how they will interact with psychotropics. For a birds-eye view of all approaches, see Figure 10 (p. 48) and the *Most Promising Therapies* for each major diagnosis (Chapter 8). Choose techniques that seem most beneficial and workable for you and your unique situation. Connect with people who have used these approaches to gain their perspective. If addictions are involved, evaluate options in *Addiction Co-Therapy* (p. 332). When you complete this step, you're ready to exit the *Preparation* stage of recovery and enter the *Rebuilding* stage.

Execute, track, and improve. This step is where you work your plan, maximizing self-determination – and this can be a lengthy effort. Start experimenting with the approaches you've selected, since that is the only way to know if they will work for you. Future steps become clearer as you put your plan into action. Keep track of how your symptoms, activities, and challenges change over time. This can tell what works for you and what doesn't. Although you need to stay close to your supporters, it's best to own and manage your plan as much as possible, letting it evolve as needed, with your practitioners' involvement.

Consider *Recovery Models & Tools* (p. 327) to help manage your recovery. Get grounded in what brings you hope, so you can act with optimism. Work diligently, but patiently. If new approaches work, keep using them. If they don't, evaluate others and move on. Calibrate your plan to your available energy and focus; trying to do too much at one time is often unproductive. Setbacks are almost inevitable, unfortunately, so you must be willing to modify your plan and continue forward. If things get too difficult, consider *Hospital, Residential & Community Care* (p. 330). Ensure *Over-Care Avoidance* (p. 257).

If you are on psychotropics and non-drug approaches are working well, talk to your practitioner about *very slowly* reducing psychotropic dosages until you find your minimal effective dosage, which may be none at all. Watch carefully for early warning signs of trouble, though, to avoid relapse.

Pay it forward. When you are strong and maintaining recovery, consider helping others with mental health issues. Your experience and success can be tremendously inspirational and helpful to someone in the early stages of recovery. "I've been there and survived and thrive" experiences make a strong positive impact on someone's life. Your support can be offered in many forms, and you'll find it offers rewards: a strong sense of *Purpose & Meaning* (p. 94) and *Self-transcendence* (p. 105).

Like everything worth doing, mental health recovery is a challenge—perhaps the most difficult challenge we'll ever face.

We must craft our recovery while navigating through a mental health system that is in many ways broken. But right now, our challenge is not to fix it, but to fix ourselves.

To be successful, we need to experiment. We need to be self-confident enough to lead our own recovery, but humble enough to accept help from others. We need to be persistent enough to make steady progress, but patient enough to give it time. We need to be the pragmatic realist and the hopeful optimist. And perhaps most of all, we need large doses of love—from ourselves and others.

Brain Basics of Recovery

Before we review the 27 non-drug options in chapters 3-7, it is helpful to first understand key terms and concepts of the brain.

Symptom types. Mental health symptoms are usually classified as either positive or negative:

- *Positive Symptoms* are behaviors or experiences that are present in those with a mental health diagnosis but are absent in general population. For instance, delusions and hallucinations are positive symptoms of schizophrenia.

- *Negative Symptoms* are behaviors or experiences that are normally present in the general population but are absent or diminished in a person with a mental health diagnosis. For instance, reduced social interaction and the lack of visible emotion are negative symptoms of schizophrenia.

Refractory situations. Sometimes treatments we try don't work for us. If a variety of treatments have been tried with little success, the situation is often called *refractory* or *treatment-resistant*. This is often used in the context of psychotropic treatment. For instance, *refractory depression* typically means that a variety of antidepressants have not significantly improved symptoms.

Neurotransmitters. Our brain is a vast network of interconnected neurons that pass chemical information (neurotransmitters) between one another at certain connection points (synapses). There are many different chemical neurotransmitters, including dopamine and serotonin. Neurotransmitters flow between neurons when one neuron releases ("fires") its chemical message into the synapse. Once fired, the chemical neurotransmitter is attracted to the receiving neuron's receptor where it can deliver its chemical message. After delivery, the neurotransmitter is released back into the synapse where it is then absorbed back into the firing neuron in a process called "re-uptake".

Increasing or decreasing the amount of neurotransmitters in the brain has little impact on mental health. Of much greater consequence is *re-uptake*. If re-uptake is inhibited, neurotransmitters linger in the synapse and may retransmit their chemical message, thereby increasing the flow of chemical messages. *Inhibiting neurotransmitter re-uptake is a key goal of many antidepressants.* Another method to moderate neurotransmitter flow involves partially blocking its transmission. Antipsychotics (drugs used to treat schizophrenia) generally block certain neurotransmissions, thus slowing the flow of chemical messages.

Inflammation and Oxidative Stress. *Inflammation* is the body's natural response to *antigens* – bacteria, viruses, toxins, drugs, and other substances that appear foreign and harmful. When the immune system is activated by one of these intruders, a specific *antibody* is released, designed to neutralize the specific antigen detected. Pro-inflammation agents cause swelling, which helps isolate the foreign substance from further contact with body tissues. When the antigens have been neutralized, anti-inflammatory agents are released, thereby beginning the healing process.

In a normal immune system, a natural balance exists between inflammation and the anti-inflammatory agents. But in some cases, the immune system continues to create antibodies that maintain inflammation. *It is believed that inappropriate inflammation over an extended period of time can lead to mental health symptoms.*

C-reactive protein (CRP) is an enzyme marker for chronic inflammation. Studies show that CRP is elevated in individuals with schizophrenia, [143] bipolar,[144, 145] depression, [146, 147] and anxiety[148] suggesting that inflammation is an important part of these disorders. Some anti-inflammatory agents have been shown to improve schizophrenia symptoms, among them aspirin, estrogen (in women), and the antioxidant *N-acetylcysteine* (p. 184).[149] In fact, in one study, patients with schizophrenia given aspirin (1,000 mg/d) for three months had a significant decrease in positive symptoms, with the best response from those with the highest inflammation markers.[150]

Inflammation is often associated with another condition, *oxidative stress.* There is an ongoing interplay in the body between oxidative free radicals (which can be harmful to the body) and antioxidants (which combat free radicals). *Oxidative stress, often caused by environmental or emotional stress, is an imbalance toward excess free radicals. Many experts believe oxidative stress is the key cause of schizophrenia, bipolar disorder, and autism.*[151]

Since mental health symptoms are linked to inflammation and oxidative stress, finding methods to reduce inflammation and oxidative stress may aid mental health recovery.

Cholesterol. One method to reduce inflammation is to ensure adequate cholesterol levels. Although we often strive to reduce cholesterol, it is an important anti-inflammatory that helps protect the brain from oxidative stress. Low cholesterol is often seen in patients with mood disorders. In fact, a large case-control study suggests that using statins, a cholesterol reducing drug, increases depression.[152] The impact of cholesterol on mood appears to differ by sex. Women with low HDL ("good" cholesterol) are more likely to have severe depression, while men with low LDL ("bad" cholesterol) are more depressed.[153]

Epigenetics. The study of gene expression is *epigenetics.* Until recently, scientists believed that a person's genetic characteristics were cast in stone at the moment of conception. Nowadays, strong evidence suggests that this is only partially true. Genes can be *expressed*—either silenced or activated—based on aspects as diverse as diet, nutrient imbalances, exposure to environmental toxins, trauma, and stress. The variability in gene expression is clear when we notice that identical twins can have vastly different mental health while sharing the exact same genetic material.

Epigenetics can be likened to a dinner party with a hot-headed guest. If you create a supportive environment, you help avoid the expression of negative tendencies. However, if you create a hostile environment, you can provoke their latent destructive tendencies and end up with a food fight. Some of us have hot-headed genes that can lead to mental health issues. But, by creating and maintaining a supportive environment–through *Wellness Basics* and *Restorative Therapies* (see Figure 9, p. 47)—we can help minimize destructive outcomes.

Research on epigenetics offers tremendous hope for those with mental health issues, since many mental disorders are thought to have epigenetic origins.[154] *Nutrient Therapy* (p. 167) is a particularly powerful approach because it alters the body's internal environment, helping to avoid the activation of genes tied to mental health issues. *Nutrient Therapy* can also address methylation issues, epigenetic abnormalities that are extremely common in people with mental health issues. [19] (See methylation discussion below.)

Methylation.[19] Methylation is a biochemical process that aids neurotransmitter synthesis, powerfully affecting neurotransmitter activity at the synapse. Abnormal methylation is common in people with schizophrenia, bipolar, depression, anxiety, and certain behavior disorders.[802] A methylation imbalance occurs in approximately 30% of the general population, but in nearly 70% of people with mental health issues. This is an important focus for new mental health research in epigenetics.

Overmethylation increases neurotransmitter activity in the synapse (less re-uptake), while *undermethylation* decreases activity (increases re-uptake). *Vitamin B9* (p. 171) and *SAM-e* (p. 188) influence re-uptake significantly. Vitamin B9 stimulates reuptake, while *SAM-e* inhibits it. For this reason, people with overmethylation often thrive on vitamin B9, while people with undermethylation do not tolerate B9 well, but can often improve depression using SAM-e. [19]

WHAT ARE ADDITIONAL RESOURCES?

- Communication Skills. https://goo.gl/iYYSMD.
- Problem Solving. http://goo.gl/ZWF1ue, https://goo.gl/x79P6N.

3 – Wellness Basics

The first category of the *Wellness Continuum* (Figure 9, p. 47) includes *Wellness Basics*, divided into groupings of body, mind, and spirit (Figure 12).

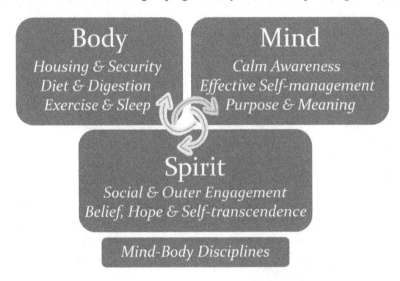

Figure 12 – Wellness Basics

According to the Substance Abuse and Mental Health Services Administration (SAMHSA), "Recovery is holistic... including mind, body, spirit, and community. This includes... housing... complementary and alternative services, faith, spirituality, creativity, and social networks."[155]

- **Body Wellness Basics** connect physical health and mental health with *Housing & Security, Diet & Digestion*, and *Exercise & Sleep*.
- **Mind Wellness Basics** are based on three interrelated approaches. *Calm Awareness* is a state of alert being, where we slow down and peacefully observe life. *Effective Self-management* is a process of pragmatic doing, where we consciously guide our thoughts, emotions, and actions to achieve our goals. *Purpose & Meaning* offers a clear and compelling direction we set for ourselves. *Mind Wellness Basics* are not only vital for mental health, but for all aspects of our lives including directly influencing our happiness.
- **Spirit Wellness Basics** establish a strong inner foundation to support recovery. *Social & Outer Engagement* means reaching beyond ourselves to interact effectively with people in meaningful reciprocal relationships. *Belief, Hope & Self-transcendence* carries that idea further, embracing a personal world view that helps us find peace and understanding. Although *Belief, Hope & Self-transcendence* can be based in religion or spirituality, these qualities can also be found in creative expression, employment, a learning environment, family, and more. Numerous clinical trials underscore the importance of *Spirit Wellness Basics* to mental health.

Wellness Basics are commonsense ways of living, shown to aid mental wellness. Some Eastern cultures combine them into *Mind-Body Disciplines* (p. 111). *Yoga, T'ai Chi Chuan,* and *Qigong* use mindful body work, calm awareness, breathing, and a spiritual connection.

The value of *Wellness Basics* is underscored in something called the *Hispanic Paradox.*

Upon arriving in the United States, Latino immigrants are generally healthier than most Americans—including mentally.[156] However, this advantage changes within a matter of years.[157] In comparison to immigrant Latinos, American-born Latinos face a significantly higher risk of depression, social phobia, post-traumatic stress disorder, anxiety, and substance abuse.[158] Many experts believe this is caused primarily by acculturation – adopting the unhealthy American lifestyle and abandoning *Wellness Basics* from their own culture.

Latino acculturation is also associated with a decline in social support,[159] greater illicit drug use, poor diet,[160] and a more sedentary life style. As immigrant Latino populations begin to mirror the unhealthier lifestyles of their neighbors, they also begin to reflect higher incidents of mental health issues.

Wellness Basics can provide great benefits, and they are the most accessible approaches to mental health recovery. The challenge lies in removing barriers to access and changing ingrained lifestyles. Fortunately, we can start with small steps, even if they seem very modest, and we gain momentum with success. Making lifestyle changes not only empowers us but helps us implement changes that can be profound and long-lasting.[1465]

Housing & Security

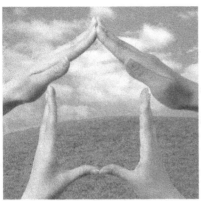

WHAT IS THE ESSENCE?

Housing & Security is the gateway to all other *Wellness Basics*. According to the Substance Abuse and Mental Health Services Administration (SAMHA), safe housing is one of the four key factors supporting a life in recovery.[1461]

Housing should be *affordable* (costing less than 30% of an individual's income), *independent* (with privacy and choice), *accessible* (near services and public amenities), *stable* (so a sense of "home" can be developed), and *safe*.[161] Housing should also help maximize *Self-determination* (p. 87) and *Social Engagement* (p. 99), both of which are vital for mental health.

Housing options. Someone suffering from mental health issues who is homeless and/or unable to earn a suitable income has options, some of which may be supported by state or federal funding. They include:

- **Emergency housing.** Many communities have homeless shelters run by civic or faith-based organizations. Housing may also be available for youth, veterans, and individuals fleeing domestic violence.

- **Housing Choice Vouchers.** Housing Choice Vouchers (also known as Section 8 vouchers) assist low-income families, the elderly, and the disabled. The vouchers subsidize a portion of the rent for conventional leases, if the housing meets program guidelines. Section 8 vouchers are administered locally through public housing agencies, but they are funded through the U.S. Department of Housing and Urban Development (HUD). Eligibility is primarily based on income.

- **Supportive housing.** Supportive housing combines housing and services (including mental health services). It is especially helpful for the homeless or those with very low incomes and/or serious persistent issues, including addictions, mental health issues, and HIV/AIDS. The goal is to maximize independence and stability, so rents are set at affordable levels.

- **Group Housing.** Group housing provides a safe home for people under one roof, often with integrated support services to help with daily living, food, and other support.

Security can take many forms: *physical security* (freedom from crime, harm, and abuse), *food security* (continuous access to nutritious food), *financial security* (having money to cover basic needs), and *healthcare security* (having access to doctors and mental health services).

Food security options. The homeless and those with mental health issues often struggle to provide themselves with a healthy diet.[162] Data from 149 countries suggest that food insecurity is associated with poorer mental health across the world.[163] In the U.S., help is available:

- **Supplemental Nutrition Assistance Program (SNAP)**. Formerly known as food stamps, SNAP is a federal program that helps people with no or low income gain access to food. The United States Department of Agriculture oversees SNAP under the Food and Nutrition Service (FNS), and benefits are distributed by each state's Division of Social Services or Children and Family Services. Funds are deposited into an Electronic Benefits Transfer debit card account that can be used at grocery and drug stores. Currently, people may qualify for benefits if they earn less than 130% of the federal poverty level for their household size.
- **Other U.S. federal programs**. FNS runs nutrition programs for Women and Infants, summer meal programs, and others. See www.fns.usda.gov.
- **Food kitchens**. Local civic and faith-based organizations may have food kitchens, meals-on-wheels, and other nutritional support for those in need.

Financial security options. The U.S. Social Security Administration offers programs with strict eligibility requirements.[164]

- **Social Security Disability Insurance (SSDI)**. SSDI pays benefits to people who can't work because they have a medical condition (including a mental health condition) expected to last at least one year. In general, to get benefits you must have worked "recently" and for a certain duration.
- **Supplemental Security Income (SSI)**. SSI pays benefits to disabled adults and children, including individuals with mental health issues, who have limited income and resources. SSI payments may continue when individuals return to work, but as more money is earned, SSI payments may be reduced or ended.

Healthcare security options. Healthcare insurance is available for purchase in the United States, in addition to other healthcare programs.

- **Healthcare.gov.** The U.S. Affordable Care Act (also known as "Obamacare") helps people find, enroll in, and receive credits to help pay for medical insurance. It includes mandatory coverage for certain mental health, behavioral health (such as psychotherapy and counseling), and substance abuse services. Specific coverage varies by plan.
- **Medicaid**. Medicaid is an American program that provides health coverage to low-income adults, children, pregnant women, the elderly, and people with disabilities (including mental health disabilities). Medicaid is administered by the states, which must cover certain mandatory benefits and can choose to provide other optional benefits. To receive services from some *Community Mental Health Organizations* (p. 36.), you may need to be on Medicaid.
- **Children's Health Insurance Program (CHIP)**. CHIP provides children with standard Medicaid benefits, including Early and Periodic Screening,

Diagnostic, and Treatment (EPSDT) services. This includes mental health services.

WHAT EVIDENCE SHOWS THIS IS EFFECTIVE?

> *"There's no place like home. There's no place like home..."*
>
> *-- Dorothy,*
>
> The Wizard of Oz

Housing and mental health. Homelessness is traumatic and disorienting, resulting in vulnerability, hopelessness, and feeling out of control. Homeless people are often sleep-deprived, thirsty, and hungry. These stressors greatly exacerbate mental health symptoms.[165] In fact, persistent poor housing is predictive of worse mental health.[166] This is especially true for schizophrenia: lower rates of owner-occupied housing is one of the strongest predictors of higher psychosis rates.[167] Minimizing stress from insufficient housing is a vital first step for recovery.

Physical Security. People with severe mental health issues are four times more likely to be a victim of crime than the general population; more than 25% have been a victim of crime within the last year.[168] Many of the victims are homeless or sheltered in unreliable facilities which make them more vulnerable. Housing offers protection from the elements and from dangerous social conditions. Within our homes, we can regulate interpersonal contact.[169] A secure environment is critical to mental health.

Economic stress and mental health issues. Research has proven that as socio-economic status declines, the risk of mental illness rises proportionally.[170] Analysis of a database with more than 100,000 people with mental health issues verifies the fact that economic stress strongly impacts mental health. According to leading researchers, "Preventive and early intervention strategies that pay particular attention to the devastating impacts of unemployment, economic displacement, and housing dislocation" help individuals with mental health issues.[171] Reducing economic stress can be an important foundation for mental health recovery.

Choice and supportive housing. Studies confirm that people with mental health issues strongly prefer living in their own place, either alone or with one or two roommates, rather than in group settings shared with others who have mental health issues.[172, 173] *Supportive housing* typically offers this independence and is more cost-effective than homeless shelters.[174]

Treatment First vs. Housing First. There are two schools of thought on homelessness and mental health. *Treatment First* approaches demand that homeless people get clean from drugs or stable on psychotropics before they are eligible for housing assistance. *Housing First* approaches, which offer stable housing without requirements for treatment or sobriety, have been shown to be far more effective because they help people gain greater control over their lives, which is a factor leading to recovery.[175] Individuals in these programs are significantly less likely to use or abuse substances[176] or to be incarcerated. Stable housing can act as a motivator for people to seek services that help them support and sustain treatment.

WHAT CONSIDERATIONS SHOULD I KEEP IN MIND?

Estimates suggest that between 20% and 25% of America's homeless population is suffering with *severe* mental health issues. *Housing & Security* and *Emotional Sanctuary (p. 101),* are prerequisites for their recovery.[177] If housing with family or friends is unavailable, individuals may find subsidized housing in many communities, although it is often in chronic short supply. The local Public Housing Agency (or Housing Commission), HUD websites, and the *NAMI Housing Toolkit* (See *Resources*, below.) are the places to begin a search. Using public support should never be considered a personal weakness or failing. It is a courageous effort of self-determination, working to create sustainable mental wellness.

We've talked about the critical need for a safe environment. Now we move on to consider *Diet & Digestion*.

REAL-WORLD EXPERIENCE

Case Study 2 – Supportive Housing

Project Renewal in New York City helps people who are chronically homeless and who have mental health issues and/or addictions by offering comprehensive medical and behavioral health services. It operates more than 750 housing units, which have case managers, a program director, peer counselors, and entitlements coordinators.

The results of the program are very promising: 90% of the people living in Project Renewal permanent housing remain housed after placement; 97% of the people living in transitional apartments for methadone maintenance have moved on to living situations that are more independent, indicating they are maintaining their health.

In addition, although services are optional, 100% of supportive housing clients have identified personal goals as part of a case management care plan.

Bottom Line*: Supportive Housing works when: 1) people have housing choices, 2) individualized services are provided with housing, 3) housing is integrated into the community, 4) housing is separated from requisite services (for example, Housing First approaches), and 5) self-determination is maximized.*

WHAT ARE ADDITIONAL RESOURCES?

- Housing Choice Vouchers Fact Sheet. http://goo.gl/mIoOhh.
- HUD home page. http://portal.hud.gov/hudportal/HUD.
- HUD Homeless Assistance. http://goo.gl/y7GECz.
- HUD Exchange for local housing resources. www.HudExchange.info.
- SAMHSA Homelessness Programs and Resources. http://goo.gl/CMFBjC.
- Fair Housing and People with Disabilities. http://goo.gl/dmgKwE.
- Recovery Within Reach, housing options. http://goo.gl/eM1zBp.
- Corporation for Supportive Housing (CSH). http://www.csh.org.
- SNAP application. www.fns.usda.gov/snap/apply.
- Social Security Disability Benefits. www.ssa.gov/disabilityssi.
- Supplemental Security Income. www.ssa.gov/disabilityssi/ssi.html.
- Medicaid. www.Medicaid.gov.
- U.S. Healthcare marketplace. www.Healthcare.gov.
- CHIP. www.medicaid.gov/chip/chip-program-information.html.

Diet & Digestion

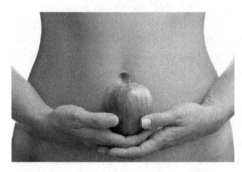

WHAT IS THE ESSENCE?

The second component of *Wellness Basics, Diet & Digestion,* focuses on the fact that a good diet provides the basic chemical elements needed for optimal brain function and mental health.

In terms of nutrition, there is no "one size fits all." Everyone has a different body chemistry, and therefore different dietary requirements. During digestion, a complex interaction between the brain and the gut occurs in the *enteric nervous system,* sometimes called the "brain in your gut." The brain/gut axis is a two-way street; a troubled gut signals the brain, just as a troubled brain signals the gut.

> *"Let food be thy medicine, thy medicine shall be thy food."*
> - Hippocrates

The digestive system is aided by probiotics, "friendly bacteria" that help maintain the digestive system and boost immunity. Dysbosis, an imbalance in gut bacteria, may be caused by antibiotic or alcohol use, stress, or high fat/sugar diets. The imbalance can cause intestinal permeability, sometimes called "leaky gut," making it easier for unhealthy substances to enter the body and cause both physical and mental issues.

WHAT EVIDENCE SHOWS THIS IS EFFECTIVE?

Diet. Population studies show that people with schizophrenia, bipolar, and depression eat more foods that produce inflammation and obesity (sugar, refined carbohydrates, and saturated fat) than the general population.[178] As a result, it may be helpful to reduce the intake of these foods while increasing the intake of anti-inflammatory foods (berries, cherries, fatty fish, broccoli, kale, avocados, nuts, green tea, peppers, mushrooms, grapes, turmeric, extra virgin olive oil, dark chocolate, and tomatoes).[179]

A diet of 40% protein, 40% carbohydrate, and 20% fat is often ideal for patients with mood and behavioral disorders.[180] Fats and oils are crucial; they help absorb vitamins, maintain cell membrane structure, and regulate the immune system. Many fats are manufactured by the body, although two are not. Those two, considered "essential" fats, are omega-3 (from fish, nuts, seeds) and omega-6 (from whole grains, cereals, vegetable oils).[181] The ratio of omega-6 to omega-3 in our bodies is important and should be about 2:1 or even 1:1 (found in prehistoric human diets). However, our Western diet overindulges in processed vegetable oils rich in omega-6, and limits fish/nut intake, thus pushing the average ratio up to about 20:1. This out-of-balance ratio is believed to contribute to psychiatric symptoms,[182] especially depression.[183]

- For *depression*. Diets rich in vegetables, fruit, meat, fish, and whole grains can reduce depressive symptoms.[184] Conversely, diets high in carbohydrates–especially refined sugar–can increase depression.[185] Countries with a tradition of eating fish (rich in omega-3s) report less general depression,[186] Seasonal Affective Disorder, and post-partum depression.[187]

- For *schizophrenia*. Populations who gain more protein from fish than red meat have a lower incidence of psychosis.[181] Refined sugar (which can cause *Hypoglycemia*, p. 203) and dairy can adversely affect people with schizophrenia. In fact, sugar consumption was the major predictor of poor outcomes in treating schizophrenia.[188] Case studies suggest that a ketogenic diet can dramatically reduce schizoaffective symptoms for some people.[189]

- For *bipolar*. Countries that consumed greater seafood have less bipolar symptoms in their populations.[190] Case studies suggest that a ketogenic diet can reduce bipolar symptoms better than medication for some people.[191]

- *More broadly*. Nutrition accounts for wide differences in cognitive ability in the elderly.[192] Those with mental health issues often eat diets high in carbohydrates.[193]

Digestion, gut microbes, and probiotics. Gastrointestinal (GI) health is vital to our mental health.[180] In fact, there are many links[194] between our gut and our brain including the vagus nerve, the immune system, brain-influencing hormones produced in the gut,[195] and neuroprotective antioxidants created by gut microbes. A study of American veterans with mental disorders reveals that they had twice the incidence of GI issues as compared to veterans without disorders.[196] See Case Study 3, p. 66 and Case Study 4, p. 67.

- For *mood disorders*. GI issues are often present with mood and behavior disorders.[180] Digestive distress can be the cause or the result of anxiety, stress, or depression.[197] Probiotics appear to lower stress[198] and improve mood significantly.[199] People given probiotics (lactobacillus and bifidobacteria) daily for thirty days reported less stress and anxiety—and no side effects.[200] In an animal study, probiotics had a significant effect on receptors that help reduce anxiety and depression.[201]

- For *major depression*. People ruminated less on bad feelings and experiences after four weeks of probiotic therapy,[202] an important finding, since rumination is one of the strongest predictive markers of depression. Probiotics appear to be a beneficial additive therapy for depression.[203]

- For *other diagnoses*. Practitioners and patients have found significant decreases in schizophrenia symptoms, tic disorders, depression, and attention-deficit hyperactivity disorder (ADHD) after antimicrobial treatment with the GG strain of the probiotic Lactobacillus acidophilus.[204]

- *More broadly*. A bacteria-free group of mice produced 60% less serotonin than a control group with normal gut bacteria. When a combination of 20 gut microbes was reintroduced to the germ-free group, their serotonin levels returned to normal.[205]

Therapeutic fasting. Studies indicate that fasting can alleviate some mental health symptoms and may improve the effectiveness of some drugs.

- For *depression*. 90% of 69 cases showed an improvement in depression using fasting therapy, and all maintained that improvement at a long-term follow-up.[211] Benefits waned, however, if people returned to high-fat diets.
- For *mood disorders*. Patients using a three-month fasting-and-calorie-restriction diet reported a significant drop in tension, anger, confusion, and total mood disturbance—along with improvements in strength and energy.[206]
- For *schizophrenia*. Clinical results from Soviet-era hospitals found that 40%-80% of patients with schizophrenia improved significantly during a fasting regime paired with increased exercise and massage. Gradually, foods were reintroduced. The shorter the duration of diagnosis, the higher the recovery rate; in fact, some patients lost all symptoms,[207] and 47% of them maintained that improvement for six years, the length of the study.[208]
- *More broadly*. One study found that fasting patients had physical symptoms associated with greater relaxation and less neurosis.[209] Also, 83% of elderly patients with mental health symptoms improved considerably using Fasting Dietetic Therapy (FDT).[210] A large clinical trial found that 87% of patients improved or eliminated symptoms for a wide variety of psychosomatic and mental disorders with a ten-day fasting therapy.[211] Ramadan fasting (a month-long day-time fast for practicing Muslims) has been shown to reduce oxidative stress and inflammation associated with mental health issues, improve brain function, and result in other psychological benefits.[212]
- *Safety*. Fasting Dietetic Therapy should be supervised by a doctor.

Substance moderation and avoidance. People with mental health issues often self-medicate with recreational drugs, alcohol, and/or tobacco. These substances can cause and/or worsen mental health symptoms.

- **Alcohol and substance abuse**. Studies suggest that alcohol consumption is unhealthy, although one glass of wine or beer daily significantly reduces the risk of developing dementia, when compared to nondrinkers or individuals who drink to excess.[18a] Substance abuse increases the likelihood of suicide.[213]
- **Caffeine**. Caffeine is associated with anxiety.[214] Individuals who wrestle with anxiety should avoid caffeine in all its forms (coffee, tea, chocolate, caffeinated sodas, etc.). Caffeine can last up to twenty hours in the system.[215]
- **Tobacco**. Studies show that smokers with mental health issues require higher doses of psychotropics than non-smokers.[216] Clinicians tend to treat psychiatric issues first and allow patients to self-medicate with cigarettes if necessary, assuming that psychiatric problems are more challenging to treat, and that quitting smoking may interfere with treatment. However, when patients quit altogether or halve the number of cigarettes they smoke, they exhibit a lower risk for mood disorders and less likelihood of alcohol and

drug problems.[217] Eating a diet rich in alkaline fruits and vegetables can reduce the craving for tobacco.[218] Unfortunately, some smokers say they are repelled by these foods and dairy products because they make cigarettes taste terrible.[219] Conversely, many smokers enjoy the taste of meat, coffee, and alcoholic beverages. A slow transition to a diet containing less meat and more fruits, vegetables, and dairy can set the stage for quitting tobacco.

WHAT CONSIDERATIONS SHOULD I KEEP IN MIND?

Because of the very strong interaction between the brain and gut, healthy diet and digestion are perhaps the most powerful controllable approaches for improving mental health. When the gut is disrupted, it fails to absorb necessary nutrients, which can cascade to imbalances in brain chemistry and the onset of mental health symptoms.

Many people today are overfed but undernourished. A significant number of studies come to the same conclusion: *a healthy diet is crucial for mental health.* It should contain plenty of fresh fruits and vegetables, sufficient fat, low-fat protein sources, probiotics for digestive health, sodium, and potassium electrolytes. The diet should be low in refined sugar (an excess can cause *Hypoglycemia,* p.203), white flour, and processed foods (especially junk foods).

A "Mediterranean diet" rich in vegetables, fruit, legumes, whole grains, lean meats, fish, heart-healthy fats and oils, with minimal animal fats and sweets is considered an excellent model. [16] It is associated with lower depression, lower anxiety, and improved quality of life.[220] Significant amounts of omega-3 foods are found in this diet.

Fish Mercury Levels

- *Low Mercury. Limit to 2 6-8 oz. portions/week of clams, flounder, oysters, perch, salmon, sardines, scallops, shrimp, sole and tuna (canned, light and yellowfin).*
- *Moderate Mercury. Limit to 1 6-8 oz. portion/week of cod, crab, haddock, herring, mahi, tuna (canned, white or albacore), and white fish.*
- *High Mercury. Limit to 1 6-8 oz. portions/month of halibut, marlin, northern lobster, orange roughy, pollock, red snapper, saltwater bass, tuna steaks, and wild trout.*
- *Very high Mercury. Avoid king mackerel, swordfish, shark, tilefish, and fish caught in local lakes (unless local advisories declare them safe).*

Figure 13 – Mercury in Fish

Although eating fish is healthy, nearly all fish and shellfish now contain mercury, so we should eat predominantly low-mercury seafood. (See Figure 13.) The ultra-low carb ketogenic diet has also been shown effective in some cases.

Although vegetarian diets have significant cardiovascular benefits, studies show that those on vegetarian diets have up to double the risk of depression and anxiety.[221] If you eat a vegetarian diet, ensure that you get healthy quantities of Omega-3 fatty acids, folate, B12 and zinc in your foods, or gain sufficient quantities by using supplements.

Nutritionists urge us to incorporate changes slowly and then maintain healthy dietary changes. And it isn't enough to simply tell people they should eat right. One study found that direct access to healthy food in the home and daily reminders are often needed for effective dietary change[222] – the barriers to dietary change should be reduced as much as possible.

As a rule of thumb, dietitians recommend taking the time for excellent breakfasts because our blood sugar levels are lowest in the morning, so healthy breakfasts get us going. It's better to eat dinners early in the evening and avoid eating when we feel stressed, since too much adrenalin shuts down digestion. Additionally, probiotics survive in the colon for no more than two weeks, so nutritionists urge us to take them regularly and eat foods with good probiotic content (yogurt, buttermilk, Kefir, tempeh, and miso, among others).

Daily Reference Indexes (DRI) establish guidelines for consuming essential nutrients. DRI values represent minimums, the lowest continuing level needed to sustain nutrition. People with mental health issues should use DRIs as a starting point for their diets and consider *Nutrient Therapy* (p. 167) to reach the nutrient levels helpful for recovery–which may be well above minimal levels recommended to avoid illness. [16]

A comprehensive medical exam (See *Biomedical Test Panels*, p. 323) can help detect vitamin/nutrient imbalances, toxins, and organism-related disorders.[223] Doctors should also evaluate for possible food allergies.[224] Often gluten and dairy are sources of allergies. (See *Food Allergy Therapy*, p. 209.)

If alcohol, caffeine, and tobacco are issues, consider *Substance Abuse Approaches* (p. 305) and *Addiction Co-Therapy* (p. 332). Drink plenty of pure water throughout the day to keep bowels hydrated, relieve constipation, and move toxins out of the system.

One common problem that interferes with digestion is a lack of sleep, which in turn affects mental health. Diarrhea can also interfere with healthy digestion, because it flushes out electrolytes and nutrients; sometimes smaller meals help with that problem. A flare-up of Irritable Bowel Syndrome may be an early warning sign for a flare-up of mental health issues. If these problems exist, consult a gastroenterologist or neurogastroenterologist (brain/gut specialist).

Diet & Digestion are critically important for our overall physical health. The next section, *Exercise & Sleep,* considers how we can treat our body wisely, to help ensure mental health.

REAL-WORLD EXPERIENCE

Case Study 3 – Probiotics (Schizophrenia)

Jack suffered from delusions (a "positive" schizophrenia symptom). His practitioners noticed he felt little motivation for socializing, and when he did socialize, he had difficulties communicating ("negative" schizophrenia symptoms). His doctor recommended a trial of probiotics (BIO- THREE®), since people with chronic schizophrenia often have digestive issues.

Before treatment, Jack's predominant gut bacterium was one associated with several physical illnesses. Thirty days after probiotic treatment, this bacterium subsided, and new, more helpful strains developed as Jack's negative psychosis symptoms improved.[225]

Bottom Line: Experimenting with a simple and inexpensive regimen of probiotics may improve psychotic symptoms.

Case Study 4 – Probiotics (OCD)

Kevin pulled clumps of hair out of his head every day for 15 years. He was diagnosed with trichotillomania, an obsessive-compulsive disorder.

He stumbled on research that suggested that probiotics might help so he started taking two capsules of 30 billion CFUs a day. In six weeks he became symptom free and found he had completely lost his obsession of hair pulling. He continues with daily probiotics and is fully in remission.[226]

Bottom Line: The causation of mental health symptoms is often murky. Sometimes, taking care of Wellness Basics can be enough to end symptoms.

Case Study 5 – Ketogenic Diet (Schizophrenia)

At the age of 70, after suffering from a variety of hallucinations, Alma was diagnosed with schizophrenia. She was also obese. At her doctor's recommendation, she committed herself to a low-carb ketogenic diet. In the year following her dietary changes, as she lost weight, the auditory and visual hallucinations disappeared. She enjoyed greater energy.

Although she would occasionally break her diet for a few days and eat pasta, bread, and other carbohydrates, she had no recurrence of her hallucinations.[227]

Bottom Line: Significant research supports the value of a low-carb diet. Eating a sensible healthy diet can not only improve overall physical health but may significantly improve mental health.

WHAT ARE ADDITIONAL RESOURCES?

- The gut-brain connection. http://goo.gl/jsQpls.
- Fasting. www.FastingExperience.com.
- Candida-Related Complex and Food Allergies. http://goo.gl/eaO273.
- Irritable Bowel Syndrome. http://goo.gl/GbJEyQ.

Exercise & Sleep

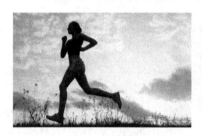 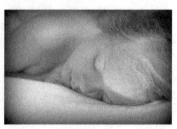

WHAT IS THE ESSENCE?

We all require *Exercise & Sleep*— the complementary acts of physical exertion and recovery. Our bodies and minds are integrated, so the state of our physical health often has a profound effect on our mental health. *Exercise & Sleep* are also two key components helping us manage stress.

WHAT EVIDENCE SHOWS THIS IS EFFECTIVE?

> *"It is exercise alone that supports the spirits and keeps the mind in vigor."*
> - Cicero

Positive effects of exercise. Exercise often decreases stress, creates energy, decreases fatigue, increases endorphins, supports self-esteem, takes the mind off anxious situations, and improves sleep.[228] These are all factors critical for mental health. Exercise can also increase serotonin,[229] acetylcholine, and norepinephrine;[230] which alleviates low self-esteem and social withdrawal.[231] Individuals with serious mental health issues are at high risk of chronic diseases associated with sedentary behavior, including cardiovascular disease and diabetes.[231] Exercise helps address these risks.

Best forms of exercise. Exercise benefits cardiovascular health, coordination, range-of-motion, agility, and strength. Mental health benefits come from a wide variety of physical activities,[232] but aerobic activity appears to provide greater benefit than resistance or flexibility training for those with anxiety disorders[233] and depression. Research has found that varying the type of exercise results in significantly less depression and stress, while significantly improving mental health and vitality.[234]

When it comes to exercise, consistency is more important than intensity. Thirty minutes of a moderate physical activity on most days (but preferably every day) delivers clear health benefits.[235] Interestingly, mental health benefits seem to be independent of the actual fitness level achieved.[236] It is better to be consistent with a lower level of activity over the long term than to have less frequent bursts of more intense activity.

Exercise and the sexes. Studies suggest that exercise seems to affect the sexes differently. It has a more positive impact on improving the mood of men than women.[237] However, older women who exercise appear to gain more benefit in avoiding dementia and Alzheimer's than men.[238]

Exercise by mental health diagnosis.

> ### A Good Mental Health Exercise Program
>
> - *Frequency. 3-5 times per week.*
> - *Time. 20-60 minutes/session.*
> - *Intensity. Achieve 55%-90% of your max heart rate (MHR). MHR = 208 − (.7 * your age).*
> - *Type. Choose a rhythmic exercise that uses your major muscle groups. Aerobic exercise is helpful for depression.*

- For *depression*. Moderate exercising two or three times per week results in significantly less anxiety and depression over a long period of time.[239, 240] Meta-analysis shows that exercise can be as effective as antidepressants, delivering moderate symptom reduction.[241] Exercise not only avoids psychotropic side effects, but often helps a person improve mental health symptoms more quickly.[242] One study found that people with major depression who followed a ten-month aerobic exercise course avoided depression significantly better than those on antidepressants.[242] Two analyses of depressed patients showed that exercise gave results similar to psychotherapy. One large study found that 12% of cases of depression could have been prevented if participants undertook just one hour of physical activity a week.[243] See Case Study 7, p. 72.

- For *anxiety and panic attacks*. Although there is little research, doctors often advise people susceptible to panic attacks to avoid exercise programs because they worry that physical activity might trigger attacks. Interviews with patients often reveal that they are concerned about having a heart attack. However, one controlled exercise program has been found to be as effective as medication in reducing or eliminating panic attacks.[244]

- *For obsessive-compulsive disorder.* After each exercise session lasting between 20 and 40 minutes, OCD patients reported significantly lower anxiety, negative moods, and symptoms.[245]

- For *post-traumatic stress disorder*. Structured exercise, including resistance training and walking, improves sleep quality and helps people recover.[246]

- For *schizophrenia*. A meta-analysis showed that aerobic exercise significantly improved attention, social cognition, and working memory. Those who exercised the most showed the biggest improvements in cognitive functioning, and exercise programs that were best for improving physical fitness were also most beneficial for cognition.[247] One smaller study found that weekly group cycling significantly increased participants' self-esteem, positive relationship, global function, and quality of life.[248]

- For *dementia and Alzheimer's*. One large study found that exercise is associated with lower rates of cognitive impairment. There is good reason to be optimistic: simple activities like walking seem to lessen cognitive impairment,[249] and regular daily walks stretching between one-quarter mile and two miles significantly reduce the risk of dementia in the elderly.

Sleep and mental health.

> ### Techniques to Promote Sleep
>
> - **Relaxation**. *Calming techniques include Controlled Breathing (p. 75), Progressive Muscle Relaxation (p. 74), Meditation (p. 78), Guided Imagery (p.79), Massage (p. 242), relaxing music, and moderate exercise.*
> - **Melatonin**. *Melatonin (p. 202) can improve sleep duration and quality by addressing sleep issues caused by disturbances to our circadian rhythms.*
> - **Valerian**. *Valerian (p. 229) is often as effective as sedative psychotropics, without the risk of dependency.*

Chronic sleep problems are common with people having mental health issues: depression (65%-90%), bipolar (69%-99%), anxiety (>50%) and attention-deficit hyperactivity disorder (5%-50%), compared to between 10% and 18% of the general population in the U.S. who report chronic sleep problems.

Studies suggest that sleep issues increase the risk of, and directly contribute to, symptoms of mental illness. Treating a sleep disorder may help alleviate associated symptoms.[250] People with depression are five times as likely to suffer from breathing problems related to a sleep disorder as those without depression.[251]

- **Good sleep hygiene**. Proper habits help sleep: restricting the time spent in bed, going to bed only when you are sleepy, getting out of bed if you are unable to sleep, reducing noise or light in the room, and getting up at the same time every morning. Moderate insomnia often responds well to improved sleep habits.[16] Avoiding caffeine, alcohol,[252] nicotine, and refined sugar[253] prior to bed will also improve chances for a good night's sleep.
- **Electronic screens can interfere with sleep.** Using a computer screen within an hour of going to bed results in poor sleep.[254] Extended use of an iPad within four hours of going to bed reduces REM sleep and melatonin production, so users feel less alert in the morning than people who read a print book for the same period. Scientists suggest that the blue light these devices emit causes the brain to think it is still day time, thereby delaying the release of the sleep-inducing melatonin. The American Medical Association indicates that nighttime electric light disrupts circadian rhythms.[255]
- **Nutrient deficiencies and sleep.** When biomedical lab testing indicates nutrient deficiencies, taking folate, thiamine, iron, zinc, and magnesium may improve sleep.[16]

Total sleep deprivation (TSD). Although sleep hygiene is a critical component in mental health, short bursts of sleep *deprivation* appear to be one of the most fast-acting antidepressants known. Treatment can be a single instance or repeated instances of sleep deprivation, either all night or partial the second half of the night. Sleep deprivation must be done under supervision, since it has been associated with an increased incidence of psychiatric disorders.[256]

- For *depression*. Approximately 60% of patients improve dramatically within hours of TSD, a finding that has been replicated in thousands of cases.[257] One study found that TSD gains were preserved in 75% of patients when it was followed by the gradual advance of the start of sleep.[258]

- For *bipolar depression*. In one study, 70% of patients with no history of drug resistance improved rapidly with TSD and *Bright Light Therapy* (p. 239) combined, and 57% remained depression-free at the nine-month follow-up. The rate was lower in drug-resistant patients; however, 44% of those patients remained depression-free, a remarkable statistic when compared with standard antidepressant drug-response rates.[259]

WHAT CONSIDERATIONS SHOULD I KEEP IN MIND?

Integrative medicine considers the body, mind, and spirit in creating wellness plans, so it is not surprising that physical activities are vital for mental health. Exercising five times a week for 45 minutes is considered ideal.

Many forms of exercise are available, though some form of aerobic exercise seems best for alleviating depression. Many people find that using large muscle groups in a rhythmic, repetitive fashion works best. Walking outdoors is one of the most accessible and beneficial exercises.

To find success with exercise, choose activities you enjoy and vary their types, intensity, and timing. Gradually increase the level and length of exercise. Working out with a partner can be helpful.[260] Exercise takes many forms: walking your dog, running, yoga, Pilates, mowing the lawn, washing the kitchen floor; they can all be adjusted for orthopedic limitations. *Mind-Body Disciplines* (p. 111) - *Yoga*, *T'ai Chi Chuan* and *Qigong* - are excellent. Their focused body awareness provides the additional benefit of *Mindfulness* (p. 74).

As with all wellness categories, our challenge is to maintain the desire and discipline to continue exercising. If we think of exercise as an important way to achieve our goals and purpose (See *Purpose & Meaning*, p. 94), we'll find it easier to exercise consistently. The self-esteem boost that comes from exercising and the simple pleasure of clearing our minds as we walk can give us a much more positive outlook on exercise—and on life.

Exercise improves sleep, and sufficient sleep is vital to good health; poor sleep makes us more vulnerable psychologically.[261] Sleep apnea can cause mental health symptoms (Case Study 6, p. 72) and is three times more common in people with schizophrenia.[262] Daylight exercise is the behavior most closely associated with improved sleep quality.[263]

Consistent restful sleep—six to eight hours every day—rejuvenates and energizes our bodies and brains.[264] Naps are good. In fact, neurologist Dr. James Gramprie recommends brief naps when needed, since they can support both mental and physical health.[265]

For ongoing sleep problems, see *Insomnia Therapies* (p. 309) and *Sleep and Insomnia Apps* (p. 328). Although tranquilizers can be used to aid sleep, non-drug approaches sustain sleep improvements, in contrast to psychotropics.[266]

Exercise & Sleep marks the last of the *Body Wellness Basics*. The next section considers the first *Mind Wellness Basic*: *Calm Awareness,* an approach that quiets life's chaos and helps create mental wellness.

REAL-WORLD EXPERIENCE

Case Study 6 – Sleep Apnea

Mel experienced almost every psychiatric symptom. "I had nightmares, psychosis, panic, anxiety, mania, depression, and seizures," he explains.

"After two and a half years, I finally discovered the true underlying biological cause – sleep apnea, which is often recognized by heavy snoring. But apnea commonly goes undetected for years. Because my brain was being deprived of adequate oxygen during sleep, I was unable to build a neurotransmitter reserve. Hence the symptoms."

After using a mechanical nasal passage expander for a week, all of his symptoms stopped—"and they have not recurred," he says.[267]

Bottom Line*: Mental health symptoms can come from unexpected causes. Leave no stone unturned when you face distressing symptoms.*

Case Study 7 – Exercise (Depression)

Thirty-three people entered a trial to assess the impact of exercise on depression. At the end, they all had different perspectives on the experience:

"Exercise has two benefits, the physical wellbeing [and] the emotional sense of challenge as I push myself."

"[Physical activity] helps distract me. I switch to positive much better thoughts, so I know it works."

"I've lost weight and that's very positive... And I'm sleeping better, which makes me feel more optimistic when I wake up in the morning."

"I am increasing my confidence [through] physical activity... I have maybe thirty years left, and I don't want to take long-term medication."[268]

Bottom Line*: Many people find benefit in exercise, though the specifics will vary. Give consistent exercise a try to see what benefits result.*

WHAT ARE ADDITIONAL RESOURCES?

- Robert Lutz on Exercise and Mental Health. http://goo.gl/VkLfYb.
- Maintaining a Healthy Sleep-Wake Cycle. http://goo.gl/aaGTPR.
- Sleep hygiene tips. https://goo.gl/cQYn8O.

Calm Awareness

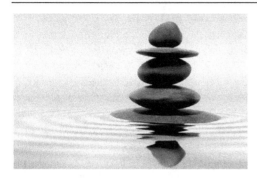

WHAT IS THE ESSENCE?

Calm Awareness is the ability to be physically relaxed, mentally alert, and emotionally centered even in stressful situations. It is a state of poise and an ability to consciously step back and watch ourselves interact with the world, enabling us to make those interactions more effective and satisfying.

With *Calm Awareness,* we can more accurately perceive and manage both the internal world of our mind and the external world of people and the environment around us. Our situations may not immediately change, but our responses to those situations can. It helps us better manage the stresses of everyday life which can have a profound positive impact on our mental health.

Calm Awareness can be cultivated, allowing us to turn off our internal auto-pilot so we can act more intentionally. We often live our lives in a fog, reacting to triggering events automatically, with worn habits. Sometimes these habits are helpful, often they are not. With *Calm Awareness,* we can begin to break unhelpful habits, so we can respond from conscious choice, instead of from unchecked impulse.

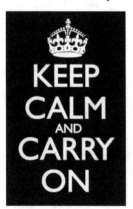

Figure 14. WWII UK motivational poster

Calm Awareness is a state of *being*, a natural companion to the state of *doing* found in *Effective Self-management* (p. 83). KEEP CALM and CARRY ON is a familiar motto coined during England's darkest days in World War II (Figure 14); it offers us all a wisdom we can use for coping in times of distress.

Calm Awareness is usually achieved in a two-step process: first *Relaxation*, then *Attention Control*.

Relaxation is slowing down and releasing tension from our body and mind. It softens muscular tightness, puts worries aside, and helps us let go of the stressors we often hold with a firm grip.

Once relaxed, we are in a more receptive state to achieve *Attention Control* – the ability to concentrate precisely, deeply, and for extended periods of time. It is a skill, and like a muscle, strengthens with use. We can use it to focus on anything of our choosing: a problem to solve, a reality to acknowledge, a moment to enjoy, or a person to love.

Relaxation techniques include *Progressive Muscle Relaxation, Autogenic Training*, and *Controlled Breathing*, but also encompass many others: a hot bath, a walk in a park, playing with a dog, or reading a good book. We all relax in different ways, and we need to find what works best for us.

There are a number of interrelated *Attention Control* techniques that include *Mindfulness, Meditation, Mantra Repetition, Affirmation, Guided Imagery, Visualization* and more.[269] These help us gently set aside racing, scattered, or unhelpful thoughts, allowing us to consciously harness our creative potential and direct it with laser focus toward something of our choosing.

Calm Awareness and happiness. *Calm Awareness* is a powerful tool that can improve our happiness by shifting our attention in time. By being grounded in the *present*, we can decrease our focus on unproductive fears, concerns, and unmet expectations about our *future*. We shouldn't disregard our future, but consciously let go of our worry about the future, so we can more clearly focus on what we need to do today to create that future.

> *"... A calm mind is key to happiness... it brings inner peace and is very important for good health... Without a calm mind we cannot see reality properly."*
>
> - Dalai Lama

In addition, focusing on the present gives us space to find happiness in today's people and realities: the smile of a child, a beautiful sunset or the satisfaction of completing an important task.

WHAT EVIDENCE SHOWS THIS IS EFFECTIVE?

Progressive Muscle Relaxation (PMR). PMR involves a simple tensing and relaxing specific muscle groups, one at a time, to create a sense of deep relaxation and calmness.

- For *anxiety and depression*. PMR is effective in helping to reduce symptoms—but it is not as effective as broader yoga practice.[270]
- For *schizophrenia*. PMR can significantly reduce anxiety with psychosis.[271] It also offers similar relaxation benefits to *Autogenic Training*.

Autogenic Training (AT) is a desensitization-relaxation technique developed by German psychiatrist Johannes Heinrich in the 1930s. AT uses six standard exercises to make the body feel warm, heavy, and relaxed by repeating a set of visualizations and verbal commands similar to *Affirmations* (p. 88). It also exerts conscious control over bodily processes that we often don't control, like our heart rate (similar to *Biofeedback*, p. 142).

- For *insomnia*. One study found that AT and *Progressive Muscle Relaxation* (p. 74) had similar positive benefits in aiding sleep.[272]
- For *schizophrenia*. The use of AT has provided good results in clinical recuperation.[273]
- For *stress*. AT is effective for chronic stress, working in ways similar to self-hypnosis and biofeedback.[274]

- *More broadly*. Analysis of sixty studies covering a wide spectrum of patient situations showed that AT had positive effects like other psychosocial interventions on relaxation, mood, cognitive performance, and quality of life.[275]

Controlled Breathing. Our breathing and emotions are closely related. Emotions influence the depth, speed, and pattern of our breathing, while conscious breath control can have a substantial positive impact on a variety of emotions including fear, anger, sadness and joy.[276] Controlled breathing typically slows down the breath rate and heart rate and induces healthy alpha rhythms in the brain.[277]

Forms of controlled breathing include Ujjayi breathing (at left) and pranayama, both from *Yoga* (p. 111) and coherent breathing (breathing at about five breaths per minute with equal inhalation and exhalation). Clinical experience has shown that these techniques are safe and effective for reducing anxiety, depression, insomnia, avoidance, and symptoms of PTSD.[15] A study of Sudarshan Kriya yogic breathing revealed decreases in depression, anxiety, stress, and PTSD.[278] *Deep Breathing Apps* (p. 328) can help.

> ### Ujjayi Breathing
>
> - *Sit with your spine erect.*
>
> - *Slowly exhale through your mouth making a "haaah" sound like trying to fog a mirror. Notice the slight tightening of the throat.*
>
> - *When ready, seal the lips.*
>
> - *Breathe through your nose on both the inhale and exhale pausing after each, to achieve 2-5 breaths per minute. Make a soft "haaah"-like sound both in and out, while gently constricting the throat.*
>
> - *Continue comfortably, with your attention focused on your breath.*
>
> *Try it when you are depressed, anxious, angry, or afraid, to promote calmness.*

Mindfulness. *Mindfulness* is a relaxed concentration – remaining fully focused and alert on whatever we choose with deliberate and sustained awareness. It isn't "zoning out" or suppressing thoughts and emotions but being fully present in the moment to clearly perceive the full nuance of our thoughts, emotions, and our environment.[279] When we are mindful, things that we previously processed unconsciously often become more conscious.

Although *Mindfulness* is a secular concept rooted in the Eastern Buddhist tradition, it has proven very effective in Western settings. Highly successful businesses use the practice routinely[280] to improve leadership. So do schools, elite sports training programs,[281] military boot camps,[282] and prison programs.[283]

Mindfulness doesn't advocate a passive or inactive approach to life. Exactly the opposite. It creates calm despite a stressful world, allowing us to actively manage our life more effectively. In fact, it is one of the most accepted techniques for helping us take charge of our own mental health.

Attitudes of Mindfulness. To gain the full benefit of *Mindfulness*, adopting a helpful set of attitudes is important. Jon Kabat-Zinn, Professor of

Medicine Emeritus at the University of Massachusetts Medical School and a leading mindfulness teacher, has defined seven attitudes of *Mindfulness* (Figure 15):[284]

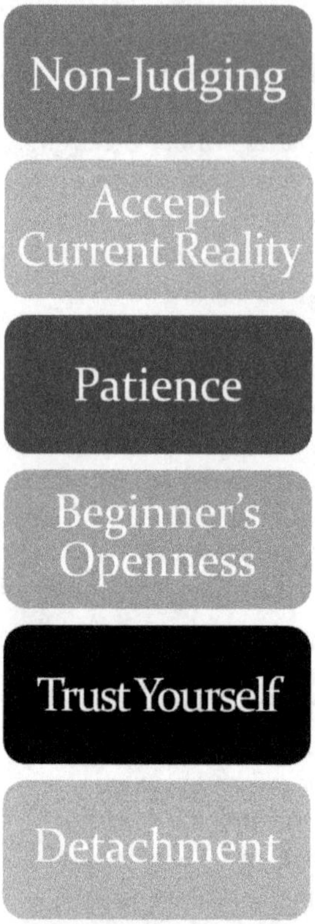

Non-Judging

Accept Current Reality

Patience

Beginner's Openness

Trust Yourself

Detachment

Non-striving

Figure 15. Attitudes of Mindfulness

- *Non-Judging* means understanding something without evaluating it as good or bad.
- *Accepting Current Reality* means embracing our current situation as we find it, without criticism.
- *Patience* means calmly waiting for things to develop, not needing them to happen immediately.
- *Beginner's Openness* offers a fresh perspective uncluttered by bias.
- *Trust Yourself* means having confidence in your personal authority and ability to address challenges.
- *Detachment* means letting go of unhelpful emotions and holding a dispassionate neutrality.
- *Non-striving* is being able to turn off the constant need for achievement.

These attitudes allow us simply to accept whatever arises. Without judgment. Without comparing our situation negatively to a far more desirable situation. We must accept where we are and find the good within it. To do this, we must relax. We can't change everything—or sometimes, anything. Thinking we can, and attempting to force immediate change, creates stress with few positive results.

As we adopt these seven *Attitudes of Mindfulness,* we learn to forgive ourselves gently for mistakes we've made. We learn to handle criticism and unkindness more effectively, without allowing them to get under our skin. We can envy people less and appreciate them more. We can more easily avoid self-condemnation and create greater mental well-being.

In addition to these attitudes of *being*, it is important to adopt attitudes of *doing*. (See Figure 17, p. 85.) The art comes in knowing how to hold these seemingly opposite attitudes at the same time.

Research on the mental health benefits of *Mindfulness* is extensive.

A Simple Mindfulness Meditation

> - *Sit comfortably in a quiet room. Relax. Forget your troubles. Slow down.*
> - *Keep your spine erect. Close your eyes. Breathe.*
> - *Allow the breath to flow naturally. Inhale energizing oxygen, exhale stress.*
> - *Notice the movements in your chest and abdomen.*
> - *Mentally scan slowly from head to toe. Notice the sensations of your body.*
> - *When your mind wanders, gently bring awareness back to your breathing.*
> - *Be patient with yourself.*
> - *After between 5 and 15 minutes, bring your awareness gently back to your whole body.*
>
> *Open your eyes and notice how relaxed you feel.*

- For *depression*. Mindfulness is especially effective for reducing anxiety, depression, and stress.[285] The U.S. Veterans Administration found that it significantly improves the depression of veterans.[286]

- For *stress and anxiety*. Mindfulness increases the ability to cope with everyday and extraordinary stressors.[287] It effectively improves mood[288] and reduces anxiety symptoms.[289] Patients with Irritable Bowel Syndrome (IBS), which is often influenced by anxiety, experienced significantly fewer symptoms of IBS and anxiety after two fifteen-minute daily sessions of mindfulness meditation.[290]

- For *schizophrenia*. Compared to untrained individuals, people practicing mindfulness perform better in conflict-monitoring tasks, orientation tasks, standardized tests, and memory. One study found that mindfulness meditation helps people live with schizophrenia symptoms better than either psychoeducation or education about mindfulness.[291]

- For *insomnia*. One study found that *Mindfulness Meditation* had a greater positive effect on sleep quality than sleep hygiene education.[292]

- *More broadly*. Mindfulness group therapy was shown to be as effective as *Cognitive Behavioral Therapy* (p. 117) for improving depression, anxiety, hopelessness, and difficulty in coping.[293] Considerable research has linked mindfulness with enhanced autonomy and self-regulation.[294]

Mindfulness-Based Stress Reduction (MBSR). The most common and documented mindfulness program is MBSR,[295] typically an eight-week training program rooted in secularized Buddhist practice. It involves weekly group meetings, homework, and instruction in mindfulness meditation, body scanning, and simple yoga postures.

- *For anxiety*. One study found that those taking MBSR therapy had a 44% decrease in anxiety.[296]
- *More broadly*. Studies found that MBSR delivers consistent and strong mental health results in situations ranging from stress reduction to serious mental disorders,[287] with improvements in quality of life, depression, anxiety, and ability to cope.

Mindful Awareness in Body-oriented Therapy (MABT). MABT incorporates mindfulness, massage, and emotional processing.

- For *substance abuse*. MABT significantly reduces the number of women's substance-use days.[297]
- For *combat post-traumatic stress disorder (PTSD)*. Women veterans using MABT experienced relaxation, reduced pain, and improved efficacy and empowerment.[298]

Meditation. Although meditation can be used as a religious or spiritual practice, in a mental health context it is a process of exerting control over our thought process. It is inner concentration that enables us to slow down and quiet "mental chatter." With sufficient practice, meditation can produce an alert inner stillness; a state of awareness with both mental clarity and emotional calm. This clarity and calm can then be brought to our daily affairs.

To quiet the mind, meditation often holds our attention on something very simple, such as an imagined peaceful scene, the breath, or a short *Affirmation* (p. 88) or mantra (below). Instead of attempting to forcefully stop thoughts and emotions, meditation gently redirects our attention continually back to our object of focus so that our thoughts and emotions naturally quiesce. Two meditation techniques helpful for mental health are Loving-Kindness[299] and Tonglen.[300]

- For *schizophrenia*. Meditation improves the management of psychotic symptoms, controls impulsive behaviors, increases self-awareness and self-acceptance, and reduces anxiety and social withdrawal.[301] Loving Kindness meditation was found broadly beneficial in decreasing negative symptoms[302] and significantly improving emotions, environmental mastery, self-acceptance, and satisfaction with life.[303]
- For *anxiety and depression*. Meditation alleviates mood disorders.[304] An eight-week meditation class is as effective as antidepressants in minimizing relapses for people with major depression.[305] These positive effects are specific to meditation, over and above simple relaxation effects.[306]
- *For OCD*, a small trial found that a kundalini meditation technique improved symptoms 38% in three months and 71% in fifteen months.[307]
- *For PTSD*. In a study of incarcerated men with moderated to high risk of trauma symptoms, those practicing transcendental meditation daily for four months achieved a 47% reduction in trauma symptoms, including anxiety, depression and stress.[308] Additionally, veterans with PTSD who had a single 90-minute meditation per week for 3 months saw better symptom reduction than veterans receiving exposure therapy or nutrition support.[309]
- *More broadly*. People who meditate exhibit more activity in the left-side anterior section of the brain (linked to positive moods).[310]

Mantra Repetition. Silent, frequent repetition of a mantra – a word or phrase often with spiritual significance – is a common element of meditation.
- For *PTSD*. A 5-week study of veteran pilots found that mantra repetition significantly reduced stress and anxiety, and improved quality of life and spiritual well-being.[311]

Controlling Expressed Emotion (EE). Expressed Emotion heightens the quality of interactions and the emotional contexts. High Expressed Emotion occurs when there is hostility, criticism, emotional over-involvement, and excessive efforts to control. Low Expressed Emotion occurs in situations where people show kindness, concern, and empathy.

High Expressed Emotion creates a negative atmosphere and triggers symptom relapses and rehospitalization for a wide range of mental disorders;[312] these emotions significantly impact illnesses.[313] In contrast, calm is a characteristic of low Expressed Emotion and low stress. Group therapy helps individuals transition from high to low Expressed Emotion.[314]

- For *schizophrenia*. High family levels of Expressed Emotion are consistently associated with higher rates of relapse.[315] The mean relapse rate was 48% for patients residing with high EE families and 21% for those in low EE families.[316]

Guided Imagery. Guided Imagery uses thoughts and suggestions to guide imaginations toward a relaxed, focused state. Imagery can be individualized to specific anxieties, and studies show it is beneficial for the immune system, physiological stress responses, and cognitive-emotional functioning.[317] When used consistently, mental imagery can reduce generalized anxiety, panic, and anxiety based upon traumatic memories.[318] It also helps people with chronic worry sleep better.[319]

Active stress management. We cannot fully eliminate stress from our lives, but we can manage it by using the "4 As" strategy. (See *Resources,* below.) We can work to *avoid* stressful situations or people, *alter* our response, *adapt* to the stress, and calmly *accept* the situation without trying to control the uncontrollable.

Open Focus. *Open Focus* meditation is a practical and effective method for reducing stress-related symptoms and enhancing well-being, using principles developed in the field of *Biofeedback* (p. 142). The technique is relatively new, so evidence is based primarily on case studies. *Open Focus* is based on our ability to change the scope of our attention, from very focused (with laser-like concentration—when reading, for example), to very broad ("taking it all in"), or somewhere in the middle. Being very focused can promote greater stress. *Open Focus* meditation helps us shift our attention more easily, moving between narrow and open focus and between higher and lower stress levels. *Calm Awareness* is a skill necessary for open focus. *Effective Self-management* (p. 83) is a skill necessary for laser focus.

Calming structure. People with mental health issues, especially bipolar,[320] often do better with a comforting structure in their lives. (See *IPSRT*, p. 132.) Structure offers predictability, which can reduce stress, avoid feelings of isolation, and expand a sense of connectedness and self-control.

WHAT CONSIDERATIONS SHOULD I KEEP IN MIND?

Calm Awareness is an important learned skill requiring time, focus, and patience. Its techniques can slow the mind and body through breathing, visualization, meditation, muscular relaxation, emotional control, and more. Some *Calm Awareness* practices combine multiple elements. For instance, *Energization Exercises,*[321] a prelude practice to one form of meditative yoga, use muscle tensing and relaxation similar to PMR and controlled breathing (pranayama) to create calmness that facilitates deeper meditation.

Mindfulness and its seven attitudes represent a strong core for achieving *Calm Awareness.*

Other *Wellness Basics* and therapies that result in calm include *Exercise* (p. 62), *Creative Engagement* (p. 137), *Sensory Therapy* (p. 239), and *Energy Therapy* (p. 159). Among the most effective and proven approaches are the three *Mind-Body Disciplines* (*Yoga, T'ai Chi Chuan,* and *Qigong,* p. 111), which rely on *Calm Awareness* fundamentals of breathing, mindfulness, and bodily control. Yoga especially has been shown to reduce symptoms of nearly every psychiatric diagnosis.

Find the *Calm Awareness* techniques that make sense for you and use them regularly. You might find it helpful to record these calming tools in a *Wellness Toolbox.* (See *Resources,* below.) Be alert to events that trigger anxiety and stress; these early warning indications signal when *Calm Awareness* tools may be needed.

One goal of *Calm Awareness* is to manage your responses to stress. Try to limit intense emotional encounters and overly-stimulating activities (everything from excessive noise to large crowds, stressful personal relationships, video games, and the internet). Create small bursts of calmness: short naps, a short break for controlled breathing, a moment to consciously appreciate your surroundings, among other methods. A supportive home environment helps tremendously. Failure to remain calm can elevate bodily *Inflammation* (p. 52),[322] which is associated with increased mental health issues.

Calm Awareness is a state of clarity, peace, and self-control. It creates an open, broad focus and a sense of immediacy. This state is extremely helpful, but the stressful demands of our lives frequently war with *Calm Awareness.* We must work, plan, problem-solve, interact, recover, and thrive, using this calm state of *being* to aid our *doing.*

Its counterpoint is *Effective Self-management* (p. 83).

Paradoxically, even though calmness is vital, a certain amount of tension – such as the stress we generate when we work toward something meaningful – is indispensable for mental well-being,[323] as we will see when we explore *Effective Self-management.*

REAL-WORLD EXPERIENCE

Practitioner's Story 1 – Mindfulness in psychiatric practice

Dr. Russell Razzaque is a psychiatrist and author based in London, England, who uses mindfulness as an important part of his practice. He has witnessed its power to aid mental health, so he not only advocates for mindfulness, he practices mindfulness. The insight gained from his personal experience helps him work with patients on their own mindfulness.

Although you can learn mindfulness from books or online, Dr. Razzaque notes that another very effective approach is to leave home for an experiential undistracted retreat, where an encouraging external environment cultivates a calm inner environment.[324]

Bottom Line*: Mindfulness is an ancient practice that has become mainstream in Western medicine. It works. The proof is substantial.*

Practitioner's Story 2 – Mindfulness in the workplace

A health services organization was failing to meet standards of care in its high-stress environment. Hoping for a turnaround, each person in the organization was asked to attend a "Mindfulness at Work" workshop.

An evaluation after the workshop found that every one of the people who attended reported that the mindfulness techniques subsequently helped them manage strong emotions. In addition, they reported an overall decrease in depression, anxiety, and stress. Some participants said that they made dramatic improvements in depression levels.

After the multi-week course, more than 90% found mindfulness techniques so valuable that they planned to continue using them.

Bottom Line*: Mindfulness is a Wellness Basic. It can help in the workplace, at home, and with mental health issues.*

Case Study 8 – Controlled Breathing (PTSD)

Mike was subject to explosive rages that worsened after serving as a first responder during the 9/11 disaster in New York City. He developed post-traumatic stress disorder, and his distress, insomnia, and rages soared. Counseling and psychotropics didn't help.

As a last resort, he tried coherent breathing, starting at ten minutes each day and gradually increasing to twenty minutes a day, using a CD to guide him.

Mike had an incredibly positive response. At a ten-month follow-up, he was using this breathing practice forty minutes twice a day, and he discovered that for the first time in his life he was able to control his temper. His anger issues disappeared, despite ongoing stresses at home and work.

By shifting to coherent breathing whenever he felt stressed, he was able to remain calm. Mike says he is happier than he has ever been.[15]

Case Study 9 - Mindfulness (Insomnia)

Maria was a "worrier". For fifteen years, she had difficulty sleeping, which meant that she always felt fatigued. Diagnosed with insomnia, she took medication on a variety of occasions, but it didn't seem to help.

Initially, Maria tried to stop the flood of thoughts that impeded her sleep, but that didn't work. Then she tried an eight-week mindfulness-based training class for insomnia that closely resembled MBSR (p. 77).

The class studied the physiology of sleep and practiced mindfulness meditation (including meditations from the book Full Catastrophe Living*). The members also discussed ways of applying mindfulness to insomnia with sleep experts. Maria learned to let go of her desire to control her thoughts; instead, she let them run their course.*

When she changed her thought patterns, Maria's anxiety dropped dramatically. She was able to fall asleep quicker, double her sleep time, and significantly improve the quality of her sleep.[325]

WHAT ARE ADDITIONAL RESOURCES?

- Progressive Muscle Relaxation. http://goo.gl/3hudjw.
- Autogenic Training. www.guidetopsychology.com/autogen.htm.
- Reduce Stress and Build Resilience. www.HeartMath.com.
- Breathing techniques. http://goo.gl/O5Df0W.
- Breathing Apps. *Android* https://goo.gl/8FCTF1.*iOs* https://goo.gl/utudcE.
- Coherent Breathing. www.Coherence.com.
- Guided Imagery http://goo.gl/L7mEPk and http://goo.gl/5cKDlL.
- Academy for Guided Imagery. www.acadgi.com.
- Center for Mindfulness. http://goo.gl/Oy913M.
- Mindfulness Training. www.bemindfulonline.com.
- UCLA Mindfulness Meditation Training. http://goo.gl/qvE5cq.
- Mindfulness 7 Attitudes. http://goo.gl/xdlo50.
- Guided Mindfulness Meditations. http://goo.gl/N6whgV.
- *Wherever You Go, There You Are,* by Jon Kabat-Zinn.
- *Meditation*, by Eknath Easwaran.
- Open Focus Meditation. www.OpenFocus.com.
- Meditation for Health and Happiness, http://goo.gl/4lPbfn.
- Loving-kindness meditation. http://goo.gl/zFYWR, https://goo.gl/HXU3AK.
- Tonglen meditation. https://goo.gl/1mmryf.
- World Meditation Directory. https://goo.gl/dXR4fK.
- Mayo Clinic "4 As" of stress management. http://goo.gl/7DlwXz.

Effective Self-management

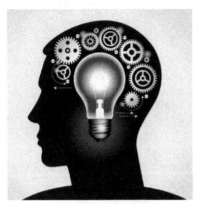

WHAT IS THE ESSENCE?

Effective Self-management is an active process of working with our thoughts, emotions, and core concepts of ourselves to create the life of our choosing. Grounded in our personal history, beliefs, and the things we value, *Effective Self-management* is an effort that requires and extends our self-understanding. It is an important process that requires considerable effort. (See quote below).

Effective Self-management is a skill of *doing* – an active companion to the more reflective skill of *being,* found in *Calm Awareness* (p. 73). Together they are powerful in helping people lead effective and healthy lives. Figure 16 (p. 84) gives a simplified view of the process that is built on two strong foundations.

The first foundation is based on 4 perspectives we hold about ourselves: *self-understanding (*knowing our personal strengths, weaknesses, needs, and core humanity); *self-compassion* (valuing, accepting, and loving ourselves); *self-efficacy* (having confidence in our ability to create a life of our choosing); and *self-discipline* (consistently making the right choices to realize that life). These perspectives are deep-seated, found at the core of our being. Maturing our sense of *self* is an evolutionary process of *personal growth,* and it has a profound effect on our mental health.

> *"One of the most important, but one of the most difficult things, for a powerful mind is to be its own master."*
> - Joseph Addison

The second foundation is our *internal grounding* (our beliefs about the world and life) and our unique *purpose and goals* within it. (See *Purpose & Meaning,* p. 94.) Our *internal grounding* acts as a compass helping us navigate toward longer-term personal goals within a sometimes-harsh *external reality*. Many people have spiritual or religious elements in their *internal grounding*.

These two foundations begin to form in childhood. They evolve over time, strongly influenced by our personal history, especially by vivid events, both positive and negative.

Although these foundations resist change, we can alter them, sometimes dramatically, to help us overcome challenges. This ability to change and grow offers tremendous hope for everyone on the path of mental health recovery.

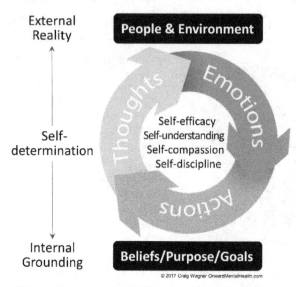

Figure 16 - Process of Effective Self-management

We all have a *Thought-Emotion-Action cycle*, in which each of the three parts influences the other two. Accepting responsibility for consciously managing this cycle is often an important starting point for recovery. Self-reinforcing and often unconscious, the cycle can propel us forward in positive directions. But it can also spiral us down in negative directions.

> *"As you think, so you become."*
> - Epictetus

For instance, when we *act* in a positive way by eating well, we tend to have *thoughts* of being in greater control of our lives, and this makes us *feel* better. Conversely, when we *think* of ourselves as incapable or unworthy, we tend to *feel* depressed and we may *act* by withdrawing from others and harboring self-doubts about our abilities and our future.

The *Thought-Emotion-Action cycle* can work extremely quickly. For instance, getting cut off in traffic can instantly elicit "Idiot Driver!" (*thought*), spawning anger (*emotion*) that can cause us to pound our horn (*action*). Becoming aware of this cycle opens the door to being able to master it, helping us to *respond* thoughtfully instead of to *react* impulsively to situations. Mastering this cycle is often a direct path to recovery. The *Thought-Emotion-Action cycle* sits at the core of one of the mental health field's most effective therapies: *Cognitive Behavioral Therapy* (p. 117).

If we continually relive the same patterns in our *Thought-Emotion-Action cycle*, we establish habits. Detrimental patterns become *limiting beliefs* – misguided ideas about ourselves in the world – that can block recovery, especially impeding us in the *Awareness* stage (p. 33). However, if we send positive patterns through our *Thought-Emotion-Action cycle*, we can progressively overcome fears and unhelpful thoughts.

> *"You need to avoid certain things in your train of thought: everything random and irrelevant. You need to get used to winnowing your thoughts..."*
> - Marcus Aurelius

Figure 16 also shows *self-determination,* our daily effort to make choices and consciously direct our life.

There are two important observations about self-determination. First, every moment is an opportunity to choose. Even in difficult situations that we can't change, we still can guide our thoughts and moderate our emotions. This isn't necessarily easy, and in some cases may seem near impossible, but we each have innate resources that help us change our inner response when we lack full external control.

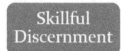

Secondly, our ability to choose is like a muscle. The more we exercise our capacity of self-determination, the stronger it becomes and the more skilled we become in using it. The opposite is also true. When we let ourselves be driven by habits, unhelpful thoughts, or emotions, our self-determination weakens and atrophies. Self-determination is what allows us to modify and hone our *Thought-Emotion-Action cycle.*

Attitudes of Effective Self-management.

Just as there are *Attitudes of Mindfulness* there are also *Attitudes of Effective Self-management* (Figure 17). Cultivating these seven attitudes helps us influence our surroundings to get what we need.

• *Skillful Discernment* means detecting the nuances and influencers in important situations.

• *Creativity* means continually working to make the best we can in each moment.

• *Enthusiasm* brings heightened energy to our efforts.

• *Expert's Decisiveness* requires applying personal experiences to make definitive choices.

• *Grow Yourself* requires continual self-improvement.

• *Commitment to Priorities* helps us attain important ends.

• And, last of all, *Action-Bias* is a preference for action rather than talk or thought.

Figure 17 – Attitudes of Effective Self-management

The basis of all seven attitudes is our strong conviction that we can create the future of our choice. We can often exert much greater influence over ourselves and our immediate environment than we ever thought possible.

Compare Figure 15 (p. 76) to Figure 17. The former attitudes are about *being*; the latter are about *doing*. One set of attitudes is not better than the other; both are necessary. In many ways, they are opposite yet complementary. For instance, we need to *commit* to the actions needed for recovery while we *detach* ourselves from the need for actions to show immediate results. Our opportunity is to develop both sets of attitudes and call upon them when needed.

Many techniques of *Effective Self-management* are found in self-improvement approaches, leadership practices, and positive parenting techniques. They also take center stage in a variety of psychosocial therapies covered in Chapter 4.

Effective Self-management and happiness. Our desires are thoughts that strongly influence our happiness. Consciously mastering our *Thought-Emotion-Action cycle* helps us exert control over our desires, so we can be happier.

Desires are neither inherently good nor inherently bad, but they can be strongly captivating. They can be beneficial when they motivate us to do things important to us. But often, unfulfilled desires, especially for material things, create a state of disappointment, envy, and unhappiness. Even if those desires are eventually fulfilled, the feeling of satisfaction is often fleeting,[326] and can soon be replaced by the tension of the next unfulfilled desire. Paradoxically, as we seek happiness by trying to satisfy our ever desire, we often create the very conditions for unhappiness: numerous unmet cravings.

> *"... I have learned to seek my happiness by limiting my desires, rather than in attempting to satisfy them ..."*
>
> - John Stuart Mills

For this reason, many traditions recommend derailing runaway desires,[327] often using techniques grounded in the three *Mind Wellness Basics*. One way to do this is to shift our thinking from a broad set of *desires* to a reduced and more consequential set of *needs*. By focusing our energy and resources on this smaller target, we are more likely to satisfy our true needs, and in the process, become happier.

WHAT EVIDENCE SHOWS THIS IS EFFECTIVE?

Self-understanding. Understanding that *our self is an active and responsible agent* is central to our recovery.[328] Self-understanding leads to a sense of identity[329] that is vital for the resilience needed in facing difficult situations in a healthy way. Self-understanding promotes kindness[330] and compassion, toward ourselves and others. *Journaling* (p. 138) and introspection assist in developing an understanding of ourselves.

Self-compassion. *Self-compassion* means being kind and understanding to ourselves when we suffer, fail, or feel inadequate. We must respect, value, and love ourselves, flaws and all, while recognizing that no one is perfect. It is an unselfish self-love. It doesn't push aside negative thoughts; it accepts them and lets them pass, a perspective of *Mindfulness* (p. 74).

- For *depression and anxiety*. Self-compassion reduces anxiety and depression.[331] A key feature of self-compassion is the lack of self-criticism, a predictor of anxiety and depression.[332]
- For *general well-being*. Self-compassion is an important source of happiness and a sense of psychological well-being,[333] life satisfaction, and feelings of social connectedness.[334] It is also strongly associated with emotional intelligence, happiness, optimism,[335] and resilience.[336]
- *Self-compassion vs self-esteem*. Self-compassion avoids judging; self-esteem judges us positively. Although high self-esteem is considered important for mental health,[337] too much self-esteem can lead to self-inflation and narcissism.[338] In fact, self-esteem is enhanced when we feel superior to others,[339] as when we are part of the "in group". This perspective impedes recovery. The importance of self-esteem varies by culture. One study found that the Japanese culture is incongruent with high self-esteem, since it envisions the individual within a web of relationships.[340]

Self-efficacy. Considerable research indicates that high self-efficacy (a sense of competence) has beneficial and therapeutic effects for individuals, and low self-efficacy (a sense of powerlessness) has a negative impact. Research identifies self-efficacy as a significant factor in overcoming phobias and anxieties, addictions, and eating disorders.[341]

Self-discipline. According to Psychiatrist M. Scott Peck, self-discipline is one of the two keys to mental health. The other is a well-developed ability to love ourselves and others.[342] Self-discipline allows us to defer immediate gratification; instead, we can focus on longer-term goals. It helps us dive into painful problems so that we can solve them. When we accept responsibility for a situation, we show self-discipline. The idea of accepting responsibility is the salient starting point for recovery from addiction.[343]

> *"Once a person is determined to help themselves, there is nothing that can stop them."*
>
> - Nelson Mandela

Self-determination. SAMHSA indicates, "Self-determination and self-direction are the foundations for recovery, as individuals define their own life goals and design their unique path(s) towards those goals."[1461] The World Health Organization regards self-determination in therapy choice as vital even in times of acute distress.[344] Regardless of the choices we make, having the freedom to make them improves our mental well-being.

Practitioners who foster self-determination by treating patients as partners, empower them to self-manage their situation in a better way.[345] Yet, some drug therapy has been shown to decrease the sense of self-determination that is so vital to recovery.[346] And the most dramatic form of denying self-determination is the ethical dilemma of forced medication. (See endnote #100.)

Guided Self-determination (p. 150) honors the individual and is one method to help people develop self-determination.

Affirmation. Affirmations impress the subconscious with positive thoughts (e.g. "I am lovable and capable.") to help replace negative ones in our *Thought-Emotion-Action cycle.* Affirmations are silently repeated, while feeling that the words are, or will become, true. The result is often calming. Choose ones that you find meaningful and powerful, and ones that directly counter negative thoughts you might harbor. Affirmations often start with "I am", since these speak to our self-identity. (See Case Study 15, p. 93.)

Visualization and Imagination. We are tremendously influenced by what we see. One negative example of this influence is found with returning veterans; they often have post-traumatic stress disorder caused by what they have seen of war. *Visualization* is a process of consciously using our "internal vision" in a positive way to imagine a detailed mental picture of a calming or affirming situation that generates positive emotions. (See Figure 18.)

Visualization can be powerful since it uses two elements of our *Thought-Emotion-Action cycle* at once. We create the *thought* of whatever we visualize, but it also has a sense of *action* since we can visualize ourselves acting in

---

5 Types of Visualization

Visualization can help us uproot unhelpful thinking and replace it with more positive thoughts and emotions.

1. **Positive Visualization** *creates an image of a new way to respond to difficulties. It is a mental rehearsal of a more helpful response.*

2. **Modeling** *recalls a vision of someone else acting effectively in a situation we find difficult. Seeing their success makes it easier for us act like that person.*[347]

3. **Sensitization** *helps with addictions. Using our imaginations, we can tie negative consequences to addictive behaviors and envision positive consequences from avoiding them.*

4. **Desensitization** *helps with fears and phobias*[348] *by imagining acting inconsistent with them. For instance, see yourself relaxing in the face of things you fear.*

5. **Pre-sleep suggestion**. *Using positive thoughts, images, or affirmations when we are half-awake prior to sleep can help break unhelpful responses. Consider using audio recordings.*[349]

Figure 18 - Visualization

---

positive ways. That action becomes even more palpable if we imagine scenes that include other senses in the picture, such as smells, sounds, tastes, and touch.

Visualization is similar to *Affirmation* (p. 88), except it uses mental pictures instead of words. Both work to create positive constructs for the mind that can help uproot and replace negative or unhelpful ones. *Visualization* is used to control pain, relax the body, and boost performance in competitive sports. It is also an important tool in *Cognitive Behavioral Therapy* (p. 117).

Cognitive Restructuring. *Cognitive Restructuring* helps identify and change unhelpful thoughts by consciously influencing our thinking instead of allowing an uncontrolled free flow of ideas. *Cognitive Restructuring* is an integral process of many psychosocial therapies, especially *Cognitive Behavioral Therapy* (p. 117). Studies show that cognitive restructuring works.[350]

---

9 Common Unhelpful Thoughts

1. *Limiting thoughts:* *"I can't do that."*
2. *All-or-nothing thoughts:* *"My politics are correct. Yours are not."*
3. *Overgeneralization:* *"Rich people are heartless."*
4. *Mental Filtering:* *Dwelling on negatives, ignoring positives.*
5. *Jumping to Conclusions:* *"He didn't speak to me. He must hate me."*
6. *Magnification/Minimization:* *"I'm an idiot since I got a 'B' on the test."*
7. *Emotional Reasoning:* *"I feel like an idiot, so I must be one."*
8. *Should Statements:* *"I'm bad since I didn't do what I should have done."*
9. *Labeling:* *"I'm a jerk."*

Figure 19 – Unhelpful Thoughts

The first step is to identify the most unhelpful and self-defeating thoughts we harbor. To make that easier, consider the common types of unhelpful thoughts in Figure 19.

Once we identify our self-defeating thoughts, we can use techniques to alter them. All these techniques share a common theme: uprooting the unhelpful thought and planting a more helpful, often opposite, thought.

Affirmation and visualization techniques include *Mindfulness* (p. 74); *Neuro-Linguistic Programming* (p. 128); gradual desensitization to the thought by repeated exposure (the basis of *Exposure Therapies*, p. 151); considering the thought as something separate from ourselves so it is easier to reject; viewing the thought as a helpful signal to an area of potential growth; and more.

Reframing. Sometimes when we subtly reframe a situation, we can improve our response to it. For instance, when people get performance anxiety before a sporting event, they are often encouraged to relax. However, reframing *anxiety* as *excitement* can improve performance more effectively than relaxing.[351] This is both a shift from a *threat* mindset to an *opportunity* mindset and a shift *from victimization* to *self-determination*.

Acting "as if". Acting "as if" is based on the idea that if you don't like the way you feel, change the things you do. It starts with the *action* element of the *Thought-Emotion-Action cycle and* is designed to create a positive feedback to combat depression. The idea is to go through unpleasant routines as if you enjoy them—while you try to enjoy them. Initially, this will feel forced, but continuing to act this way can result in real happiness. We need to genuinely attempt to develop the new skill and attitude, rather than simply enacting a charade, for this to work. Alcoholics Anonymous and *Dialectic Behavioral Therapy* (p. 120) use this technique, which is sometimes called "fake it until you make it."

Managing desires. Research underscores the value of "trimming desires" and suggests that people driven by materialistic wants are less happy than their peers,[352] experience fewer positive emotions, are less satisfied with life, and suffer higher levels of anxiety, depression, and substance abuse.[353] In addition, these same people feel less satisfied with their day-to-day life.[353] Some of the things we desire to do, like shopping, eating well, and making money, do not lead to a long-term sense of fulfillment.[354]

WHAT CONSIDERATIONS SHOULD I KEEP IN MIND?

Effective Self-management is a framework grounded in our core beliefs and colored by our deep-seated concepts of ourselves. It is closely tied to the other *Mind Wellness Basics* (Figure 20).

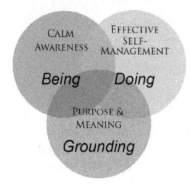

Figure 20 – Interlocking Mind Wellness Basics

- *Calm Awareness* (p. 73) creates an unruffled sense of *being*.
- *Effective Self-management* propels us with strong skills of *doing*.
- *Purpose & Meaning* (p. 94) provides *grounding* and a vision of our future.

At the core of *Effective Self-management* is gaining conscious mastery over our *Thought-Emotion-Action cycle* as well as our self-determination. A process of *personal growth*, this mastery grows with diligence and helps us identify, de-energize, and potentially eliminate unhelpful thinking that can cause fear, anger, hatred and other troubling emotions. Although *Effective Self-management* is often difficult for people in psychiatric crises, it can be grown incrementally after stabilization.

The laser-focused, future-orientated, active *Effective Self-management* complements the wide-lens, now-oriented, contented person we strive to become in *Calm Awareness* (p. 73). Both skill sets help us craft the best responses to our challenges and opportunities.

Hundreds of studies of *Cognitive Behavioral Therapy* (p. 117) testify to the validity of many *Effective Self-Management* techniques. Many of the most effective psychosocial therapies attempt to change *Thoughts*, *Emotions*, and *Actions* to help the *Thought-Emotion-Action cycle* operate more effectively. For example, *Dialogue & Exposure Therapy* (p. 146) starts with *action* by confronting troubling mental constructs in an effort to break them down; *Cognitive Behavioral Therapy* (p. 117) starts with unhelpful *thoughts* and replaces them with positive thinking patterns; and the cathartic approaches of *Individual Psychotherapy* (p. 126) elicit deep *emotions* to aid recovery.

Effective Self-management is a powerful engine for personal growth and self-determination, and it must be used wisely. To find our greatest happiness, we need to apply passion and precision toward our goals, whatever we consider most important. The next section, *Purpose & Meaning,* explores this personal vision, which we can use as a compass to guide our engine of self-determination toward the opportunities and challenges inherent in mental health recovery.

REAL-WORLD EXPERIENCE

Case Study 10 – Self-determination

Stephanie Heit (her real name by permission) was diagnosed with bipolar disorder as a young adult. She has been in and out of psychiatric hospitals for many years. To help quiet her manic symptoms and elevate her depressive symptoms, she worked with many psychiatrists, therapists, and an Integrative Mental Health physician. She tried an endless variety of therapies: psychotropics, electroconvulsive therapy, transcranial magnetic stimulation, ketamine treatments, acupuncture and herbs, meditation and yoga, and more.

The game changer was when she fired her psychiatry team at a leading university after four years of countless treatments that made her worse, not better. She went into a different hospital and luckily had an inpatient integrative psychiatrist. She began on EMPowerplus and continued on a path that led her to working with an outpatient integrative psychiatrist specializing in functional medicine.

It is two years since her last hospitalization and instead of daily suicidality she enjoys being alive. She takes an orchestra of supplements along with calcium channel blockers and thyroid medication, and she has regular tests and treatment for gut balance. The key has been addressing the underlying causes for her condition rather than treating symptoms. Stephanie works hard to be self-aware and a strong advocate for herself. She refuses to waste time with practitioners who don't help her progress.

__Bottom Line__: Your practitioners work for you. Find those you trust and give them a chance to help you. But if they don't help, find others who can. Your recovery is too important to do otherwise.

Case Study 11 – Self-determination

Sixty-four people in a mental health recovery program talked about what helped them achieve and maintain recovery. They all said the key to their success was having a sense of control and self-determination in their lives. "If you're not making choices, you're not taking responsibility. And then you start becoming a victim," one participant reported.

Many mentioned that personal growth and internal change were vital elements of recovery. So were adjustments to their attitudes and beliefs about themselves. This identity shift motivated them to start their recovery journey.

For some, the shift meant redefining themselves apart from their condition. For others, it meant embracing their diagnosis. Crucial to the shift in self-perception was the growth of self-confidence.[355]

__Bottom Line__: People thrive when they feel in control and can make choices. Honor self-determination whenever possible.

Case Study 12 – Accepting Responsibility

Kristina was working with a peer support specialist on her recovery. "It is your job to recover," the specialist stated emphatically. Kristina disagreed. "No," she told the specialist. "That's not my job. It's your job. You're supposed to fix me."

The specialist explained that Kristina was incorrect, that she had the process and the responsibility reversed. Kristina was in total shock. She was waiting for someone else to fix her.

Learning that it was her responsibility to recover was terrifying, she said later. But it also showed her that others believed in her. It awoke a feeling of confidence in herself that had been missing for a long time.

She used this confidence to learn new recovery skills. She wasn't doing it alone, but she was accepting the responsibility of self-determination.[356]

Bottom Line: *Accepting responsibility for recovery and believing that recovery is possible are acts of self-determination—and key steps in the Awareness stage of recovery (p. 33).*

Case Study 13 – Accepting Responsibility

"I've had schizophrenia for more than twenty-five years," explained one man who agreed to participate in a new therapy. "Taking responsibility for my life has been crucial to my recovery. As a first step, I learned that we must look within ourselves for our strengths. These are the tools for rebuilding our self-image and self-esteem. We must convince ourselves of our worthiness. Then, as we effectively manage our illness, we endow ourselves with an ongoing sense of mastery and control.

"Unfortunately," he added, "progress is often measured with concepts like 'comply' (with a doctor's prescription) instead of 'choose,' implying that we can't take an active role in our recovery.

But I've learned that if we build on our assets, if we confront our illnesses with courage and struggle with our symptoms persistently, we will successfully manage our lives and can bestow our talents on society."[357]

Bottom Line*: Self-reflection in the Awareness stage of recovery (p. 33) is one of the first steps toward wellness.*

Case Study 14 - Visualization (Anxiety)

Paul experienced a recurring nightmare three to five times a week for fifteen years. Desperate for relief, he went to a therapist to find help. The therapist's diagnosis was anxiety. By using a desensitization form of visualization, Paul was taught to visualize the dream while relaxing through its various scenes – a response that was inconsistent with his usual routine.

After thirteen sessions, the dream ended. Within three weeks, the dream didn't recur in any form.[358]

Bottom Line*: Even long-held troublesome thoughts can be neutralized with visualization and Exposure Therapy (p. 151), since both can directly confront these thoughts and rob them of their strength.*

Case Study 15 - Affirmation (Audio Hallucinations)

For over thirty years, Luisa tried drugs and electroconvulsive therapy to help her cope with voices that were her constant companion. Nothing worked, so she took a step back and reassessed.

"Sometimes you just have to put your foot down and know you are more powerful than your voices," she explained later. She put her foot down by repeatedly focusing her mind on deeply spiritual affirmations. Her favorite is from St. Teresa of Avila... Let nothing disturb you; nothing frighten you. All things are passing. God never changes. Patience obtains all things. Nothing is wanting to him who possesses God. God alone suffices... *She also used much more mundane approaches, like setting a timer so she could focus for ten minutes on an important project.*

In the end, Luisa advises, "Make your weaknesses your strengths, one step at a time, and one day the voices will fall silent." By putting her foot down, Luisa stopped 98% of her voices without increasing her medication. [359]

Bottom Line*: Luisa found success by repeatedly focusing her mind on spiritually inspiring affirmations and the next task at hand, directly influencing her Thought-Emotion-Action cycle (Figure 16, p. 84).*

WHAT ARE ADDITIONAL RESOURCES?

- Self-Compassion (Dr. Kristin Neff). www.self-compassion.org.
- National Gateway to Self-determination. http://goo.gl/v2pqOi.
- Self-determination in Mental Health Recovery. http://goo.gl/CjHbXC.
- Getting out of thinking traps. http://goo.gl/6wD1m3.
- Tools for changing cognitive distortions. http://goo.gl/YZBM8Y.
- Mental Health Affirmations. http://goo.gl/zgto0Q.
- Visualization. http://goo.gl/MNEJIW.
- Responding instead of Reacting. http://goo.gl/YNVfHB.

Purpose & Meaning

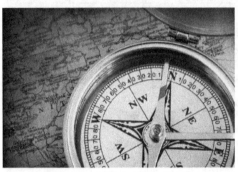

WHAT IS THE ESSENCE?

Nietzsche said, "He who has a *why* to live for can bear almost any *how*." Our *why* is our *Purpose*, the reason we do the things we do, the thing that we determine is most worthy of our time, effort, and passion. (See quote, below).

Our *Purpose* clarifies the destinations of our life and how we want to progress toward them. It defines both what we want to *do* and who we want to *be*. It offers a stable and clear beacon that guides us, and a benchmark against which we can measure progress.

> *"Every life needs a purpose to which it can give the energies of its mind and the enthusiasm of its heart."*
> - St. Francis of Assisi

Our *Purpose* is also uniquely personal. It can be grounded in family and community, artistic expression, nature, employment, religious ideals, achievement, volunteer work, and much more.

Paradoxically, our *Purpose* represents both an opportunity to choose what is most important, and a responsibility to make and enact that choice. No one can choose it for us. Viktor Frankl, psychiatrist and Holocaust survivor, emphasizes this choice.

> *"... We need to stop asking about the meaning of life, and instead think of ourselves as the ones being questioned by life–daily and hourly.... Each person can only answer to life by answering <u>for</u> their own life... We ultimately must accept responsibility to find the right answer to life's problems and to fulfill the tasks which it constantly sets for each individual..."* [360]

Our *Purpose* has several tangible benefits. It:
- *Provides direction* to keep us doing what is most important to us.
- *Motivates* us to action to address our challenges and opportunities.
- *Clarifies* the difference between our wants and needs.
- *Propels* us out of our own heads and into the world.
- *Frames* our lives and helps us create our own unique narrative.

Leading a life of *Purpose* often creates *Meaning* – a feeling of contentment and significance spawned from doing what is important to us. Both *Purpose & Meaning* are vital for mental health.

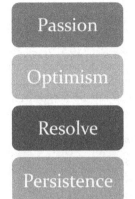

Figure 21 – Attitudes of Purpose & Meaning

Attitudes of Purpose & Meaning. As with the other *Mind Wellness Basics*, important attitudes support *Purpose & Meaning* (Figure 21), motivate us, and help us look forward in anticipation. Like all attitudes, they are molded from our experiences, but we can learn new attitudes and enhance the ones we have.

- *Passion* drives us toward our purpose.
- *Optimism* is the hopeful belief that our purpose will be realized.
- *Resolve* is the willful effort to make the choices necessary to achieve our purpose.
- *Persistence* is the tireless effort to push through adversity until we achieve our purpose.
- These attitudes are not only helpful in establishing and enlivening our purpose, but vital if we want to make steady progress in mental health recovery.

Story Telling. *Story Telling* is a universal method of encapsulating *Purpose & Meaning*. Humans love a good story. We crave yarns in theater, books, and films. We are drawn to myth and allegory in our religions. In many ways, we urgently need a narrative for our own lives that affirms our unique value and attributes meaning to our lives. Personal narratives are often vital in mental health recovery; they honor our experiences and attest to the fact that we can rise above the challenges we face. Happy endings aren't just reserved for fairy tales.

***Purpose & Meaning* and happiness**. *Purpose & Meaning* can make us happier in a variety of ways.

> *"(Happiness) is attained... through fidelity to a worthy purpose."*
> - Helen Keller

- Our *Purpose* is grounded in what we find most important. We are happier when we work on and succeed with things that are significant.
- Our *Purpose* gives us a long-term view that helps us look beyond life's inevitable rough patches. Instead of being unhappy over today's problems, we can find happiness in working to solve them, knowing we are making progress toward important ends.
- Our *Purpose* allows us to find happiness in the process of life, not just in its favorable outcomes. For example, if our *Purpose* is to create beauty through our art, we can find happiness in each expression of our creativity. We don't have to wait to win an art prize.

> *"It is the very pursuit of happiness that thwarts happiness... It must ensue as the side effect of one's personal dedication to a cause greater than oneself."*
> - Viktor Frankl

A final observation is important. Oddly, the more we focus on trying to be happy, the less happy we often become.[361] (See quote at left.) Happiness isn't something we can force into our life. Rather, it is something that often emerges from our ongoing efforts to realize our *Purpose*.

WHAT EVIDENCE SHOWS THIS IS EFFECTIVE?

Purpose & Meaning strongly influences mental health.

- For those exposed to *trauma*. A purpose is the key predictor of the victim's ability to maintain mental health or recover from a psychiatric illness.[362]
- For *college students*. Their purpose in life is one of the best predictors of their mental health.[363]
- For the *elderly*. Those with a strong sense of purpose are more than twice as likely to avoid Alzheimer's disease,[364] are apt to live significantly longer than those with low purpose,[365] and experience slower cognitive decline.[366] Purpose also appears to protect the brain's memory centers from normal age-related shrinkage; in men, it helps to grow memory centers modestly.[367] The elderly also show the ability to reverse this brain shrinkage and improve memory by engaging in meaningful activity.[368]
- *More broadly*. People experiencing meaning show diminished stress, while those experiencing short-term self-gratification have increased pro-inflammatory gene expression, similar to people experiencing chronic stress[369] and loneliness.[370] In addition, seeking this personal gratification has little impact on meaningfulness and happiness.[326]

Stories and personal narrative. Stories help people make sense of their lives, including making sense of mental health issues. Storytelling is considered the most powerful human method for recording and preserving the unique path each person forges toward growth and goals.[371] Personal narratives have the power not only to encapsulate an individual's values and philosophies, but to shape their future—and serve as a model for others.

- **Recovery narratives**. Recovery stories often feature themes that match the broader paradox of life: challenge versus hope, stigma versus assertiveness, limitations versus new possibilities, and struggle versus empowerment. In fact, many recovery stories come surprisingly close to the quest narrative of the "Hero's Story."[372] (Case Study 16, p. 98.) Being able to tell your story is akin to "finding your voice." Both experiences are empowering and strongly self-affirming. For schizophrenia, preliminary evidence indicates that people who improve the richness of their personal narratives can make sense of their experiences.[373]
- **Encouraging individual narratives.** Severe mental illness often blunts the ability to narrate personal life stories. Constructing and developing a

meaningful life story promotes recovery. In fact, it may be crucial to helping people define their identity beyond their illness.[374]

- **Narrative as therapy.** The art of creating and telling personal narratives to others is the core of *Dialogue Therapies* (p. 147) and *Journaling* (p. 138).

WHAT CONSIDERATIONS SHOULD I KEEP IN MIND?

Purpose & Meaning are grounding perspectives that give direction and significance to our life. Our *Purpose* is our unique statement of what we will do and be. *Meaning* naturally flows from our efforts to realize our *Purpose*.

Establishing a *Purpose* is essential to everyone. It makes our struggles matter. It helps us clarify the difference between our wants and needs – a realization that can lead to deep-seated happiness. It inspires the resolve, persistence, and patience needed by those who seek recovery. It also creates a useful structure for our lives, something especially important for people with bipolar.[320] Regrettably, 40% of Americans have not found their *Purpose*. [375]

For some, *Purpose* may come as a flash of clarity, but most of us find that it evolves over time. Some arrive at it through a process of discovery, others through more of a willful choice. Sometimes it becomes clear only when we face significant challenges—like those found in mental health recovery. To arrive at our *Purpose*, it is helpful to become grounded in *Mindfulness,* and review the things we find most important, based on our deeply-held beliefs and values.

> *"It's not enough to be busy. So are the ants. The question is, what are we busy about?"*
> - Henry David Thoreau

To make your *Purpose* feel tangible and attainable, write it in a short, clear sentence that is hopeful and inspirational. Make it worthy of your time and effort. Consider turning it into a compelling personal *Affirmation* (p. 88) that you use daily.

For even greater impact, define your *Purpose* in the context of a broader *Personal Narrative* – a bold statement of who you have been, who you are now, and who you will become. Those with mental health issues can include specifics of their challenges. But it should be much more: a hero's story of standing apart from, rising above, and finding meaning in these challenges.

Purpose & Meaning interact closely with the other two *Mind Wellness Basics* to profoundly influence our happiness and our mental health. (See Recommitment, p. 344, for a poetic perspective.)

The most deeply rewarding *Purpose* we can define–the one often associated with the greatest *Meaning*–is rarely selfish. In fact, many people find that their *Purpose* is most compelling when they decide to live for people or reasons beyond themselves. The next section, *Social & Outer Engagement*, explores the first step in "looking beyond" by reviewing the importance of human connectedness and creative interaction in mental health recovery.

REAL-WORLD EXPERIENCE

Case Study 16 – A Hero's Journey (Bipolar)

After she earned her Ph.D. and launched a successful career, Alice experienced the chaos of bipolar for twelve long years. She was in and out of hospitals, often living on the streets.

She started her recovery when she balked at a doctor's bleak prognosis. She cobbled together her recovery plan as she began experimenting with what would ultimately be more than fifty different approaches. One of the most important things she did to heal was to reframe her experience, she said later. She looked at her suffering as a purifying experience after reading Carolyn Myss' Spiritual Madness. *She identified with its message deeply.*

She also saw her effort as a "Hero's Journey," and her stages of recovery as steps on a universal spiritual path that required an exit from "normal suffering" and ultimate renewal, investing her life with new meaning. She reported that she found a deep sense of empathy, compassion and gratitude. She has been in remission for four years.[376]

Bottom Line*: Reframing your experience may offer renewal and recovery.*

Case Study 17 – Finding Purpose

Before his diagnosis of schizophrenia, Milt Greek felt messianic, certain that he was in contact with God and Jesus. His path to recovery has been long, but ultimately rewarding. Despite its difficulties, with the help of psychotropics and a therapist, he has improved significantly. To stay well, he says he must work toward the clear purpose that he established for himself: "To better the world, or at least my own community."

Although no one would ask for a diagnosis of schizophrenia, Milt says, "The diagnosis gave me purpose, and that purpose has been very much a part of my recovery." The author of Schizophrenia, a Blueprint for Recovery, *Milt speaks to community groups and peers about mental health topics.*[377]

Bottom Line*: Everyone needs a strong purpose to flourish—both people who are healthy and those seeking recovery. Purpose helps us transcend difficulties and find meaning in our difficulties.*

WHAT ARE ADDITIONAL RESOURCES?

- *Man's Search for Meaning*, by Viktor Frankl MD PhD.
- *The Act of Will*, by Roberto Assagioli MD.
- *On Purpose*, by Victor Strecher. www.dungbeetle.org.
- Mobile app for your purpose. https://goo.gl/GN6TpS, https://goo.gl/ji3frM.

Social & Outer Engagement

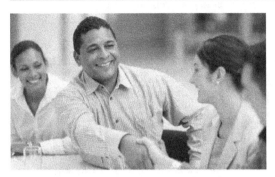

WHAT IS THE ESSENCE?

Social & Outer Engagement, the first *Spirit Wellness Basic,* is a set of techniques that propel us into meaningful interaction with people and our environment.

Social Engagement can take two forms: close *human companionship* with family and friends, and *social networks,* which typically are more casual but involve a broader set of people. In both situations, trust and meaningful cooperative relationships marked by empathy are important. *Social Engagement* is vital to recovery, since it can be a source of hope, love, and many varieties of support.

Outer Engagement is connecting with nature, music, arts, hobbies, or other things we enjoy. This interaction often has a creative element that provides grounding and meaning.

WHAT EVIDENCE SHOWS THIS IS EFFECTIVE?

Sense of Belonging. Building strong social memberships in a group provides a sense of "belonging", which is vital in helping clinically depressed patients recover and prevent relapse.[378] In fact, end-of-life conversations[379] affirm that that many people count their relationships as the most meaningful part of their lives. For women, networks of friends (but not family) are most important for mental health. For men, networks of friends and family both appear to improve mental health.[386] For those with mental health issues, one of the crucial themes for quality of life is a sense of belonging achieved principally by positive quality relationships and a lack or rejection of stigma.[380]

Human Companionship. Companionship is found in close relationships with friends or family where there is mutual acceptance and trust. Adults who are isolated and lack friends and companionship have the worst psychological outcomes.[381] In fact, adults who had emotionally supportive and close relationships were four times more likely to overcome their depression than those without

> *Companionship is vital for people with mental health issues since they often feel isolated, alone and vulnerable...*

such relationships.[382] A person with mental health issues describes true *Human Companionship* as "being able to talk to someone without fear of being judged, made fun of, lectured... yelled at, bossed, disregarded, or invalidated."[383] Companionship practices[384] include:

- *Hospitality* (spending time together in a safe space)

- *Neighboring* (finding common ground)
- *Side-by-side stance* (treating the other as an equal)
- *Listening* (to both the words and the emotions behind them)
- *Advocacy* (encouraging and assisting in a spirit of giving)

> *"Like everyone, I feel the need of relations and friendship, of affection...*
>
> *"I cannot miss these things without feeling a void and a deep need ...*[385]
>
> -- Vincent Van Gogh, who experienced frequent depression and anxiety

Social Networks. Social networks are less-intimate relationships with a broader set of people (work mates, friends, et cetera). Social networks are needed for human development and help avoid mental ill-health.[386] The frequency of social interactions with friends (but not family) is associated with better long-term outcomes for those with psychosis.[387]

Social Engagement and Loneliness. Studies suggest that social engagement and absorbing leisure activities help delay or prevent dementia.[388] They also help avoid loneliness—which is important, since lonely individuals report higher levels of stress and worse sleep. Both conditions are associated with mental health issues.[389] A meta-analysis of more than three million people found that loneliness, social isolation, and living alone are a greater threat to longevity than obesity, and they are on the same level as smoking fifteen cigarettes a day.[390]

Social Isolation and Stigma. The importance of *Social Engagement* is evident when we see the negative impact of its opposite: social isolation created by stigma. Often people with mental health issues are stereotyped, discriminated against, and isolated because of social stigmas. Stigmas can be debilitating and can impede recovery. (See Case Study 13, p. 102.) Studies indicate that stigmas have a strong and enduring negative impact on psychological well-being.[391] Stigmas decrease self-esteem,[392] cause anxiety and depressive symptoms, and lower satisfaction with our lives.[393]

Giving, Volunteering and Service. Volunteering is an act of *Self-transcendence (p. 105)* that can help us feel appreciated and needed, and improve our psychological well-being. Analysis of 73 studies found that people who engaged socially by volunteering reported less depression and better overall health than those who did not volunteer.[394] The "sweet spot" appears to be at about two or three hours per week. The value of volunteering appears to be age related: young adults gain little, a marked benefit occurs for those over 40, and an even larger positive impact occurs for those over 70 years of age.[395] Not surprisingly, those who seem to gain the greatest mental health benefit from volunteering are people who were previously the most socially isolated.[396]

Unconditional Love. At the broadest level, companionship practices can be considered an expression of love – being able to think and act with someone else's best interests in mind. This understanding is often experienced as a shift from the narrower self-fulfilling desire found in *passion*, to the broader acceptance, respect, and giving found in *compassion*.

Mental Health America indicates that *unconditional love* is a fundamental requirement for mental health.[397] *Unconditional love* is based in the same sentiment as *Self-compassion* (p. 86), except the love is externalized to others. Love is much more than sentimentality, and the lack of love is debilitating. Children who do not receive parental love and acceptance are much more likely to experience four vital mental health side effects: difficulties in psychological adjustment, depression, behavior problems, and substance abuse.[398]

Emotional Sanctuary. Often people with mental health issues feel emotionally vulnerable and need an emotional sanctuary, a refuge that can provide peace and escape from what they perceive as a hostile world. The sanctuary may be a physical place or anything or anyone else who provides solace: special individuals, nature, music, art, exercise, prayer, and meditation, among many others. This reflects the Jewish refrain, *May the place comfort you*, an acknowledgement of the universal need for a refuge of support and encouragement.[399] Some people connect a sense of emotional sanctuary with particular places, and they look for ways to expand the number and variety of places where they can experience this sense of control and comfort.[400]

Nature Engagement. Experiencing nature has many health benefits. It can encourage physical activity, reduce chronic stress, and provide meaning. Simply visiting a garden or walking in the woods improves our mood, quality of sleep, and ability to concentrate--particularly for the elderly with depression.[401] These positive effects are especially important since nature-based recreation is in steep decline.[402] It has also been suggested that our decreasing exposure to nature helps explain the high levels of mental illness in urbanized areas.

- For *depression*. The greening of blighted vacant lots in urban settings is associated with significantly reduced depression and thoughts of worthlessness by residents, especially in the poorer neighborhoods.[403] Also, people living near green areas as children have less depression later in life.[404] Nature experiences can reduce negative thinking patterns (rumination) associated with depression.[405] One study found that spending 30 minutes a week in nature can reduce the occurrence of depression by as much as 7%.[406]
- For *schizophrenia*. Swedish adults living in the most densely populated areas had a 70% higher risk of developing psychosis than controls.[407]
- For *stress and anxiety*. One Japanese study found that people who took forest walks had a 12% decrease in cortisol (a stress hormone) and a 6% decrease in heart rate as compared to people who took walks in cities.[408]
- For *attention-deficit hyperactivity disorder*. Children improve by spending time in nature.[409]
- *More broadly*. A meta-analysis found nature activities are broadly beneficial, especially for improving self-esteem.[410] One study found that people with a large green space near their homes are less likely to be impacted by stress and had better overall mental health than those who did not.[411]

WHAT CONSIDERATIONS SHOULD I KEEP IN MIND?

The external focus of *Social & Outer Engagement* is a healthy counterpoint to the more internal focus of *Mind Wellness Basics*. These perspectives are complementary, and both are correlated with better mental health outcomes.

Skills in *Social Engagement* are first built within the family and gradually cascade to friends and larger communities. The sense of belonging and cooperation found by becoming a member of a supportive group aids the recovery process and can be developed using perspectives of *Self-transcendence* (p. 105), *Support Groups* (p. 131), and *Peer Support Specialists* (p. 131). In addition, many *Psychosocial Restorative Therapies* are based on a strong sense of respectful and individualized personal interaction, including *Open Dialogue* (p. 147) and *Soteria* (p. 148).

Close relationships and social networks that provide support, friendship, love, and hope are considered by SAMHSA to be one of the four key dimensions of recovery.[1461] People in mental distress crave companionship, where people truly care for and unconditionally value them. The reverse can be true, too: when a person with mental health issues steps away from focusing on their own needs to help others, their sense of satisfaction affirms their own self-worth.

A key aspect is to engage in meaningful activities, diverting the focus away from personal mental distress to something external. The best activities are often creative. (See *Creative Engagement,* p. 137.) Animal companionship can also be very helpful in recovery; pets are often a source of unconditional affection.

Social interaction can provide vital recovery support and grounding. It leverages *Self-understanding* (p. 86) and *Self-compassion* (p. 86), but takes us beyond strict self-interest. It reorients these skills, from an inward perspective to an outward perspective. The next section, *Belief, Hope, & Self-transcendence* takes an even larger step. It explores how our core beliefs and outlooks for the future can have a significant impact on mental health.

REAL-WORLD EXPERIENCE

Case Study 18 – Overcoming Stigma (Schizophrenia)

"I have had schizophrenia for more than twenty-five years," one man reported. "There are many obstacles for people with a psychiatric disorder. We are seen as weak, but we are among the most courageous. We struggle with raging fears, brutal thoughts, and the misunderstanding, distrust, and stigma we experience in the community.

"There is nothing more devastating, discrediting, and disabling than social stigma when we are in the process of recovery from a mental illness. To have a diagnosis is to be discounted. Your label never leaves you. It gradually shapes an identity that is hard to shed.

"We did not choose to be ill. But we can choose to confront our illnesses. As we do, we become more able, and we can bestow our talents on the society that has abandoned us.[357]

> ***Bottom Line****: Stigma cannot survive when the art of human companionship is fully practiced.*

Case Study 19 – Feeling Needed and Valued

In one study, sixty-four people in mental health recovery told their stories of what helped them achieve and maintain recovery.

They cited social networks as important factors. "They offered many benefits beyond friendship and socializing," one individual explained. "They allowed me to be creative and productive."

Others mentioned the ability to contribute. Social interaction "..made me feel accepted and less isolated," another participant said. "The fact that my efforts were needed, appreciated, and valued gave me confidence and a sense of fulfillment. It motivated my recovery."

"Mixing with the public makes me feel good about myself and helps me feel valuable and worthwhile..." another person reported, adding that relationships requiring responsibilities—as a parent, guardian or pet owner—provided considerable motivation for recovery.[355]

Bottom Line*: We are social beings who thrive on social interaction. And we also want to contribute. Both make us happier and aid recovery.*

Practitioner's Story 3 – Recovery via Dialogue (Schizophrenia)

Dr. Daniel Fisher, a psychiatrist and MD, has schizophrenia. His passion is to use voice and dialogue to spur recovery. He co-founded the National Empowerment Center (www.power2u.org) to do just that.

"According to Finnish psychologists, psychosis is the result of a person retreating into monologue, or their own world. I can relate," he said. "I retreated into complete monologue."

His experience inspired him to create a "dialogical space" between the therapist and his patient, "a space into which life can come," he explained. "This is the space that I believe our peer movement has been creating.

"Recovery is [living] a free and fulfilling life in the community—a life in which we are the authors, not the subjects, of our destiny."[412]

Bottom Line*: See Dr. Fischer's blog at (http://goo.gl/AWRPny).*

WHAT ARE ADDITIONAL RESOURCES?

- 9 Habits of extraordinary relationships. http://goo.gl/IYf9mh.
- Building and sustaining relationships. http://goo.gl/a7euMJ.

Belief, Hope, & Self-transcendence

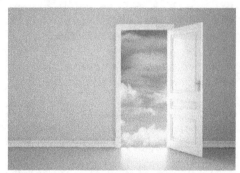

WHAT IS THE ESSENCE?

Everyone has beliefs, core concepts of how we think the world works and how we can best live in it. Our beliefs evolve over time, sometimes adopted from our parents or modeled by other people, sometimes more consciously chosen.

Our beliefs put a framework around what we think is possible, and they strongly influence our expectations about life and our mental health.

> *"Whether you think you can, or you think you can't — you're right."*
>
> - Henry Ford

The starting belief for recovery is this: *I can recover*. First, we must realize that we have the capacity to change our lives, to persevere through setbacks, and muster the energy to create our own recovery. Belief and hope are crucial—not because they are magical, but because they get us moving. They motivate us to do the hard work needed to recover—and they provide the calm to deal with adversity. Henry Ford captures the creative nature of our thoughts and beliefs in the quote, above.

The belief that we will recover, and the hope in our ability to recover, are so important that the combination is often considered a turning point for the entire recovery process. (See the *Awareness* stage of recovery, p. 33.) They provide the important transition from passively *wishing* you could recover to actively *knowing* you can recover if you are willing to work for it.

But, in addition to belief and hope, recovery is enabled by a perspective of self-transcendence. The crux of the matter is this:

If you think only of yourself, significant challenges (like mental health recovery) can be all-consuming, since what you value far and above all else is under siege. If, however, you find importance in things beyond yourself – in family, friends, community, the arts, nature, religion, etc. – even when personal challenges arise, you have additional sources of peace and meaning to help you address your current experience.

Transpersonal Psychology closely examines self-transcendence. It rests on the idea that there are 3 stages of human development.[413]

Identification is the first stage. Here we develop a strong sense of self-identity (sometimes called a strong ego), raise self-esteem, and abandon negative patterns of thought, emotions, and behaviors. *Effective Self-management* (p. 83) offers core techniques and perspectives for Identification.

> *"The thought of death accelerates the living... Death is a teacher and mentor, a disturber of selves and minister to souls in <u>this</u> life."*[414]
>
> - Søren Kierkegaard

Disidentification is the second stage, in which we seek to grow beyond the self-centered ego. Here we confront life's bigger questions. It is often helpful to consider our mortality at this point, since it helps reduce excessive attachment to our roles, possessions, and activities; we recognize that they are all temporary. (See quote at left). We retain a strong sense of self, but we stop fixating on our every desire. *Purpose & Meaning* (p. 94) and *Social & Outer Engagement* (p. 99) offer approaches for Disidentification.

> *"Only to the extent that you live (a life of) self-transcendence, are you truly human... The more you forget yourself – by giving of yourself to a cause or a person to love – the more human you are."*[360]
>
> - Viktor Frankl

Self-transcendence is the third stage, where we find great meaning in things larger and more enduring than ourselves. Interacting with family, community, nature, the arts, spirituality, and our passions are approaches to Self-transcendence. (See quote at left) With this orientation, we hold, but move beyond a deep respect for ourselves, to a broader sense of interconnection and respect for others. This is often motivated by a significant experience or shift in identity—which may be incomprehensible to people who have not had such an experience.[415]

Self-transcendence, like any significant human change, means disruption. In some cases, this disruption is labeled mental illness, when it is actually a byproduct of the growing pains of personal growth. As one example, 41% of Americans claim to have had a profound self-transcendent or religious experience that changed the direction of their lives.[416] Their experiences might have similarities to psychosis,[417] but there is little value in labeling them so.

There are attitudes that help promote *Belief, Hope & Self-transcendence* (Figure 22, p. 106). These attitudes are helpful perspectives based on real-life human experiences, as well as philosophies, religions, and spiritual traditions.

- *Respect* values ourselves and the people and things beyond us.
- *Humility* asserts that our humanity is no greater than that of others.
- *Love* means supporting the best interests of others, but also ourselves.
- *Gratitude* is appreciation for the good that life and people offer us.

Although these four attitudes are found in religious and spiritual perspectives, they are effective tools available to everyone. They help us deal with our present challenges and help us on the path to recovery.

Importance of language. The words we use are critical. Subtleties of language can create stigma and steal hope. (See Case Study 21, p. 109.) Use language that those in mental distress use to describe their experience. This shows respect (p. 38). And only by showing respect will supporters be allowed to come close enough to truly help.

WHAT EVIDENCE SHOWS THIS IS EFFECTIVE?

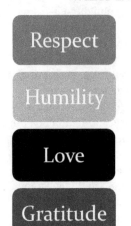

Figure 22 – Attitudes of Belief, Hope & Self-transcendence

Positive impact of grounding beliefs. Many studies show that people with strong grounding beliefs achieve better mental health outcomes than those who don't have them, irrespective of what those beliefs are. Strong grounding beliefs are associated with lighter levels of depression, faster recovery from depression, lower suicide rates, less anxiety, less substance abuse, and a greater sense of well-being, hope, and optimism.

Grounding beliefs provide hope and empowerment[418] as well as a heightened sense of purpose and meaning in life.[419] One study found that people with more than a slight belief in a higher power were twice as likely to gain symptom relief as those who didn't believe in a higher power.[420]

Individuals with serious mental health issues who said they had higher levels of spirituality and religiousness exhibited a better sense of well-being and reduced psychiatric symptoms.[421] (See Case Study 15, p. 93.) There is considerable evidence that a religious life offers significant protective and positive implications to mental health, and this evidence is consistent with accepted behavioral and psychodynamic theories.[422]

> *"...It is our job to form a community of hope... It is our job to create rehabilitation environments that are charged with opportunities for self-improvement... It is our job to ask people... what it is they want and need to grow and then to provide them with good soil in which a new life can secure its roots and grow.."*[423]
>
> *- Patricia Deegan*

Positive impact of hope and expectation. People who expect to recover often do. In fact, people with schizophrenia who expressed high and moderate expectations of recovery saw a significant reduction in negative symptoms, while people with low expectations saw none.[424] Additionally, a study found that those who expected depression treatment to be effective had better outcomes than those who didn't.[99]

The impact of expectation extends even further. When practitioners express their positive expectation of recovery, patient outcomes improve.[99] Hope plays an important role. People who have recovered from severe mental health issues indicate that hope was an extraordinarily important part of it.[425] In fact, SAMHSA has declared that hope is the catalyst for recovery.[1461] Practitioners who expect your recovery and who offer of proven solutions to help you achieve it, can be a tremendous source of well-founded hope.

Belief as a coping technique. Eighty percent of the people in persistent mental distress use religion to cope, and many reported spending as much as half of their total coping time in religious practices such as prayer.[426] According to researchers, "Religious activities and beliefs may be particularly compelling for persons who are experiencing more severe psychiatric symptoms… [serving] as a pervasive and effective method of coping, thus warranting its integration into psychiatric and psychological practice." Some suggest that religious practices provides a sense of meaning and purpose in difficult circumstances, promotes a positive world-view, and promotes acceptance of the suffering encountered.[427]

Limiting beliefs impede recovery. Beliefs influence outcomes. Believing that mental distress keeps us from fulfilling our needs, impedes recovery.[428] Also, research found that defeatist beliefs – common in those with schizophrenia – had significant impact on negative symptoms (see Glossary).[429] Helping people dislodge these beliefs and replace them with beliefs that emphasize personal competence was a significant aid to recovery. (See Case Study 31, p. 124.)

Positive impact of disidentification. We naturally identify with the things we hold most important: our families, our close friends, our jobs, and our life passions. Although this identification can provide meaning, a challenge arises: When we identify with something, we relinquish a measure of control over our wellbeing. How? When we identify with a person, we connect our thoughts and emotions to that person, and we allow our thoughts and emotions to fluctuate with the person's own ups and downs. If we closely identify with our job, we feel good when our job goes well and depressed when it doesn't.

Psychology summarizes this quandary: We are controlled by the things with which we identify. But we can control those things if we dis-identify ourselves.[430] This same idea is found in Eastern thought: we control our well-being by avoiding attachment to the results of our efforts.[431] The core message is this: minimize identification and attachment to things outside of ourselves.

At first blush, this might sound absurd. Does this advocate not caring about those things important to us? No, it doesn't. Rather, it advocates caring deeply about these things, but not tying our sense of well-being to them. It advocates working hard to support or achieve those things but retaining our peace and equanimity if things don't turn out as expected. We should work toward specific *results*, but transfer our identification from results to something larger, like our journey of recovery, self-compassion, and deeply-held beliefs, among others.

Positive impact of self-transcendence. Studies show that self-transcendence is essential for mental well-being,[432] and is correlated with mental health in older adults and those facing the end of life. There is a dramatic correlation between self-transcendence and positive mood[433] and emotions.[434] In fact, those with elevated self-transcendence are five times more likely to be happy than those with low levels.[432] This is even true for people in the most difficult situations: a study of people with severe schizophrenia found that the self-transcending act of helping others was an important part of their recovery.[435]

Positive impact of gratitude. Studies suggest that gratitude is helpful in creating enthusiasm and motivation[436] as well as instilling an expectation of success[437] – perspectives important for mental health recovery. In one study, participants who "counted their blessings" reported fewer physical symptoms of illness and spent up to 1.5 more hours exercising each week.[438]

Faith/hope/compassion. The World Health Organization reports, "Health professions have largely followed a medical model, which … [focuses] on medicines and surgery, and gives less importance to beliefs… [This] mechanistic view … is no longer satisfactory. Patients and physicians have begun to realize the value of … hope, and compassion in the healing process."[439]

WHAT CONSIDERATIONS SHOULD I KEEP IN MIND?

Belief, Hope, & Self-transcendence are three gates to recovery. *Belief* that you can recover can inspire you to get on your feet and work toward recovery. *Hope* sustains your efforts with a heightened expectation of success. *Self-transcendence* finds meaning and peace even in the difficult times when recovery seems far off. All three outlooks can be learned and adopted through practical clinical methods,[432] social interactions, and other means.

When people in mental distress, as well as their practitioners and loved ones, expect a full recovery in their minds and hearts, a vital step toward recovery has begun. A positive expectation can stimulate energy, commitment, and actions toward recovery. A negative expectation suffocates the spirit of self-determination and convinces the patient to accept the current situation as inevitable. (See Case Study 23, p. 110.) The bottom line is this: **Expect to recover—and work with practitioners who expect you to recover.**

One of the most disempowering things that can be said to a person in mental distress is, "Your situation is incurable." Sources as varied as WebMD[440] and the United States Library of Medicine[441] make such misguided claims about schizophrenia, even though cases of full remission abound. Such statements steal *hope* from people when they need it most. They also stigmatize, which can lead people to adopt a "why try?" mentality.[442] SAMHSA[155] and the large body of recovery literature are clear that *hope* is a critical turning point in the *Awareness* stage of recovery (p. 33). *Hope* should be firmly based in scientific realism but *hope* and the lack of hope can become powerful self-fulfilling prophecies.

How we perceive the world through our beliefs impacts recovery. Research suggests that embracing our religion, spirituality, or other core grounding aids mental health recovery and can be a significant source of *hope*. This grounding can take many forms: family, service to others, communing with nature, community, prayer, affirmation, *Bibliotherapy* (inspirational books and poetry, p. 138), *Mindfulness* (p. 74), *Meditation* (p. 78), and more. Religious and spiritual affiliations offer support consistent with mental health therapies: *Companionship* (p. 99), advice, emotional support, *Problem Solving* (p.45), positive role models, emotional release, and reality testing.[443]

At a broader level, twelve-step programs based on models with a self-transcendent/spiritual component show clear success. Mental health recovery models (See *Recovery Models & Tools*, p. 327) are becoming increasingly prevalent,*[444]* and some include a self-transcendent dimension.

Belief, Hope, & Self-transcendence puts mental health in a larger context, one that views the body, mind, and spirit as integrated into a larger significance. The next section, *Mind-Body Disciplines*, considers three approaches that integrate many mind and body techniques into a cohesive practice.

REAL-WORLD EXPERIENCE

Case Study 20 – Never Say "Incurable" (Schizophrenia)

When Patricia was diagnosed with schizophrenia, she was told that it was incurable and that she would be disabled for the rest of her life. She raged against this bleak prophecy, but eventually gave into despair.

"But there were those who loved me who didn't give up," she said after her recovery. "They remained hopeful. Gradually I began to respond to their loving invitation. The small and fragile flame of hope and courage illuminated the darkness of my despair.

"Those of us who have recovered know that this grace is real. Hope does not come as a sudden bolt of lightning, but is the turning point that must quickly be followed by the willingness to act. I rebuilt my life on hope, willingness, and responsible action. I learned to say: 'I am willing to try'"[445]

Bottom Line: *Find hope in the scientific evidence supporting non-drug approaches and the reality that many people have recovered. Patricia's affirmation, "I am willing to try" is the essence of prudent experimentation.*

Case Study 21 – Avoiding Hopeless Language

In one study, sixty-four people in mental health recovery told their stories of what helped them achieve and maintain recovery.

Many people acknowledged that recovery was a complex process of adjusting personal attitudes and beliefs, adopting an optimistic outlook, and having hope for their potential to live a meaningful and healthy life.

They pinpointed social stigma and hopeless language as significant factors hindering recovery.[355]

Bottom Line: *Although not always easy, we can choose to be positive and hopeful. Finding hope gives incentive to work toward recovery.*

Case Study 22 – Hope in Support Groups (Schizophrenia)

Akiko Hart manages a series of projects for people who hear voices.

She notes that it is often hard to hold hope for ourselves and receive it from others. It can often feel like a burden to carry. But she found that one of the strengths of support groups is that they can help us hold hope.

". . . In a Hearing Voices group, I'm not sure that hope even needs to be articulated with words. It's there in the room because the group exists. . . the very fact that there is a group means there is hope. . . And sometimes within a group, we are able to hold hope together, briefly, in that hour. . ."[446]

Bottom Line: *Hope doesn't need to be a solitary effort. Come together with others to find how simple sharing can elevate hope for the entire group.*

Case Study 23 – Belief in Recovery

Amy was hospitalized over forty times for mental health issues. Her doctors told her about all the things that she would never be able to do again, and in despair, she said, "I finally gave up."

But something changed during her last hospitalization.

"The psychiatrist told me she believed I could get better," Amy recalled. "She said that it would be the hardest thing that I would ever do. This was the first time that someone believed in me and I began to glimpse a possible future. This helped me take steps to get out of the hole I was in."

Another important event occurred when a psychologist asked her to talk about her hopes and dreams. "I couldn't tell her," Amy said. "I was so used to living a life without hope. I cried. And in that moment, something changed. I started seeing life as possible. I started to talk about things I wanted to do. Every time I came up with something, a little bit of life was breathed into me.

"The doctor believed in me, which allowed me to start believing in myself. My last hospitalization was fifteen years ago. I'm now the peer support recovery coordinator at the very hospital where I was hospitalized. My diagnosis is not who I am. Who I am is Amy."[447]

Bottom Line*: Believing you can recover and having practitioners who believe the same is vital. This expectation is a very real catalyst, offering hope and incentive to do the hard work of recovery.*

Case Study 24 – Hopelessness of a Life-Long Diagnosis

Sara Knutson is a mental health survivor-activist. "The medical model message is that people have little to live or hope for; our brains are defective and there is no cure." she writes. "Whether or not the 'disease' is deadly, the message certainly is. It literally kills."[448]

Bottom Line*: The message of life-long disability offered by the medical model can cruelly rob people of an essential ingredient of recovery: hope.*

WHAT ARE ADDITIONAL RESOURCES?

- Association of Transpersonal Psychology. www.atpweb.org.
- Interfaith support for mental health. www.pathways2promise.org.

Mind-Body Disciplines

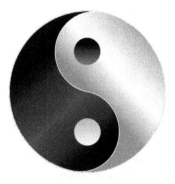

WHAT IS THE ESSENCE?

The three primary *Mind-Body Disciplines* are *Yoga, T'ai Chi Chuan,* and *Qigong*. Each has been practiced for centuries.

These disciplines integrate body work (movement or postures), breathing, and focused awareness. People who practice these disciplines often consider them to be *Wellness Basics,* since their use is designed to create and maintain well-rounded health. These practices contain many of the fundamentals of *Wellness Basics,* including *Mindfulness* (p. 74), *Controlled Breathing* (p. 75), and Exercise/Movement (p. 62).

Mind-Body Disciplines may be practiced individually or in a group, but to learn their complexities and nuances and to reap the greatest health benefits, a trained teacher is needed, and daily practice is encouraged.

Each *Mind-Body Discipline* has a spiritual element that can be integrated or disregarded. For instance, *Spiritual Qigong* seeks to integrate the mindfulness of *Qigong* into daily life, while spirit aspects of yoga are oriented toward a transcendent experience. There is no need to ascribe to, or consider, the spirit element to gain mental health benefits from *Mind-Body Disciplines*.

Yoga. Yoga is an ancient Indian philosophy and discipline covering six major systems of wellness. The most common form of yoga in Western culture is hatha yoga, which itself has many forms, including Iyengar, Ashtanga, Vini, Kundalini, Bikram, and Sudarshan Kriya (SKY). Yoga typically uses postures with active muscular control, intentional breathing and focused body awareness. Another branch of yoga, Raja Yoga, also strongly emphasizes meditation.

T'ai Chi Chuan. T'ai Chi Chuan is a martial art sometimes called a moving meditation. This low-impact, weight-bearing aerobic form of exercise requires relaxed, graceful movements, coordination, balance, gentle stretching, focused awareness, and controlled breathing. In traditional Chinese Medicine, Tai Chi is thought to benefit many chronic medical conditions, both physical and mental.[449] Tai Chi form (the flow of one posture into another) is designed to balance one's *chi* (life force).

Qigong (pronounced "chee gung"). Qigong is an ancient Chinese health system that combines physical postures (moving or stationary), breathing, self-massage, and *Mindfulness* (p. 74). It focuses on the awareness of stimuli originating inside the body and of the body's movement and alignment (posture, orientation, and balance). Qigong cultivates energy to heal and increase vitality. There are two types of medical Qigong. The first is *Self-healing Qigong,* whose exercises vary from the slow movements of Tai Chi to the more vigorous styles of Kung Fu. The second is *External Qigong,* in which Qigong practitioners emit Qi to others with the intention of healing.

WHAT EVIDENCE SHOWS THIS IS EFFECTIVE?

Yoga. Yoga is broadly therapeutic across nearly all mental health diagnoses.

- For *anxiety and depression.* An eight-week SKY Yoga class using asanas, meditation, and *Ujjayi Breathing* (a form of *Controlled Breathing*, p. 75) significantly improved anxiety and reduced panic attacks.[450] In this study, the significant majority of patients continued their practices, and over the course of three years, they maintained significantly reduced levels of anxiety and depression. Many studies of people with anxiety and depression reported positive findings, although yoga does not fit RCT trial designs.[451] Two studies of *Iyengar Yoga* found significant improvement in class members' depression when attending sessions several times a week.[452, 453] Regular yoga practice reduces the need for conventional drugs in most anxious patients.[454]
- For *obsessive-compulsive disorder.* One study found that those taking Kundalini yoga had significantly greater improvement of OCD symptoms than the control group given relaxation and mindfulness training.[455]
- For *PTSD.* SKY Yoga effectively relieves symptoms.[456] In a study of recent war veterans, SKY Yoga was found to reduce PTSD symptoms, including anxiety, respiration rate, and the startle reflex, both initially and at the one-year follow-up visit.[457]
- For *bipolar.* Although clinical testing has not been extensive, an online survey of those with bipolar who practice yoga showed an overwhelmingly positive improvement, with one in five calling it "life changing". Reduced anxiety and calm were also common responses.[458] However, yoga should be used with caution by people with bipolar who are prone to rapid-cycling.[16]
- For *schizophrenia.* A meta-analysis[459] found that both asanas (yogic postures) and pranayama (yogic controlled breathing) are an effective add-on therapy to drug therapy. Yoga can improve a variety of psychopathological symptoms,[460] including psychosis, depression, and cognition,[461] as well as giving people a greater sense of quality of life and neurobiological changes. Mindfulness meditation (p. 74), which is sometimes a part of yoga, helps people cope with psychotic symptoms at a level superior to psychoeduation.[291] Ujjayi breathing is associated with rapid improvement in mood, energy, and attention in patients predominantly diagnosed with schizophrenia,[462] although research shows that *prolonged intense* meditation may worsen psychosis.[463]
- For *insomnia.* A small trial found that controlled breathing, visualization, mindfulness, and body postures improved the quality of sleep.[464]
- For *substance abuse.* Practicing SKY breathing techniques for forty-five minutes every other day improved detoxification symptoms in alcohol-dependent patients.[465]

- *More broadly.* One yoga session can significantly improve anxiety, anger, depression, and confusion.[466]

T'ai Chi Chuan. T'ai Chi Chuan is associated with reduced stress, anxiety, depression, and mood disturbance, while significantly increasing self-esteem and stress management capabilities.[467] It appears to increase brain volume and positively influence neuropsychological factors.[468] A study of older adults with major depression found that the complementary use of Tai Chi augments the results of psychotropics.[469]

Qigong.

- For *depression.* In a double-blind trial, the mood of those receiving qigong improved and their anxiety was reduced, compared to a control group.[470] In another trial, geriatric patients significantly improved their depressive symptoms after a sixteen-week Qigong class.
- For *anxiety and stress.* A comparison of qigong to biofeedback found that qigong better reduces the frequency and intensity of stress factors.[471] Evidence suggests that qigong offers several health benefits and there is a growing appreciation for the similarity of Qigong and Tai Chi.[472]
- For *heroin abuse.* Between two and two-and-one-half hours of daily practice significantly reduced withdrawal symptoms and accelerated detoxification.[473]

WHAT CONSIDERATIONS SHOULD I KEEP IN MIND?

The controlled breathing, mindfulness, and body work of *Mind-Body Disciplines* have proven widely beneficial, both historically and clinically. Proper training by a skilled teacher is essential, although people with social phobias can learn from online sources or videos. Of all approaches to mental wellness, yoga seems to be one of the most broadly beneficial. This may be due to the tight integration of mind and body in these disciplines.

The major challenge of *Mind-Body Disciplines* is that people must maintain a regular discipline to get sustained benefits. Often this discipline is easier to maintain in group practice.

Many *Mind-Body* and *Energy Therapies* use *Controlled Breathing* (p. 75) to promote relaxation and calmness. One possible reason for the effectiveness of controlled breathing is that it may stimulate the vagus nerve, which can elevate moods. (See *Vagus Nerve Stimulation,* p. 251.)

REAL-WORLD EXPERIENCE

Case Study 25 - Qigong (Anxiety)

After a woman experienced chronic anxiety for six years with chest and nasal congestion, she was prescribed psychotropics.

During an exam, a traditional Chinese doctor diagnosed the woman as having qi stagnation in the middle of her body, and he recommended acupuncture plus a calming qigong practice. She received a total of four treatments. After each, her anxiety and physical congestion improved.

Following the fourth treatment, she stopped psychotropics and experienced anxiety only in the evenings. Seven weeks after the initial diagnosis, she went in for a checkup. By that time, she had been off psychotropics for two months. She reported no ongoing anxiety. [16]

Bottom Line: *Don't avoid therapies just because they are foreign to you. Their origin doesn't matter. Their effectiveness does.*

Case Study 26 – Ujjayi Breathing (Anxiety)

Ed had been a popular student but felt overwhelmed in his first semester in college. He became increasingly anxious and depressed, using alcohol to calm himself. One day he drank so much that he had to be rushed to the hospital. He left college feeling ashamed, insecure, and a failure.

Psychotherapy helped slightly. He told his practitioner that he wanted to avoid psychotropics. He decided to try Ujjayi breathing. Ed learned Ujjayi and felt relief within a few minutes. He liked the way it relaxed his body and quieted his thoughts. Ujjayi gave him a sense of control over his anxiety – a much more positive prospect than being dependent on medication.

Ed's anxiety improved without medication. He returned to school with a much greater sense of self-control and peace. [15]

Bottom Line: *Consciously controlled breathing can heal the mind.*

Case Study 27 – Uddiyana Bandha Yoga (PTSD)

Esther survived sexual abuse. Her traumatic experience appeared to be a causative factor in her later development of bulimia, purging several times a day. She was advised to practice Uddiyana Bandha - a Yoga technique that uses the diaphragm in ways similar to regurgitation - twice daily away from food. With this practice she was able to reduce purging and uses psychotherapy to further aid her recovery. [474]

Bottom Line: *Our mind and body are tightly entwined. Intentional physical movements can help reduce the distress of trauma.*

WHAT ARE ADDITIONAL RESOURCES?

- Iyengar Yoga. http://www.bksiyengar.com.
- SKY Yoga. www.ArtOfLiving.org.
- Ujjayi Breathing. http://goo.gl/55WKL7.
- Yoga for Depression. www.YogaForDepression.com.
- National Qigong Association. www.nqa.org.
- Qigong Institute. www.QigongInstitute.org.

4 – Psychosocial Restorative Therapies

Psychosocial

Cognitive Behavioral Therapy
Individual Psychotherapy
Interpersonal, Family & Peer Therapy
Cognitive Enhancement Therapy
Creative Engagement Therapy
Biofeedback
Dialogue & Exposure Therapy
Energy Therapy

Mental Focus

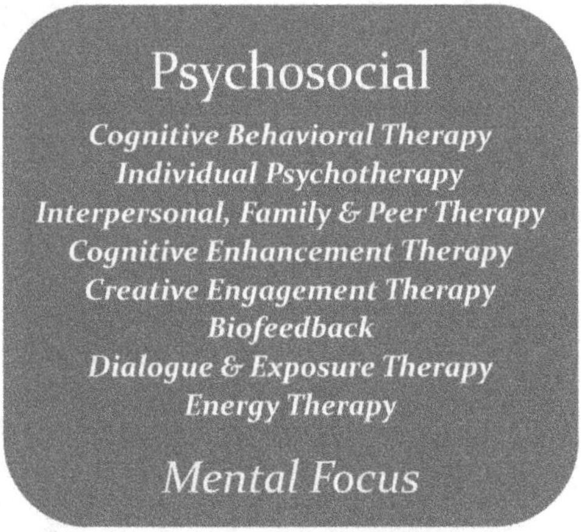

Figure 23 – Psychosocial Restorative Therapies

The second category of the *Wellness Continuum* (Figure 9, p. 47) offers *Restorative Therapies* that seek to address underlying causes and influencers of mental distress. They are either *Psychosocial* (related to the mind and social interaction) or *Biomedical* (related to the body). Helping one often helps the other.

Psychosocial therapies examine thoughts, emotions, motivations, and self-identity, seeking to understand and address underlying trauma, stress, grief, obsessive/unhelpful thinking, and more.

Psychosocial Restorative Therapies (Figure 23) can reduce or eliminate symptoms, improve functioning in the community, decrease relapse, and reduce hospitalizations. [475] Research shows them effective across all diagnoses (Figure 24) including in cases of persistent mental distress.[476] They have the added benefit of minimizing exposure to the risks and side effects of psychotropics.

However, psychosocial therapies are underused. The British Psychological Society notes, "It remains scandalous that... still only a minority of people [in mental distress] are offered talking therapy."[477]

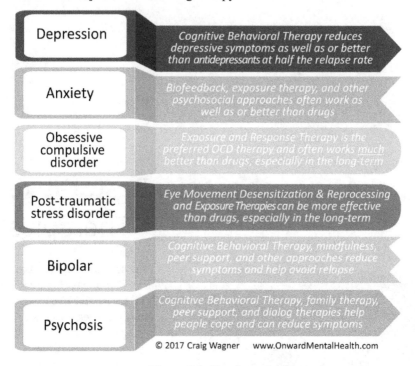

Depression	Cognitive Behavioral Therapy reduces depressive symptoms as well as or better than antidepressants at half the relapse rate
Anxiety	Biofeedback, exposure therapy, and other psychosocial approaches often work as well as or better than drugs
Obsessive compulsive disorder	Exposure and Response Therapy is the preferred OCD therapy and often works *much* better than drugs, especially in the long-term
Post-traumatic stress disorder	Eye Movement Desensitization & Reprocessing and Exposure Therapies can be more effective than drugs, especially in the long-term
Bipolar	Cognitive Behavioral Therapy, mindfulness, peer support, and other approaches reduce symptoms and help avoid relapse
Psychosis	Cognitive Behavioral Therapy, family therapy, peer support, and dialog therapies help people cope and can reduce symptoms

© 2017 Craig Wagner   www.OnwardMentalHealth.com

Figure 24 - Psychosocial Therapies

The wide variety of *Psychosocial Therapies* can be delivered in different ways. One-on-one "talking therapy" is common, but support groups, family therapies, online tools, mobile apps, and self-initiated formats are available. Self-managed *Recovery Models & Tools* (p. 327) are also useful. Although these therapies can be used independently, best results are often found when they are provided by, or coordinated through, a trusted psychiatrist, psychologist, social worker, psychiatric nurse, or counselor. Often the quality of the relationship with the therapist is as important as the specific therapy chosen.

Testing is underway using ketamine (an anesthetic drug) and MDMA (a variant of the street drug, ecstasy) to boost feelings of trust and compassion that make psychosocial therapies more effective. Preliminary positive results caused the FDA to grant "breakthrough" status to MDMA-assisted therapy for PTSD.[478]

Mind Wellness Basics (p. 55) share common elements with *Psychosocial Restorative Therapies*. The former uses the techniques in a preventive manner; the latter use them to reinstate wellness once issues arise.

Cognitive Behavioral Therapy

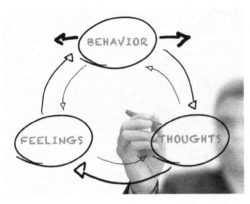

WHAT IS THE ESSENCE?

Cognitive Behavioral Therapy (CBT) is an evolving cluster of therapies that examine the relationships between thoughts, feelings, and behaviors. CBT is the most widely used and one of the most effective of all psycho-social approaches.

CBT was invented in the 1960s by psychiatrist Aaron Beck. It grew from his experience with psychotherapy, where he noticed his patients seemed to have an unconscious internal dialogue that could cause rapid changes in emotions. He designed CBT to make that dialogue conscious. First wave CBT was based on early 20th-century behavioral concepts. Second wave CBT (the most commonly studied and "classic" form) expanded to include a focus on maladaptive thinking. Third wave CBT adds principles of *Mindfulness* (p. 74), emotions, acceptance, relationships, and goals.[479]

> *"Both thought and feeling are determinants of conduct, and the same conduct may be determined either by feeling or by thought."*
>
> - William James

CBT is based on the idea that thoughts drive our emotions and actions, and behaviors and emotions influence how we think. By exploring unhelpful *Thought-Emotion-Action* cycles (see Figure 16, p. 84), people can learn how to modify them. As a result, they become happier and more able to weather adversity and create meaningful lives for themselves.

CBT teaches people not so much how to control their world, but how to control the way they interpret and respond to their world. It is predicated on the belief that events don't cause our emotions; emotions are caused by the way we interpret and give meaning to events. CBT can help break vicious cycles of negative thinking, feelings, and behaviors that influence mental health symptoms. CBT therapies often emphasize *Mindfulness* (p. 74), a technique well-validated by psychological research. The four broad steps of classic CBT are found in Figure 25 (p. 118).

Cognitive Behavioral Therapy can be delivered in a variety of forms, with the help of a therapist, in a group or family setting, with computer-aided tools, phone apps, and by self-help books.

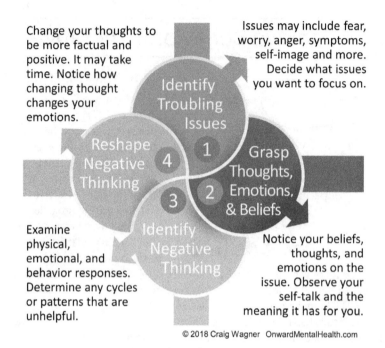

Change your thoughts to be more factual and positive. It may take time. Notice how changing thought changes your emotions.

Issues may include fear, worry, anger, symptoms, self-image and more. Decide what issues you want to focus on.

Identify Troubling Issues

Reshape Negative Thinking 4

1 Grasp Thoughts, Emotions, & Beliefs

3 2

Examine physical, emotional, and behavior responses. Determine any cycles or patterns that are unhelpful.

Identify Negative Thinking

Notice your beliefs, thoughts, and emotions on the issue. Observe your self-talk and the meaning it has for you.

© 2018 Craig Wagner OnwardMentalHealth.com

Figure 25 - Steps of CBT

Regardless of the delivery format, CBT is a guided self-help process, teaching skills for people to use on their own.[480]

CBT is generally short-term and structured, with homework between sessions. It uses a problem-solving and goal-directed approach to address mental health issues.

There are many off-shoots of CBT, most of them tailored to specific diagnoses. This cluster of therapies is most useful for mood, anxiety, personality, and psychotic disorders, but also effective with nearly all diagnoses.

CBT is often considered a "first-line treatment" for many anxiety disorders, including generalized anxiety disorder, post-traumatic stress disorder, panic disorder, obsessive-compulsive disorder, and specific phobias.

WHAT EVIDENCE SHOWS THIS IS EFFECTIVE?

CBT for specific diagnoses. Generally speaking, all off-shoot forms of CBT have shown benefits for the specific diagnoses and groundings they address. In addition, core CBT has been found effective for a wide variety of diagnoses.

- **CBT for psychosis (CBTp)**[481] CBTp targets psychosis and schizophrenia, helping to identify delusional or paranoid beliefs and their negative impact to help create better coping responses. A meta-analysis[482] found that CBT was effective in reducing symptom severity, and it appears to be more effective than any other treatment in reducing depression in people with psychosis. The size of the impact of CBTp appears to be small[483] to moderate[484] on psychosis symptoms (with less impact on audio hallucinations).[485] CBTp also can result in less malevolent voices[486] and help people better manage their symptoms.[487] The National Institute for Health and Care Excellence recommends[488] offering CBT to all people with psychosis or schizophrenia.

- **CBT for insomnia (CBT-I)**. CBT-I involves psychoeducation, behavioral strategies, cognitive therapies, and relaxation training. Three meta-analyses and one major review concluded that CBT is effective in the treatment of primary insomnia (insomnia not attributed to a medical, psychiatric, or environmental causes),[489] with a medium to large impact on symptoms.[490] It also can be more effective in both the long- and short-term than sleeping medications.[491] (See Case Study 29, p. 123.)

- **CBT for anxiety**. Studies comparing CBT to psychotropics found comparable benefits between the two. Those taking CBT saw anxiety levels drop significantly as compared to treatment-as-usual.[492] The combination of CBT and pharmacotherapy was slightly more effective than CBT alone.[493]

- **CBT for obsessive-compulsive disorder**. A meta-analysis suggests that CBT significantly reduces OCD symptoms, as opposed to those receiving standard care (typically psychotropics).[494]

- **CBT for bipolar**. CBT is most effective during the maintenance phase.[495] Although CBT has little power to prevent relapses, it improves quality of life, social adjustment, and the chances that people will continue taking their medication. It also diminishes clinical symptoms.[496]

- **CBT for depression**. In both group and individual forms, CBT appears to be highly effective with depression. In fact, it compares favorably to the results of psychotropics. [12] CBT offers better long-term outcomes than psychotropics and half the relapse rate. CBT results are comparable to other active individual psychological therapies (See *Interpersonal Psychotherapy*, p. 132.) and short-term psychodynamic psychotherapy.[12] For mild and moderate depression, brief CBT therapy (six to eight sessions over ten or twelve weeks) is effective. For moderate to severe depression, sessions range from sixteen to twenty sessions over six to nine months.[497] (See Case Study 28, p. 123.)

- **CBT for dissociative disorders**. Evidence suggests that CBT reduces symptoms of dissociation, depression, general distress, anxiety, and post-traumatic stress disorder, and it allows a decrease in dosages of medication while improving work and social functioning.[498]

- **CBT for PTSD**. Trauma-focused CBT was found to be effective in the treatment of post-traumatic stress disorder symptoms as well as anxiety and depression when they occur simultaneously, thereby enabling people to improve their quality of life.[499] A meta-analysis of 23 studies indicates CBT had better PTSD remission rates than *Eye Movement Desensitization and Reprocessing* (EMDR, p. 152).

Recovery-Oriented Cognitive Therapy (CT-R). CT-R is a collaborative behavioral therapy for people with chronic schizophrenia. It is based in the *recovery model* (See *Mental Health Care in Transition*, p. 19) and emphasizes attainment of personal goals, removal of roadblocks, and self-determination. CT-R helps people change their dysfunctional attitudes and beliefs while increasing their motivation to improve competencies. It does so by creating a positive cycle. When people prove they can do one small thing well, their motivation increases and distracts them from their psychosis; this creates time and motivation to tackle bigger things, which results in greater competencies, higher motivation, and the gradual elimination of defeatist beliefs. (See Case Study 31, p. 124.)

- For *schizophrenia*. One randomized trial found that CT-R given weekly for eighteen months significantly improved negative symptoms in low-functioning individuals.[500]

Spiritually-Oriented Cognitive Therapy (SO-CBT). Based on CBT principles, SO-CBT helps people identify unproductive thoughts and replace them with helpful thoughts by incorporating a spiritual component to the process. SO-CBT has been used successfully to address anxiety, neurosis, OCD, schizophrenia, and depression. Christianity, Islam, Mormonism, Taoism, and non-traditional spirituality have been successfully incorporated into SO-CBT.[501] Still considered experimental except for Christians, SO-CBT evidence is scant, except for depression. A meta-analysis[502] confirmed that SO-CBT is at least as effective as standard CBT in improving depressive symptoms.

Computer-aided CBT (CCBT).[503] Internet-enabled CBT relies on a mobile or internet-based app that is effective but is understandably considered more impersonal[504] than face-to-face sessions. (See *Mental Health Apps*, p. 328.) When CCBT includes therapist support by phone or email, outcomes are stronger[505] and mental improvements are considered equal to face-to-face CBT.[506] Personal preferences should be evaluated when considering CCBT; people with social phobias and those who are embarrassed about seeking help are the strongest candidates.[507] CCBT has been proven to alleviate anxiety symptoms and patients report it improves their quality of life.[568]

Dialectic Behavioral Therapy (DBT). DBT views change within the context of opposing forces that must be balanced and synthesized. It is typically delivered in 4 modes of therapy:[508] 1) dialogue with the therapist; 2) developing skills in *Mindfulness* (p. 74), regulating emotions, interpersonal effectiveness, and tolerance of distress; 3) transferring these new skills to every-day life, increasing the motivation to change and building a structure that reinforces effective behavior;[509] and 4) group sessions. It often requires homework. DBT differs from CBT because it seeks a balance between changing and accepting your beliefs and behaviors.[510] (See Case Study 33, p. 125.)

- For *borderline personality disorder* (BPD). DBT is the most commonly chosen therapy; it especially helps people who are suicidal and self-injurious. Substantial evidence shows that DBT has a significant lasting impact for BPD cases.[511]

- For *depression*. DBT was found more effective than psychotropics, with reports that it significantly improved depressive symptoms within six months.[512]
- For *attention-deficit hyperactivity disorder*. Two studies show significantly reduced symptoms post-treatment.[524]

Acceptance and Commitment Therapy (ACT). Not to be confused with *Assertive Community Treatment*, ACT helps people notice, accept without judgment, and cope with distressing thoughts, beliefs, sensations, and feelings. ACT does not seek to alter or change inner experiences, but it helps people accept them and move on. Originally developed for non-psychosis mental health issues, ACT does not see clients as damaged, but focuses on psychological flexibility to improve functional behavior. The Substance Abuse and Mental Health Services Administration (SAMHSA) considers ACT an evidence-based approach.

- For *OCD and anxiety*. Evidence exists to prove that ACT is useful in these diagnoses.[513]
- For *depression*. ACT can provide significant symptom improvement, like that of CBT.[514]

Mindfulness-Based Cognitive Therapy (MBCT). MBCT links mindfulness meditation with cognitive therapy by interrupting patterns of unhelpful thinking and changing a person's relationship to unhelpful thoughts. Instead of challenging negative thoughts, MBCT teaches people to release them, thereby reducing their impact. While CBT is geared to people who are ill, MBCT can be used to help people stay well.[515] (See Case Study 30, p. 123.)

- For *bipolar*. Patients participating in MBCT showed such improvement in executive functioning and memory that their levels became comparable to the general population, and the improvements in many cognitive areas (particularly memory and task monitoring) were maintained for at least three months.[516] MBCT also significantly reduced anxiety (which can trigger mania).[517, 518] Other improvements were improved mindfulness and the ability to regulate emotions.[519]
- For *depression*. MBCT is used primarily as an aid to avoid relapse, although it is successful in helping prevent depressive episodes[520] and reduce anxiety,[521] especially with people who have suffered three or more bouts of depression.[522] In fact, it can prevent a recurrence of depression as effectively as antidepressants, particularly in people with histories of childhood abuse.[523]
- For *attention-deficit hyperactivity disorder*. MBCT has been used successfully for ADHD. Group programs report a significant decrease in symptoms from pre- to post-treatment; 31% of the participants showed immediate improvement after treatment, and 97% self-reported at least moderate benefit.[524]

Mindfulness Based Sobriety (MBS). MBS is like MBCT for depression; it integrates mindfulness with cognitive-behavioral techniques to prevent relapses.

Rational Emotive Behavior Therapy (REBT).[525] REBT is a form of CBT whose goal is to solve emotional and behavioral problems by focusing on a person's perceptions, attitudes, and maladaptive behaviors (such as procrastination, addictive behaviors, aggression, unhealthy eating, et cetera). Various methods help people transform dysfunctional beliefs into more realistic and helpful beliefs. Little conclusive evidence supports REBT effectiveness, aside from the ample evidence supporting CBT.

Behavioral Activation (BA). While CBT focuses on thoughts in *Thought-Emotion-Action cycles* (see Figure 16, p. 84), BA is a depression therapy that urges us to action. "If you don't like how you feel, change the things you do" is a phrase that captures the essence of BA. It helps people engage in activities that can improve mood like exercising, going out to dinner and learning new skills.

- *For depression.* A review of three meta-analyses found BA to be as effective as CBT for depression, and potentially more effective in avoiding early termination of treatment.[526] One study found BA to be simpler to deliver than CBT, resulting in less cost and the need for less-thoroughly trained staff.[527]

WHAT CONSIDERATIONS SHOULD I KEEP IN MIND?

One of the most effective psychosocial therapies for mental health, *Cognitive Behavioral Therapy* encompasses a large family of related therapies focused on breaking free of unhelpful thoughts, emotions, and behaviors. All forms of CBT are broadly applicable across diagnoses. CBT gives people a measure of direct control over their symptoms—without the side effects psychotropics might have.

Therapist rapport and support are important in all therapies, including CBT. Its relatively short-term format (one session per week for anywhere from several weeks to several months) is easier to manage than long-term talking therapy.

Like many other forms of psychosocial therapy, the cost and availability of CBT resources is often a problem. Using a little creativity, however, can often help you gain access. CCBT, free online self-help and PDF-based CBT materials, as well as online therapist-to-client matching services can help. (See *Resources*, below. One example is www.MindQuire.com.) CCBT is considerably less expensive and easier to schedule than therapist-led CCBT and is as effective as face-to-face CBT therapy if therapist support is provided. Also, Android and iOS devices have *Cognitive Behavioral Therapy Apps* (p. 328).

You might also consider forms of therapist-led psychosocial therapy, which appear to be as effective as CBT.

Although CBT is a mental health therapy, its concepts apply broadly to anyone working to improve personal effectiveness. Its success is, in part, due to its grounding in two *Wellness Basics* that are vital to mental health: *Calm Awareness* (p. 73) and *Effective Self-Management* (p. 83).

REAL-WORLD EXPERIENCE

Case Study 28 – Cognitive Behavioral Therapy (Depression)

Mr. B is a gay man, 61, who suffered from spiraling depression after being diagnosed with early-stage bladder cancer.

"I was a queer kid, and I've gotten lifelong messages that big parts of me, even my core, had to be hidden if I wanted to be loved—or even survive. This takes a toll," he told his practitioner.

Mr. B attended twenty CBT sessions over a year, working to disentangle his depression from his cancer and positive-HIV status. He kept a thought diary and recorded his progress in changing his automatic thoughts, to "chip away at [his] bedrock of self-hate." He restructured his mental models from self-blame and hopelessness to "fighting for the top-notch care I deserve."

Mr. B achieved full recovery from depression and is now in remission.[528]

Bottom Line*: Beating depression is often an internal struggle. Drugs can mask symptoms, but they cannot replace the challenging internal effort required to heal self-defeating thoughts and attitudes.*

Case Study 29 – Cognitive Behavioral Therapy (Insomnia)

For more than six months, Tim, 38, felt fatigued during the day and had difficulties falling and staying asleep at night. He took 10 mg zolpidem, a sedative, at bedtime to help him sleep. During CBT for insomnia, he was educated about the sleep process, basic sleep hygiene, and what activities and stimulants to avoid before going to bed.

Tim then started sleep restriction (forcing sleep into a specific time window) and stimulus control (using bed only for sleep and getting out of bed if awake for more than twenty minutes). He was also trained in relaxation techniques.

The cognitive behavior therapy then focused on modifying his negative beliefs about sleep, particularly one Tim expressed frequently: "Since my sleep is not going to improve, I can't be the best I can be at work."

After Tim completed six CBT-I sessions, he was able to increase his total sleep time and improve his sleep efficiency, which resulted in less fatigue during the day. He was also able to taper his zolpidem dosage.[529]

Bottom Line*: CBT-I can help people learn how to regain control over their sleep through an integrated set of commonsense practices.*

Case Study 30 – Mindfulness-Based Cognitive Therapy (Depression)

Di, 53, had been taking antidepressants for fifteen years. In an eight-week MBCT class, Di learned meditation techniques. Two years later, he was still practicing those techniques four or five times a week for as much as an hour. He plans to continue it for the rest of his life.

"It's helped me immensely. It's given me the ability to come up against something that would have previously thrown me, think it through, come up with a solution, and then move on. It's helped me deal with recurrent thoughts. I look at life in a new light. I'm much more cheerful and positive. My friends and family noticed a change and improvement," he reported.

"[MBCT] was very worthwhile. It's a very sound way of combating mental illness and promoting mental health."[530]

Bottom Line: *Through mindfulness meditation from MBCT, people can develop a positive attitude, which helps us all cope with the difficulties of life.*

Case Study 31 – Recovery-Oriented Cognitive Therapy (Schizophrenia)

Kathy made daily phone calls to local authorities seeking help for threatening voices she believed would kill her. The result was agonizingly consistent: she was hospitalized over 100 times in a twenty-year period.

Finally, she was offered Recovery-Oriented Cognitive Therapy. With her therapist, she collaboratively identified meaningful personal goals that were broken down into tasks she could accomplish, starting with learning how to make a cup of coffee. Slowly, she began to challenge her negative beliefs and replace them with beliefs of personal competence.

Within six months, the phone calls stopped. She had a growing sense of personal empowerment, her psychosocial and neurocognitive functioning increased, and her psychotic symptoms decreased. She was not hospitalized once in 24 months.[531]

Bottom Line: *If you continually do the same thing, you continually get the same result. So it was with Kathy's 100 hospitalizations. She broke her negative cycle by starting a positive one: doing something small and parlaying success to things successively more difficult. Sometimes recovery is found in simple ideas.*

Case Study 32 – Behavioral Training

Nathan was in prison. "When you're there, there's not a lot of treatment unless you're dying. This leads to wondering where you can find hope," he reported. "I was introduced to the Jericho Project, a reentry program for people with mental illness who repeatedly return to jail."

The therapists made certain that he faithfully got to his doctor and therapy appointments. They taught him new behavioral techniques that worked for him: life skills, budgeting, eating healthy—"a lot of things that are really important," he said later. "I learned that [success] is about finding ways to be fulfilled."

After his release from prison, he was placed at 'Lending a Hand', a program run by a director whose experiences were like Nathan's. "He never gave up on us," Nathan said. "The Jericho Project helps you stay straight."[532(a)]

Bottom Line: *Sometimes a big part of mental health is knowing how to cope. Behavioral training, like CBT, teaches life-long coping skills.*

Case Study 33 – Dialectic Behavioral Therapy (BPD)

Z was 27 when she was diagnosed with borderline personality disorder. A victim of severe childhood abuse, she also suffered from severe depression, obsessive-compulsive disorder, and post-traumatic stress disorder.

By that time, she had become the county's most frequent user of emergency services. She spent half of her twenty-seventh year in psychiatric hospitals or in jail on drug or prostitution charges. She attempted suicide weekly and cut herself daily. Desperate for help, Z entered a DBT program, where she received individual therapy and group skills training. She also worked with a case aide to find housing.

Gradually, Z began to solve her problems. She started drug treatment, entered transitional housing, and landed a part-time job. At the end of her two-year DBT program, she had gone a year without one hospitalization, one attempt at injuring herself, or an attempted suicide.

Bottom Line*: DBT can help even those who show the most self-destructive behavior.*

WHAT ARE ADDITIONAL RESOURCES?

- Free Online CBT. https://moodgym.anu.edu.au.
- CBT apps and online tools. http://goo.gl/Iv5nQN.
- DBT Skills Handbook. http://goo.gl/5TMvSg.
- Multi-language CBT Self-help site. www.getselfhelp.co.uk.
- US CBT Assoc. www.nacbt.org, UK CBT Assoc. www.babcp.com.
- Mindfulness-Based Relapse Prevention. www.mindfulrp.com.
- CBT for Psychosis Resources (Ron Unger). https://goo.gl/rUhXAN.

Individual Psychotherapy

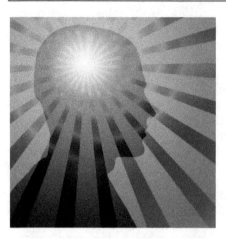

WHAT IS THE ESSENCE?

Individual Psychotherapy (IP) encompasses a broad overlapping set of mental health approaches that often rely upon one-on-one therapist sessions to understand, manage, and/or resolve mental distress.

Extensive evidence testifies to the fact that psychotherapy is effective in addressing a wide range of mental health conditions. Therapists can be a gateway to a broad set of *Psychosocial Restorative* therapies, including *Cognitive Behavioral Therapy* (p. 117). Therapies listed below are typically broader than the other categories of *Psychosocial Restorative* therapies (p. 115), which have a more specific targeted purpose.

WHAT EVIDENCE SHOWS THIS IS EFFECTIVE?

Psychoeducation. Although not strictly therapy, psychoeducation combines education and (often) peer support, to teach mental health fundamentals and provide recovery strategies for individuals with mental health issues and their families.[533] Psychoeducation should be started at the beginning of the recovery process and continue through the *Awareness stage* (p. 33), building hope and confidence.

Face-to-face classes offer personal interactions and support, but online classes have the advantage of being available anywhere and anytime; personal interactions take place via discussion forums, live chat, and conference calls. The National Alliance on Mental Illness (NAMI)[534] offers personal training in larger cities, with a therapeutic focus on psychotropics. For a broad exposure to non-drug options, see self-directed *Recovery Models & Tools* (p. 327). It is important to *Educate Yourself* (p. 50) and learn *Skills in Self-Care* (p. 46).

Trials found that patients combining medication with family psycho-education during the first two years of diagnosis have relapse rates 50% lower than those on medication alone.[127] However, another study showed that for depression, psychoeducation provided only marginal benefits at one year.[535]

Motivational Interviewing (MI). Often employed with *Cognitive Behavioral Therapy* (p. 117), MI is brief individual counselling (usually two to four sessions) that focuses on a person's motivation to change. It is most commonly used for alcohol and substance abuse.

Acknowledging that recovery is grounded in free choice, the MI goal is to motivate patients to choose recovery. MI practitioners act as partners in the change process, offering empathy, optimism, encouragement, and hope while supporting *Self-efficacy* (p. 87). They help patients understand the differences between their current behaviors and personal goals, validating the need for change.

Motivational challenges occur at each of the *Stages of Recovery* (p. 33).[536] For instance, individuals in the *distress* stage need to understand the need to change, so MI highlights the benefits of change. People in the *preparation* stage need to learn potential change strategies and choose the one most appropriate for them.

- For *substance abuse*. MI was found to be an effective stand-alone intervention for alcohol abuse and substance abuse, including marijuana.[537]
- For *schizophrenia*. MI is valuable in the *Awareness* stage, since lack of awareness is common in schizophrenia.[538] (See Case Study 34, p. 129.)
- For *anxiety*. Using MI before *Cognitive Behavioral Therapy* substantially benefitted people with severe anxiety.[539] In fact, those who received the two therapies were five times more likely to recover from anxiety within one year after treatment ended.[540]
- *More broadly*. When MI is combined with a healthy diet and exercise, it improves the chances of successful recovery, most especially for individuals dealing with addictions.[541]

Narrative Therapy (NT). Narrative Therapy helps people reframe the stories they tell about their lives, so they can focus on the positive instead of the negative. NT helps people identify and apply their skills and abilities, so they can address their problems effectively.

Solution-Focused Brief Therapy (SFBT). Solution-Focused Brief Therapy is resource-oriented and goal-focused, helping people change by helping them construct solutions. In the first year, the SFBT is significantly more effective than long-term therapy; however, the differences are not noticeable after two years. After three years, long-term psychodynamic psychotherapy is far more effective than SFBT.[542]

- For *depression*. SFBT is effective in reducing depressive symptoms.
- For *schizophrenia*. A small study found that some people using SFBT dramatically lowered the degree in which they believed in their delusions.[543]

Psychodynamic Psychotherapy (PP). Based on the work of Freud and others, Psychodynamic Psychotherapy helps patients identify the underlying influences of their mental and emotional issues and then eliminate them. PP's effectiveness is like that of other psychosocial therapies, including CBT.[544] *Short-term* PP helps people explore and work through specific psychological and interpersonal conflicts. *Long-term* PP is open-ended, intensive, and explores unconscious conflicts as well as developmental and psychological issues.

- For *anxiety*. CBT appears to be more effective than short-term PP.[545]
- For *depression*. A meta-analysis of short-term PP for depression showed that symptoms changed dramatically after treatment, and the changes were maintained for at least a year.[546] Psychotherapy is as effective as medication in treating depression and is more effective than medication in preventing depressive relapse.[10] When short-term PP was combined with psychotropics for depression, people were far more likely to sustain remission than the control group taking psychotropics only.[547]
- For *bipolar*. Evidence suggests that, as an adjunct to mood-stabilizing medication, individual psychotherapy can significantly reduce relapse rates and improve overall functioning and well-being.[10]

Hypnotherapy. During hypnotherapy, practitioners plant positive suggestions in the minds of patients who are in a hypnotic state–a state of focused attention and reduced peripheral awareness where people have an enhanced capacity to respond to suggestions. Little trial evidence supports hypnosis,[548, 549, 499] which defies Randomized Controlled Trial studies, but many positive case studies exist. (See Case Study 37, p. 130.) There is insufficient data to assess the effectiveness of hypnosis for schizophrenia.[550]

Neuro-Linguistic Programming (NLP). NLP maintains that changing our beliefs gives us control over our inner lives and behaviors. Little evidence supports NLP at present.[551] However, case studies suggest its effectiveness. (See Case Study 35, p. 129.)

- For *anxiety*. NLP can significantly improve mental health and enable patients to reduce dosages of psychotropics. One study found it can reduce symptoms of anxiety, aggression, paranoia, compulsive behaviors, and depression.[552] Another noted its efficacy with phobias.[553]
- *More broadly*. NLP has also proven effective in alleviating the symptoms of post-traumatic stress disorder[554] and certain phobias.[555]

Recovery Models. Effective *Recovery Models & Tools* (p. 327) can be used within a therapist-client relationship. Typically, they revolve around a theme of *Effective Self-Management* (p. 83). One of the most widely implemented is the *Wellness Recovery Action Plan*™ (p. 329) for broad mental health recovery and the *Matrix Model* (p. 328) for substance abuse.

WHAT CONSIDERATIONS SHOULD I KEEP IN MIND?

Extensive evidence indicates that psychological interventions can provide substantial functional improvements for people suffering from mood disorders, anxiety, and related disorders.[10]

Since IPT requires work with a therapist, it is important to find a trustworthy, empathic therapist—and that may take time. The therapist helps select the specific form of psychosocial therapy that seems most appropriate. (See Case Study 121, p. 294.)

REAL-WORLD EXPERIENCE

Case Study 34 – Motivational Interviewing (Schizophrenia)

Carl, 45, was diagnosed with chronic paranoid schizophrenia. He had a drug abuse problem, a history of violence, and he smoked 100+ cigarettes a day.

When he began motivational interviewing with his case worker, they determined that one of his major problems was a lack of strength and energy.

With his case worker, he set a plan, which included a modest exercise goal and a slow withdrawal from the psychotropics he had been prescribed. Additionally, the case worker helped broker housecleaning and shopping support and took Carl to dental appointments for his badly decaying teeth.

Carl reduced his psychotropics from 80 to 4 mg/day and started walking his dog. He quit smoking, aided by nicotine patches and daily case worker calls. He plans to follow a similar process to end his drug abuse.[556]

Bottom Line: *Recovery should start with what is important to the individual hoping for change. Look for ways a person's issues interconnect. Structured problem-solving and close support can produce success.*

Case Study 35 – Neuro-Linguistic Programming (Depression)

Belinda was diagnosed with depression, which was spiraling out of control. She couldn't relax; her body felt tired constantly. Her self-esteem was at rock-bottom, and she felt anti-social, unable to trust people. She had been taking antidepressants and had scheduled counselling off and on for three years.

"I'd almost given up. I didn't think it was possible to change," she recalled.

Her therapist gave her nine sessions of Neuro-Linguistic Programming over a three-month period. The first few sessions focused on healing emotions. Together, they talked through the challenges in her life. Next, they worked to transform Belinda's limiting beliefs and negative perceptions. Later sessions focused on developing skills for communicating with family members and colleagues. Within six weeks, Belinda could stop taking antidepressants.

"I've left a lot behind, and I've come through the other end stronger emotionally," she said. "I feel at peace with everything."[557]

Bottom Line: *The biggest lesson Belinda learned was putting past events into perspective, making sense of them, and forming more realistic views.*

Case Study 36 – Psychoeducation

Herb is a cop. While he was growing up, his mother had behaviors he didn't understand. As an adult, he decided to learn about them—and her.

"NAMI [National Alliance on Mental Illness] Family-to-Family training was eye opening. Wonderful. A personal learning experience for me," he said. "I learned the important message: my mom is still my mother, the person that I dearly love. The illness is also present, and it causes behaviors that used to upset me."

During his psychoeducation, he learned to set boundaries with his mother. "I also learned not to argue," he continued. "I can't expect her to do what I want. Nor can I fix her. I asked, 'Is she happy?' and 'How do I help her become happy?' Did that change her illness? No, but it helped our relationship blossom."

Education benefits entire family and community dynamics, Herb said. "Everyone can do better when educated — that's why we train officers and why we teach families."532(b)

Bottom Line: *Education focused on mental health issues and appropriate responses can make a tremendous difference for supporters of people in crisis. The best results occur when psychoeducation occurs early in the recovery process.*

Case Study 37 – Hypnosis (Anxiety)

Simon, 23, could not eat in public for fear of being sick. The anxiety increased ten-fold if any women were in the group. He was diagnosed with anxiety. His therapist tried hypnosis and other psychosocial techniques.

Under hypnosis, the therapist suggested Simon could be calm and relaxed at any time, that he could eat comfortably with friends, and that he didn't need to strive for perfection constantly. The therapist also regressed Simon to the first time he had felt this anxiety (an early childhood bullying experience) and to two different experiences of anxiety with women, especially a troubling recent relationship.

Work on the most recent relationship was perhaps the breakthrough. After the fifth session, Simon could appear in public in a calm and confident way and eat without problems. He also started a relationship with someone he had always kept at arm's length. His fear of criticism was reduced.558

Bottom Line: *By identifying and confronting past life events that triggered anxiety, we can begin to neutralize their power. Therapies that are unique in their implementation, like hypnosis, defy proof with Randomized Controlled Trials, but that doesn't mean they don't work for some people.*

WHAT ARE ADDITIONAL RESOURCES?

- Society of Clinical Psychology. www.psychologicaltreatments.org.
- EMDR. http://goo.gl/qtGti0.
- Motivational Interviewing. www.motivationalinterviewing.org.

Interpersonal, Family & Peer Therapy

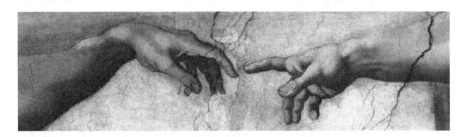

WHAT IS THE ESSENCE?

Interpersonal, Family, & Peer Therapy is a cluster of therapies that relies on family, friends, peers, and community members to help individuals struggling with mental health issues. This therapy leverages the fundamental human benefits of *Social & Outer Engagement* (p. 99). It acknowledges that recovery is fundamentally a personal, self-determined process, but rarely a solitary effort. Recovery is accomplished more quickly when we accept help from people who are skilled, accepting, concerned, and willing to become involved.

In many ways, "it takes a village" to achieve lasting recovery. This section helps identify the villagers and how they can be most helpful.

WHAT EVIDENCE SHOWS THIS IS EFFECTIVE?

Peer Support. Peer support offers assistance from others who are on their own journeys to mental health recovery.[559] With their unique "experts-through-experience" credibility, peers can serve as practical and inspiring role models, providing invaluable first-hand experience and counseling. Peer support often uses self-management approaches. (See *Recovery Models & Tools*, p. 327.)

- **Peer Support Specialists (PSS).** A PSS is a person who has progressed in recovery and is willing to help others with serious mental health concerns. They help improve recovery, as well as social inclusion, empowerment, quality of life, and hope.[560] The Center for Mental Health Services calls peer support "a key to recovery."[561] PSSs have been successful in convincing their peers to enter a treatment program.[562] Despite these benefits, little research exists to support its effectiveness,[563] although ample evidence is validated by case studies. (See Case Study 38, p. 134.)

- **Peer Support Groups.** Support groups are interactive sessions where people openly share their histories, concerns, and progress with peers. Group members learn from one another, connect, and offer advice. The most common support groups are for individuals with mental health issues, but groups are also available for their supporters. They often include a leader who is sometimes a therapist. In one meta-analysis, group therapy was as effective as individual treatment in 75% of the cases, and more effective in 25%.[564] A second study showed significant reductions in depression following group psychotherapy.[565] Support groups, particularly those led by Certified Peer Specialists, can have strong results: diminished symptoms, increased coping skills, and increased satisfaction with life.[566] People in one study[567] who combined support groups with face-to-face psychotherapy reported significant benefits, although another study found no benefits.[568] (See Case Study 39, p. 134 and Case Study 40, p. 134.)

- **Peer Respites.** Peer respites, also known as crisis residential programs or crisis respites, are supportive peer-run home-like settings for people experiencing psychiatric crises. These are a less traumatic alternative to care in a psychiatric emergency room. Many patients who have experienced both psychiatric hospitalization and peer respites strongly prefer peer respites. Although few respites are available in the United States, their numbers are rising. Initial studies show they can achieve better results than in-patient facilities,[569] and at lower cost. (See Practitioner's Story 5, p. 133.)

Interpersonal and Social Rhythm Therapy (IPSRT). IPSRT establishes daily routines and sleep cycles, using activities and social stimulation designed to moderate moods and relieve symptoms. When IPSRT is used during acute bipolar episodes, individuals have significantly longer periods of stability,[570] far greater regularity in daily routines, and improved functioning at work.[571]

Interpersonal Psychotherapy (IPT). Predicated on the belief that mental health issues and interpersonal issues are interrelated, IPT's brief, structured approach aims to improve relationships and interpersonal skills. People learn to evaluate and improve their interactions with others using specific tools.

- For *depression*. IPT (both in-person and over the phone) offered people struggling with depression benefits on par with stand-alone *Cognitive Behavioral Therapy* (p. 117) and stand-alone antidepressants.[572] There doesn't seem to be an additive benefit of IPT to psychotropic therapy.[573]

Family-Focused Therapy (FFT). Family-Focused Therapy works within a family's unique personality to create problem-solving methods that will improve family dynamics. FFT is a hybrid of two forms of psychotherapy: *psychoeducation* (teaching patients and their families about mental health issues) and *family therapies*.

- For *schizophrenia*. A meta-analysis of 94 studies found that FFT appears to be an effective treatment for psychosis by reducing relapse; one study showed a 28% relapse rate for patients using FFT and a 48% rate for those who did not.[574] It also improves social functioning and insight.[482]
- For *bipolar*. Using FFT with medication consistently yields faster mental health recovery and longer intervals of wellness than without FFT.[575] Several studies show that FFT reduces relapse rates.[576]

Family Constellation Therapy (FCT). Based on the work of German psychotherapist Ben Hellinger, FCT's goal is to reveal family dynamics that span generations, then eliminate their harmful effects by encouraging people to accept their history and move on. Used in more than twenty-five countries, primarily in Europe, the therapy relies on family role-playing to identify and find solutions. Although there are more than 2,000 FCT practitioners, data about its efficacy is insufficient.

Twelve-Step Programs. Twelve-step programs, which originated with Alcoholics Anonymous, offer a structured approach to recovery in most substance-abuse treatment programs. The choice of a sponsor (a peer counselor to support a person going through the steps) is vital to success. Findings suggest that attending at least one meeting a week is effective in maintaining abstinence from both illicit drug and alcohol use, with about the same success rates.[577] Less-than-weekly participation does not result in favorable outcomes.

WHAT CONSIDERATIONS SHOULD I KEEP IN MIND?

Interpersonal, Family, & Peer Therapy expands a person's network of supporters. These therapies draw people out of social isolation and open them to help from others. Support from peers is especially helpful, since they have valuable and similar life experiences. These therapies have both stand-alone value and additive value to psychotropic therapy.

REAL-WORLD EXPERIENCE

Practitioner's Story 4 – The Power of Peer Respites

Yana Jacobs received a Substance Abuse and Mental Health Services Administration (SAMHSA) grant to study the Second Story (SS) Peer Respite in Santa Cruz, California, which had been active for four years at that time. Based on Soteria (p. 148) concepts, SS is open to people in any recovery stage when they are in crisis.

When SS was evaluated by the Human Services Research Institute (HSRI), researchers found SS guests were significantly less likely to use in-patient and emergency services than others with similar mental health issues. Also, SS guests had statistically significant improvements in wellness, quality of life, personal relationships, and connection to a community of peers.

A guest reported that if her choice relied upon hospitals and a crisis house, "I would feel very mentally ill and labeled—like, 'These are mentally ill patients.' But I'm not a patient. I'm a person. At SS, I get treated like a full human being."

Second Story was promised state funding following the report.[578]

Bottom Line*: Peer respites work by relying on constant human contact and the use of medical intervention only when necessary. They offer a better experience for the individual and cost much less than hospitals.*

Case Study 38 – Peer Support Specialist

Ed was admitted to the hospital after a frightening psychiatric episode. After his discharge, he was introduced to a peer support worker, whom Ed regards as "probably the single most important factor in my recovery," explaining, "Working with him over many months, I was able to slowly get some perspective on my life, and then design what might be my future. His story was inspiring. I felt that I could trust him more than any other mental health worker because of his own experience of mental illness."[579]

Bottom Line*: People need to work with people they trust—practitioners and peers. Peer support specialists can build tremendous trust because of the experiences they share with someone struggling with mental health issues. There is no stigma when a peer is involved.*

Case Study 39 – Unconditional Acceptance in Support Groups

Andrea was diagnosed with bipolar. She attends a Bipolar UK peer support group and engages with their online eCommunity.

"At the Support Group, I am always accepted for who I am and how I am right at that moment", she says. "I don't need to apologize or make excuses for anything; that is truly priceless."[580]

Bottom Line *Unconditional acceptance is an attribute of successful support groups. This safety encourages people to engage, helping both themselves and other group members.*

Case Study 40 – Support Groups Improving Self-worth

Roger, 60, suffers from depression, alcoholism, and anger issues. He saw a notice about a weekly mental health support group offered by United Way and supported by Mental Health America, and he decided to attend.

Over the next three years, Roger's ability to manage both his depression and his anger improved. He believes the group has played a substantial role in his improvement, and he feels that he, in turn, contributes insights that help others. These feelings of worth helped reduce his depression, he told his therapist.

Because of his participation in the group and the friendships he made, Roger joined in social activities with members outside of meetings—"and that helps me think more positively."[581]

Bottom Line*: You can both give and receive help in support groups, thereby contributing to your own and others' personal growth and recovery.*

WHAT ARE ADDITIONAL RESOURCES?

- IPSRT Overview https://www.ipsrt.org, http://goo.gl/MYedeP.
- Peer support: National Empowerment Center www.power2u.org.
- Families Therapy. www.family.practicerecovery.com, www.familymentalhealthrecovery.org.

Cognitive Enhancement Therapy

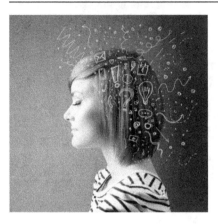

WHAT IS THE ESSENCE?

For schizophrenia and related disorders, Cognitive Enhancement Therapy (CET) enhances the brain's cognitive abilities and improves social functioning by capitalizing on the brain's ability to heal itself through enriched cognitive experiences.

CET and similar therapies, including Cognitive Remediation and Cognitive Rehabilitation, seek to improve vigilance, attention, mental processing speed, working memory, and planning, thereby improving social and vocational issues that resulted from cognitive impairments.

CET is geared to people whose mental health is stable, but who have not fully recovered. It consists of simple systematic cognitive exercises on computers, with weekly group sessions lasting one to two years. Although CET's initials may be confused with *Cognitive Behavioral Therapy* (CBT, p. 117), they are very different. CBT focuses on the *accuracy of the content* of cognition (For example, "Is it true that everyone hates me?"), while CET focuses on improving the brain's *information processing* (For example, "How can I focus my attention better, so I can remember things?").

WHAT EVIDENCE SHOWS THIS IS EFFECTIVE?

A meta-analysis[582] found that although CET appears to significantly improve psychosocial functioning, it seems to have little effect on the symptoms of schizophrenia – a finding consistent with studies showing that cognitive impairment is relatively independent of other symptoms. CET programs that included strategy coaching related to functioning were more effective than programs that focused only on drill and practice.

In a two-year randomized study of 121 persons with schizophrenia or schizoaffective disorder, CET had strong and enduring benefits in neurocognition, mental processing speed, cognitive style, social cognition, and social adjustment.[583]

In one study, 54% of CET participants were actively engaged in paid and competitive employment at the end of two years of CET, as compared to 18% of those who received enriched supportive therapy (EST); plus, they earned significantly more money and were more satisfied with their employment. CET improved many negative symptoms, as well as anxiety and depression.[584]

A long-term study found most of the effects of the CET on cognition and behavior were maintained one year after treatment ended.[585] CET can avoid gray matter loss in key brain areas and the increase in gray matter in others.[586] Although the computer component is important, graduates believe the social interactions (See *Social Networks*, p. 100) of CET are invaluable.[587]

Cognitive symptoms for bipolar can closely mirror those of schizophrenia. A small trial of CET for bipolar found that 70 hours of computer-based neuroplacticity exercises resulted in significant improvements in cognitive performance, including cognitive speed, visual learning, and memory. Participants maintained these improvements six months after the end of the treatment, and in some areas showed continued improvements.[588]

CET is recognized by the Substance Abuse and Mental Health Services Administration (SAMHSA) as an evidence-based practice. Additionally, the Center for Cognition and Recovery (CCR) was awarded the 2011 SAMHSA Science and Service Award for its work with CET.[589]

WHAT CONSIDERATIONS SHOULD I KEEP IN MIND?

If we consider our mental faculties a muscle, CET doesn't seek to explore why the muscle may have been weakened in the first place but accepts the current situation and works to make the muscle stronger and more functional by putting it to work. CET is complementary to other forms of psychosocial therapy, since it addresses the functional dexterity of the brain (such as processing speed and working memory), while the other therapies examine the thought and emotional content of the brain.

While medication has been shown to improve some positive symptoms of schizophrenia (for example, hallucinations and voices), no current medications address cognition (a negative symptom), although CET is showing promising results in addressing some negative symptoms. One of the difficulties with CET is the prolonged time commitment, often 48 weeks or more.

WHAT ARE ADDITIONAL RESOURCES?

- Center for Cognition and Recovery http://cetcleveland.org/default.aspx.
- Hogarty G, Personal Therapy for Schizophrenia and Related Disorders, a Guide to Individualized Treatment, Guilford Press, 2002.

Creative Engagement Therapy

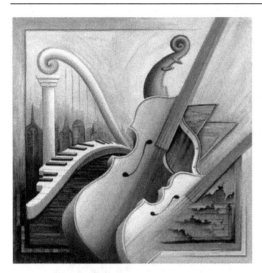

WHAT IS THE ESSENCE?

Creative Engagement Therapy encompasses a family of approaches that help people connect with and improve their inner world and functioning through self-expression and engagement in the outer world.

Each therapy in this group involves direct contact with things that contain beauty, order, or wonder—and the result is often calming, meaningful, and inspiring. *Creative Engagement* is an opportunity to hone skills and find enjoyment, relaxation, and socialization. It emphasizes the process of creation and the quality of the interaction, rather than the final product.

WHAT EVIDENCE SHOWS THIS IS EFFECTIVE?

Music Therapy. Music therapy can encompasses creating music, singing, listening, moving, or dancing to music as a means of improving mood, emotional awareness, and calmness. It can also open communication for those who find it difficult to express themselves in words. (See Case Study 44, p. 140, and a related approach, *Sound Therapy,* p. 240.)

- For *schizophrenia.* Adding a music therapy component leads to greater improvement in symptoms, when compared with standard care alone.[590, 591]
- For *depression.* Researchers found that music therapy reduced depression in those with dementia[592] and helps improve mood.[593] Participants in a drumming circle experienced significant improvement in depression, anxiety, and social resilience; and their blood chemistry altered toward an anti-inflammatory profile associated with greater well-being.[594]
- For *childhood development and behavioral issues.* A test of 251 children showed that those who received music therapy had significantly improved self-esteem and significantly reduced depression, as compared with those who received treatment without music therapy.[595]

Art Therapy. Art therapy, which can include drama and music therapy, encourages self-expression through artistic expression.

- For *schizophrenia.* Art therapy does not seem to help.[596]

- For *bipolar*. Art/music therapy helps stabilize those with bipolar,[597] a group that represents significant numbers in the creative arts.[598]
- *More broadly*. One study found that art therapy improved self-esteem and self-confidence, provided a safe space for reflection, and was a cathartic springboard for future engagement.[599]

Bibliotherapy. Bibliotherapy uses books, poetry, self-help materials, and other forms of the written word as an aid to recovery.

- For *depression*. Two meta-analyses[600] found bibliotherapy as effective as individual or group therapy for unipolar depression.
- For *PTSD*. Writing therapy can help confront fears and traumatic memories. One study found that writing compared favorably to the exposure therapy known as *Eye Movement Desensitization and Reprocessing* (p. 152).[601]
- For *alcohol abuse*. Analysis of twenty-two studies found that bibliotherapy has a modest rate of success for decreasing at-risk drinking.[602]

Writing/Journaling Therapy. Journaling about stressful or traumatic experiences can be therapeutic—provided emotional expression and cognitive processing can make sense of the experience.[603] Journaling and building *Stories and Personal Narrative* (p. 96) increases *Self-Understanding* (p. 86) which are both helpful in the larger process of *personal growth,* a vital component of *personal recovery.* (See *What is Recovery?*, p. 31.)

The narrative process of writing poetry, journaling, or "storytelling to ourselves," helps us interpret our lives.[604] Although research is not significant, evidence suggests that journaling improves physical and mental health functioning; consequently, it is becoming a common practice in the criminal justice system, where it has been integrated into preconviction and postconviction efforts to reduce recidivism.[605] (See Case Study 42, p. 140.)

Wilderness/Adventure Therapy. *Wilderness Therapy* is an intense form of engaging with *Nature (p. 101)*, pushing people beyond their typical limits and calling on greater self-sufficiency, courage, and self-management. It is particularly effective in dealing with substance abuse situations.

- **Peer Outdoor Support Therapy (POST)**. POST brings both outdoor therapy and peer support together to address the well-being of military veterans. Although POST programs have operated for many years, they have not yet been evaluated systematically.[606] However, qualitative research available on POST's approaches supports its use.
- **Outward Bound**. Outward Bound, a *Wilderness Therapy*, provides opportunities for personal growth, self-reliance, and teamwork. Veterans who attended Outward Bound improved their mental health, interpersonal relations, and sense of purpose; they also showed greater interest in their personal growth, investigating their emotions, and seeking help.[607]

Animal Therapy. Pets can make all the difference in a person's outlook, engagement, and happiness, as countless people will attest. But animal therapy can mean more than just caring for a pet. *Emotional support dogs* provide affection and companionship. *Service dogs* are task-trained, to signal the onset of anxiety, remind people to take medication, and accomplish other tasks.[608] Pet owners are less likely to suffer from depression than those without pets; researchers have found that playing with a pet can elevate serotonin and dopamine levels, which calm and relax us.[609] Caring for an animal can help us feel needed, diverting our concerns about mental health issues. *Equine-Assisted Therapy* uses horses to help people deal with depression, anxiety, ADHD, and other chronic mental health issues.[610] (See Case Study 43, p. 140.)

Dance & Sport Therapy. Dance appears to increase happiness and EEG activity in psychiatric patients.[611]

- For *depression*. If you want to reduce your stress levels, learn to tango. Research shows it is significantly more effective in dropping stress levels than, for example, a mindful meditation class—which has its own values. Dance is a significant predictor for the increased levels of mindfulness.[612]

- For *schizophrenia*. Participating in sports has a positive effect on psychiatric symptoms in schizophrenia.[613] Research has shown a 20% reduction in negative symptoms.[614] (See Case Study 41, p. 139.)

WHAT CONSIDERATIONS SHOULD I KEEP IN MIND?

Creative Engagement complements other approaches to recovery. A more active form of *Sensory Therapy* (p. 239), both invite people to step away from their challenges and find opportunities to relax and engage. When practiced by therapists, it is a directed activity to enhance cognition, socialization, motor skills, emotional development and other domains.

Creative Engagement can to bring joy and pull us out of ourselves. Physical movement with a captivating new focus is central to these therapies. Simple creative acts offer us a sense of normalcy, joy, and refuge.

REAL-WORLD EXPERIENCE

Case Study 41 – Sports Engagement (Schizophrenia)

Eric is a single dad with schizophrenia who discovered the life-giving benefits of cycling. "On my journey…the sport has saved me," he said. "Each race, no matter the size, is an accomplishment for me, win or lose."

Before he climbed onto a bicycle, Eric had times when he was afraid to leave his home. Now the opposite is true: he finds joy, solace, and healing in the outdoors. "Just to get out there and participate in cycling competitions surprises both me and my doctor," he said. "I know my sport isn't for everyone, but it doesn't have to be cycling. Just find something you enjoy and do it. It's good to focus your mind on an activity you enjoy."

When a friend shared her regrets about not being athletic, Eric pointed out that she already had a passion: cooking. "I believe doing any enjoyable activity can lead to a more rewarding life," he told her.[532] (f)

> ***Bottom Line***: *To escape mental difficulties, engage in enjoyable and meaningful activity. When we focus our energies on something captivating, we forget our challenges and find a sense of inner peace, even joy.*

Case Study 42 – Poetry (Bipolar)

Yashi suffered from bipolar. Writing poetry became an entirely new focus—"It's my lifeline and helpline," she said. "Poetry helped me tap into places and leave behind the horror of hopelessness. I could cry for help. It unleashed my ability to communicate with the world while trying to cope with my bipolar. Poetry was the only place in my brain where I liked myself, where I could feel special.

"Prayer, positive thinking, poetry, family therapy, and medical treatments helped recovery rear its wonderful head and empower me. I had to share my hope with others, through my words."[532 (c)]

Bottom Line: *When we find a creative outlet that inspires us, like Yashi, we can explore an interior place that is healing and affirming.*

Case Study 43 – Equine-Assisted Therapy (PTSD)

Tim was a sergeant in Operation Desert Storm. He came back from war with post-traumatic stress disorder. "I spent twelve years out of society," he recalled. During that time, he refused to leave his house. Doctors prescribed psychotropics and talking therapy. They were only marginally effective.

Tim then found a different kind of counselor: Jack, a coal-black Percheron with an Equine-Assisted Therapy program called Horses for Heroes. Jack convinced Tim to leave his house and experience an entirely new form of treatment. "I wouldn't trade this place for anything," he said. "Instead of sitting around and feeling sorry, it got me out."

When asked what the program does for him, he says, "I can actually talk without crying now. Surrendering yourself to a big monster [is a challenge]—you have to trust he isn't going to go wild. I had to put myself out there. Bonding with the horse really helped. When you're on a horse, you focus, you're in the moment... This is hands-on and real."[615]

Bottom Line: *Find something activity that will draw you out of your head, so you can concentrate on the present moment.*

Case Study 44 – Music Therapy (Dementia)

By the time Rose, 80, was diagnosed with dementia, she was speaking in single-word sentences, apparently unaware of her surroundings. She was unable to take care of herself. However, when a music therapist visited her and sang, "You are my Sunshine," Rose joined in, and her words were clearly understood. She sang with recognizable pitch and emotional expression, her face brightening. During the therapy, she made eye contact, and for several hours following therapy, nursing home attendants reported that she seemed to be in a better mood, less agitated and more relaxed.[616]

__Bottom Line__: Never be dismissive of people with Alzheimer's. They can still find joy.

WHAT ARE ADDITIONAL RESOURCES?

- MH service dogs. www.petpartners.org & http://usdogregistry.org.
- Equine-assisted Therapy. www.therapeuticridinginc.org.
- Nature Therapy. www.discoveryquest.org.
- Music Therapy. www.musictherapy.org.

Biofeedback

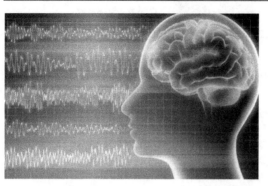

WHAT IS THE ESSENCE?

Biofeedback uses devices to monitor physical functions that are normally outside of our awareness— such as blood pressure, heart rate, and body temperature.

In most forms of *biofeedback*, people train themselves to exert influence intentionally over a monitored function to help them relax. Benefits from biofeedback are like those of *Calm Awareness* practices (p. 73).

Five major forms of biofeedback each monitor a biological function in a different way.

- **EEG Biofeedback.** Also known as *Neurofeedback*, EEG Biofeedback monitors brain waves using electroencephalograms by placing sensors on the scalp; video displays or sounds measure the results. With practice, individuals can learn how to create specific brain waves that are considered beneficial.[617]

- **Low-energy Neurofeedback System (LENS).** LENS monitors brain waves using a very low-power electromagnetic field. A single set of wires attached to the scalp carries signals from the brain to the monitor and carries feedback signals back to the brain. Although feedback signals are very weak, they can change brainwaves without conscious effort.[618]

- **Electromyographic (EMG) biofeedback** monitors muscle contraction, measured through electrodes placed on the skin.

- **Heart Rate Variability Biofeedback (HRVB)** monitors the beat-by-beat heart rate, allowing people to adjust their heartbeat until it is in sync with their breathing—which is called *respiratory sinus arrhythmia (RSA)*. RSA seems to be associated with greater heart and lung efficiency, and it can influence the vagal nerve[619] which is strongly associated with mood. (See *Vagus Nerve Stimulation Therapy*, p. 251.) RSA is often achievable within seconds, even in people who have never tried it before.[620]

- **Thermal feedback** monitors and allows people to adjust their body temperature, which is measured by a sensor attached to a finger.

WHAT EVIDENCE SHOWS THIS IS EFFECTIVE?

EEG Biofeedback. EEG Biofeedback has been studied most extensively for people with attention-deficit hyperactivity disorder, who often show low levels of arousal in frontal brain areas. Neurofeedback helps them increase arousal levels.

- *For attention-deficit hyperactivity disorder.* Results for EEG neurofeedback are mixed. One analysis found that it is likely to improve ADHD symptoms, but more extensive testing is needed.[621] Two small Randomized Controlled Trials (RCT) found that both EEG neurofeedback and sham neurofeedback can significantly improve ADHD symptoms in similar degrees.[622, 623] The American Academy of Pediatrics approved biofeedback and neurofeedback as a Level 1 or "best support" treatment option for children suffering from ADHD.
- For *anxiety.* Biofeedback helps manage many anxiety symptoms and is probably as effective as conventional relaxation techniques;[624] when they are used in combination, anxiety symptoms improve more than using relaxation techniques alone.[625]
- For *substance abuse.* A test using EEG Biofeedback with 120 patients who had multiple addictions showed an abstinence rate of 77% at the end of one year.[626]
- For *schizophrenia.* In one study, 98% of the patients who undertook sixty neurofeedback sessions guided by qEEG (see *Glossary*, p. 337) showed clinical improvement.[627] In another, neurofeedback for treatment-resistant schizophrenia improved cognitive and behavioral patterns that were sustained for at least two years.[628] Benefits also include consistent increases in attention/vigilance, working memory, processing speed,[629] and social competence,[630] results that were similar to those in *Cognitive Enhancement Therapy* (p. 135).
- *More broadly.* In one study, patients experienced improvements in both visual and auditory attention levels, and, most notably, MRI scans revealed that their brains changed structure in areas linked to attention skills.[631] In another, functional changes occurred in a key brain network after a thirty-minute session of noninvasive, neural-based training.[632]

LENS. Evidence for LENS is small and growing. Anecdotal evidence suggests results occur in fewer LENS sessions than in the traditional neurofeedback model.

- For *depression.* A case series involving twenty people found that over the course of twenty LENS sessions, they reported a significant drop in depression.[633]
- For *PTSD and Traumatic Brain Injury.* Two case studies enlisted Afghanistan and Iraq war veterans for twenty-five LENS sessions; all symptoms improved dramatically.[634]
- For *anger.* Two case studies suggest that LENS can provide significant benefit in anger management.[635] (See Case Study 48, p. 145.)

Heart Rate Variability Biofeedback. A literature review found HRVB to be a very promising intervention for hypertension, depression,[636] anxiety, PTSD, and insomnia.[637] (See Case Study 45, p. 144.)

WHAT CONSIDERATIONS SHOULD I KEEP IN MIND?

Biofeedback takes advantage of the close alignment between our bodies and minds; the mind's ability to control bodily conditions is something that we normally don't consider. One major benefit of biofeedback is its ability to reduce stress, which aids recovery in all diagnoses.

REAL-WORLD EXPERIENCE

Case Study 45 – Heart Rate Variability Biofeedback (PTSD)

David, a 46-year-old craftsman, developed post-traumatic stress disorder after he was injured in an explosion at work. Six months of psychotherapy didn't help him; during that time, he developed agoraphobia and started drinking.

He was encouraged to accept his anxiety instead of suppressing it. To help, David wrote a story about his experience. As a form of exposure, he read his story in the present tense, reliving the emotions while receiving Heart-Rate Variability biofeedback. He also related his story while he used a breathing practice.

With continued repetition, David's symptoms dropped by more than one-third. His agoraphobia was no longer an issue, and he could control his drinking.[638]

__Bottom Line__: Trauma is often self-perpetuating, if we don't address it head-on.

Case Study 46 – EEG Biofeedback (Anxiety)

Karen, 31, was diagnosed with chronic anxiety. For more than three years, she tried a variety of psychotropics and psychosocial therapies that provided little relief. Then, following a brain wave analysis, she started weekly EEG biofeedback to decrease alpha waves and increase beta waves.

After fifteen sessions, Karen had significantly decreased anxiety. Treatment was cut back to twice a month. At a three-year follow-up, she was symptom free.[639]

__Bottom Line__: EEG biofeedback can help us develop conscious control over our brain waves. Since our body and mind are closely connected, brain wave control can reduce the mind's anxiety.

Case Study 47 – Handheld Biofeedback (Insomnia)

Francis was a medic deployed in an Iraqi combat zone. During and after his service, he had recurring sleep problems. Cognitive Behavioral Therapy and sleep hygiene education did not help. His doctor recommended using StressEraser, a handheld biofeedback device that uses an infrared signal to monitor HRV at the finger pulse. The device displays HRV as a wave that increases when we inhale and decreases when we exhale.

After one week of using the device, Francis slept much better. At a six-week assessment, his sleep remained good, so he stopped his treatment.[640]

Bottom Line: We can consciously relax ourselves through a variety of Calm Awareness (p. 73) techniques and biofeedback. Experiment to find what works for you.

Case Study 48 – LENS (Head Injury)

For two years after being struck by a hit-and-run driver, Evelyn was a different person. Her brain injury made her hypersensitive to both sound and sights, which gave her splitting headaches. Consequently, she had problems with memory, focus, and attention. Her intellectual abilities after the accident tested far below what her academic background predicted.

Her practitioner gave her cognitive development exercises to help desensitize her sensory abilities. He also gave her a series of Low-Energy Neurofeedback System (LENS) sessions. By the twelfth session, she began to improve, and by the twentieth session, her cognitive functioning returned to normal.[641]

Bottom Line: Did LENS therapy or cognitive exercises help Evelyn? In the end it doesn't really matter. What matters is that she recovered. Diligent and prudent experimentation with a variety of therapies may deliver what works for us.

WHAT ARE ADDITIONAL RESOURCES?

- HRVB. Heartmath Institute. www.HeartMath.org.
- Neurofeedback overview. www.eeginfo.com.
- Neurofeedback research and resources. http://goo.gl/1qj6gI.
- EEG education and research. www.eegspectrum.com.

Dialogue & Exposure Therapy

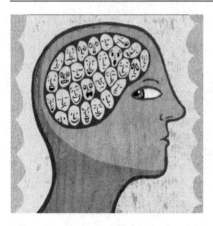

WHAT IS THE ESSENCE?

Dialogue & Exposure Therapy combines two sets of therapies that target different diagnoses but share numerous similarities.

Dialogue Therapies are a cluster of interventions targeting the auditory verbal hallucinations (AVH) of schizophrenia. A common thread in many of these is the art of dialogue: talking directly to voices, peers, and supporters as a means of reducing the frequency and impact of AVHs—this runs directly contrary to previous thought, which considered any acknowledgement of voices harmful or counterproductive.[642] However, dialogue has shown strong success in some cases and is a valuable way to understand and accept an individual's experience as a first step in recovery. (See Practitioner's Story 6, p. 154.)

Language is an important tool in recovery, since it conveys each person's unique recovery experience.[92] *Dialogue Therapies* can give us a growing mastery over AVHs. In some cases, this mastery can eliminate the voices.

Exposure Therapies confront troubling or obsessive thoughts and emotions that can result from trauma or other causes. Trauma is a vital consideration since it is not only associated with PTSD, but also with psychosis[643] (see Figure 26), and OCD (30-82% of people with OCD have experienced trauma[644]).

All Diagnoses	Schizophrenia
69% of female & 59% of male psychiatric inpatients have experienced childhood sexual or physical abuse.	The childhood experience: 47% emotional abuse, 51% emotional neglect, 41% physical neglect.
Average of 46 studies	Average of 6 studies

Experiencing this childhood adversity...	...has this psychosis risk multiplier	Analysis size
Sexual Abuse	2.4X	20 studies
Physical Abuse	2.9X	13 studies
Emotional Abuse	3.4X	6 studies
Neglect	2.9X	7 studies
Bullying	2.4X	6 studies
Parental Death	1.7X	8 studies
Mother's Death	12.3X	6 studies
3 forms of adversity	7X - 18X	14,362 people
5 forms of adversity	30X - 193X	14,362 people

© 2017 Craig Wagner – www.OnwardMentalHealth.com

Figure 26 - Childhood adversity & mental health

Exposure Therapies re-expose the victim to the trauma in a controlled and repeated manner, to reduce or eliminate its impact.

Exposure can be *in vivo* (direct confrontation of the feared situation), *imaginal* (mental imagery), and *virtual* (artificial experience often computer-based). *Exposure Therapies* are based on the idea that going to the heart of a problem, although painful in the short-term, can release the negative grip of the problem and aid long-term healing. The Substance Abuse and Mental Health Administration (SAMSA) indicates, "Trauma is often a precursor to… mental health problems. (Mental health) services…should be trauma-informed."[1461]

A common thread in *Dialogue & Exposure Therapy* is the acceptance and direct engagement with the compelling force (a voice, traumatic memory, or intrusive thought).

WHAT EVIDENCE SHOWS THIS IS EFFECTIVE?

Dialogue Therapies

Voice Dialoguing.[645] Voice Dialoguing is predicated on the belief that voices often reflect different aspects of ourselves or our experiences. In this process, a therapist directly engages with the voice to help patients understand, and possibly change, their relationship to their voices. For some people, voice dialoguing illustrates their awareness of underlying emotional and social problems, and helps them improve communication; ultimately, it should develop a more peaceful and productive relationship with the voices—if not eliminating them entirely.[646] Voice Dialoguing can be a powerful experience, only undertaken with a trusted trained therapist. (See Case Study 50, p. 155.)

Open Dialogue[SM] **(OD).** Open Dialogue is an early-intervention family/team-oriented approach for dealing with psychosis that could be one of the most exciting advances in the care of psychosis. Using a language grounded in the patient's perspective, a strong and supportive network of people will speak with the individual suffering with psychosis. Everyone involved is present with the therapist and the person in distress.[647] The central emphasis of OD focuses on "being with the individual in crisis" more than "solving the immediate symptomatic problem."[648]

Dialogue helps break through the sense of isolation that individuals feel when their experience seems to defy normal description. This immediate patient-centered response leverages the benefits of interpersonal interaction that are rooted in *Social Engagement* (p. 99).

- For *psychosis*. A five-year study found that OD reduced the need for psychotropics; 82% did not have any residual psychotic symptoms and 86% had returned to their studies or a full-time job.[649] Longer term studies found that those receiving antipsychotics are over three times more likely to be on disability income than those receiving OD.[650] In a small US OD pilot, half of the participants stopped using antipsychotics and saw outcomes similar to those who remained on drugs.[651]

Soteria.[652] Soteria is a 24/7 early-intervention approach for psychosis carried out in a protective and tolerant home-like environment rather than a hospital. A trained nonprofessional staff expresses and demonstrates empathy and nonintrusive behaviors, such as "standing by attentively," while few if any psychotropic drugs are used. The staff builds bridges to the individual to help with recovery. The original Soteria residential experiment showed that between 85% and 90% of acute schizophrenia patients can be returned to the community without hospitalization. The Soteria principles are being leveraged in other non-hospital crisis environments like *Peer Respites* (p. 132).

Voice Coping Strategies. People with schizophrenia often need coping strategies for Auditory Verbal Hallucinations (AVHs), since they can persist, even with the use of intensive and prolonged antipsychotics.[653] Experimenting is the best way to find strategies that work best for you. The following have been effective for some. See "Additional Resources" (p. 158) for more.

- **Subvocalization Interruption.** Growing evidence suggests that AVHs are related to speech and language. When healthy people think and read, muscle activity called subvocalization can be detected in the throat and tongue.[654, 655] "Talking to ourselves" or "inner speech" when reading are common examples of this. One study found that AVHs are often preceded by subvocalization. If these movements can be interrupted, hallucinations often decrease markedly. In one study, fourteen of eighteen patients with schizophrenia were able to eliminate their auditory hallucinations by interrupting their subvocalization.[656] Humming a single note can reduce auditory hallucinations by 59%.[657] Singing and reading aloud may also be helpful. Another study found that when individuals held their mouths open during AVHs, they stopped in 72% of the cases.[656]

- **Modulate the "Degree of Listening."** A common coping strategy is to select which voices to listen to or ignore. About one-third of voice hearers can completely ignore the voices,[658] though this approach may cause the voices to become more hostile. (See Case Study 49, p. 154.) From limited evidence, a better method may be to listen to "positive" voices only. Some found this offered a greater control over the voices, while others found it a process of learning to think more positively.

- **Modulate Sound.** Anecdotal cases testify that people using sound-generator treatments (designed for tinnitus) for one month find complete remission of audio/visual hallucinations.[659] Others found that listening to a stereo[660] or radio with headphones[661] can decrease or eliminate the severity of AVHs. These approaches appear to provide sound interference or distractions that disrupt the hallucination. Interestingly, preventing sounds from entering the ear can be successful. One study found that patients who wore an earmuff on their left side showed a 50% reduction in AVHs.[662] One possible explanation for this is that AVHs appear to be related to stress, and the ear muff may reduce anxiety by reducing distracting auditory input. A high-quality musician's ear-plug will reduce even more sound and be less noticeable.

- **Modulate Social Engagement.** Either increasing or decreasing social interaction can be helpful. One study[663] concluded that increasing social contacts and conversing can reduce AVHs. This can be as simple as calling a supportive friend on the phone. This may distract the mind from voices. Others find that they need to withdraw from social interaction, since it may be a source of stress that can increase AVHs. Once again, individuals must discover what works for them.
- **Frustrate Voices with Repetition.** Try repeating to yourself everything your voice says, word for word, in your mind. This may cause voices to stop or become calmer. For loud voices, slowly reduce the "volume" as you repeat the words; this can often reduce the volume of the voice itself.
- **Take Initiative with Voices.** Asking voices about themselves may help. Ask their age, why they are pestering you, their recreational activities, anything that comes to mind. This puts you in a more assertive relationship with voices and may help you more willfully control them.
- **Reframe Voices.** Try assuming that voices are present to help you but are clumsy in their helping. Analyze their words and reframe their negative language into something constructive. For example, if voices say you are an incapable person, acknowledge that you have improvement areas, like everyone. Then put positive focus on an improvement area of your choice.
- **Draw Limits for Voices.** Some find it helpful to accept a voice, but to constrain or structure its expression (for example, setting certain times of day or topics for the voices).[658]
- **Anxiety Reduction Techniques.** A variety of *anxiety reduction techniques* (p. 294) have been effective in reducing the impact of AVHs.[664]

Avatar Therapy. Avatar Therapy allows patients to choose a digital face (or "avatar") for their voice. A therapist who understands and mimics the voice then sits in a separate room and "talks" with the patient.[665]

- For *schizophrenia*. A small study of those receiving *Avatar Therapy* reported a significant reduction in the frequency and volume of the internal voices, and 10% reported that the voices had disappeared altogether.[666] In another study, patients in *Avatar Therapy* reported a significant reduction in the frequency, intensity, omnipotence, and malevolence of the voices.[667] (See Case Study 56, p. 157.)
- For *depression*. One small study of avatar-based self-management in young adults found a significant reduction in depression over three months.[668] Another found that Help4Mood, a virtual agent for engaging patients in depression monitoring and treatment, also resulted in meaningful improvements of depression when used regularly over a four-week trial.[669]

Hearing Voices Network (HVN). This network is a collaboration of support groups for people who hear voices. The movement challenges the notion that hearing voices is necessarily a symptom of mental illness. Instead, the network regards voices as meaningful and understandable, although unusual. (See Case Study 51, p. 155, and Case Study 52, p. 156.)

Instead of a clinical group or treatment program, HVN is a social group that comes together to discuss common issues. The United Kingdom Hearing Voices Network maintains that developing a compassionate relationship with troubling voices is helpful, suggesting, "Softening feelings toward the tormenting voice can be reflected back to the voice-hearer, bringing a starting point for the alleviation of suffering."[670]

Interestingly, showing this compassion to voices is similar to simple *Self-Compassion* (p. 86), a *Wellness Basic* associated with mental health. If the voice is considered an element of the individual's psyche, kindness and acceptance can have logical merit.

Many people who attend HVN support groups attest to its value. A study of HVN attendees found that the sessions provide support that is unavailable elsewhere and foster both social and clinical positive outcomes.[671] Aspects of HVN's approach are also supported by clinical evidence:

- Although voices can be viewed as meaningless, it doesn't help hearers if someone insists that they must accept a particular framework for understanding their mental health symptoms.[104] Failing to respect or accept an individual's experience is a roadblock to recovery.[674] HVN accepts members and what they say about their voices without judgment.
- Investigations have shown that if listeners accept hallucinations as an aspect of the normal human condition without resistance—although, admittedly, this is difficult—they can adapt to hearing voices and change their responses to the voices.[672]
- Voice hearers want to talk about the content and meaning of their voices,[673] and HVN groups allow them to do that. *Support Groups* (p. 131) have proven helpful to recovery, and HVN groups are essentially supportive for voice hearers.

Guided Self-determination. Guided Self-Determination (GSD) is a shared decision-making and problem-solving method that helps people become self-determining. It values both patient and practitioner opinions and guides the patient through problem solving, honoring the patient's perspective rather than immediately trying to change it. A lack of respect for a patient's opinion can be a roadblock to recovery,[674] so when the practitioner honors and accepts a patient's perspective, the patient is likely to honor and accept the practitioner's perspective. A unique insight of GSD is that delusions are sometimes most effectively unseated if they are addressed tangentially, since direct approaches often meet with strong resistance to change.[675] GSD helps dissolve people's resistance to change by allowing them to be in charge of their recovery. One trial found that GSD improved clinical insight, symptom severity, and social functioning of those with schizophrenia.[676] (See Case Study 55, p. 157.)

Lucid Dreaming. Lucid dreaming is a hybrid state between sleeping and wakefulness, when we are aware that we are dreaming as we dream. This offers the potential for re-experiencing traumatic thoughts in an environment where the dreamer has a measure of control over the experience. Most people need progressive training to develop the skill to dream lucidly.

- For *PTSD*. Research shows that nightmares are among the most common symptoms, and an integral part, of PTSD; up to 80% of people with PTSD have them. Therefore, addressing nightmares while they occur via lucid dreaming shows promise, but few studies have explored that possibility.[677]
- For *schizophrenia*. Brain analyses have shown similarities between brain activity in lucid dreaming and psychosis, suggesting that dream therapy may be useful in treatment for psychosis.[678]
- For *depression*. Early evidence suggests that lucid dreaming may help improve depressive symptoms and mental health, perhaps by giving people a greater sense of self-control.[679]
- For *insomnia*. Preliminary research suggests that if insomnia is caused by anxiety, confronting the source of anxiety while lucid dreaming can not only improve wakeful anxiety, but also sleep quality.[680]

Exposure Therapies

Exposure and Response Prevention Therapy (ERP). In ERP, an individual is carefully exposed to things that trigger obsessive thoughts or reactions to a previous trauma, among them thoughts, images, objects, and situations. Response prevention is making a choice not to do a compulsive or unhelpful behavior once the anxiety or obsessions have been "triggered." Although ERP should be launched with a therapist's guidance, it can evolve to self-management. ERP is a form of Cognitive Behavioral Therapy (p. 117). (See Case Study 57, p. 158.)

- For *obsessive-compulsive disorder*. On study found that at three- and six-month follow-ups, those who received ERP showed significantly more improvement than the control group.[681] Another trial found ERP was much more effective than stress management in improving OCD symptoms when both were an add-on therapy to psychotropics.[682]
- For *PTSD*. The International Consensus Group on Depression and Anxiety supports ERP as the most appropriate approach for PTSD,[683] although little data exists related to the treatment of combat-related PTSD. Studies generally indicate ERP typically results in a 60% remission of PTSD.[684]

Exposure, Relaxation, & Rescripting Therapy (ERRT). ERRT targets chronic nightmares of people exposed to traumas. It uses physiological, behavioral, and cognitive methods. People write detailed accounts of their nightmares and read them aloud. After identifying themes, people re-script their nightmares to make them more positive and self-empowering. The patients then imagine their rescripted dream in a manner similar to *Guided Imagery* (p. 79) each night before bed. Three relaxation techniques are involved, among them *Progressive Muscle Relaxation* (p. 74).[685]

Within a week of practice, ERRT can improve sleep and reduce chronic nightmares and related psychopathology; this improvement was maintained through the six-month follow-up.[686]

Virtual Reality Exposure Therapy (VRET). VRET contains parts of two evidence-based therapies: *Cognitive Behavioral Therapy* (CBT, p. 117) and *Exposure and Response Prevention Therapy* (above). VRET uses computer-based delivery to help people confront and process traumatic memories by simulating these traumatic events. VRET controls the emotional intensity of the scenes and does not demand that the patient actively access his/her experience through memory retrieval.[687] (See Case Study 54, p. 156.)

- For *psychosis*. VRET should not be used in confronting psychosis. Immersion in a virtual environment can increase delusions.
- For *PTSD*. An open clinical trial resulted in positive clinical outcomes while treating twenty veterans suffering from PTSD.[688] Three patients with PTSD who had been unresponsive to previous exposure treatments responded successfully to VRET.[687] The gaming aspect of VRET, which is identified as a key requirement in many analyses,[687] offers a way of breaking down barriers to mental health care in the military by offering an experience similar to what many veterans already know.
- *More broadly.* Of the three types of exposure therapy *in vivo* and *virtual* are the most effective,[689] and VRET was found as effective as standard CBT, but it required one-third of the number of treatments.[690]

Eye Movement Desensitization and Reprocessing (EMDR). EMDR[691] seeks to minimize the impact of previous traumas or disturbing memories through an eight-step protocol that processes these memories by focusing on past traumas, current situations that trigger dysfunctional emotions, and the positive experience needed to enhance future behaviors. While recalling disturbing memories, the patient focuses on an external stimulus – most often repetitive visual tracking of a moving object, but it could also involve hand-tapping, audio stimulation, and other methods. EMDR may be effective because it is related to rapid eye movement (REM).

- For *PTSD*. A meta-analysis of PTSD treatments found that EMDR was as effective as other trauma therapies, but patients reported EMDR was significantly better than others.[692] Results suggest that *EMDR* and *ERP* tend to be equally effective.[693] (See Case Study 53, p. 156.)
- For *schizophrenia*. EMDR significantly reduced auditory verbal hallucinations and delusions in those who also had PTSD.[694]

Somatic Experiencing. Somatic Experiencing (SE) is a body-oriented approach to the healing trauma. It is based on the premise that people may be "stuck" in the fight, flight or freeze responses that leads to dysregulation of the nervous system and a continuing state of trauma. SE is designed to facilitate the release of traumatic energy through physical, cognitive, and emotional self-discovery.

- For *PTSD*. A small study found SE effective, providing a large benefit to those with PTSD. After SE, 44% no longer had a diagnosable disorder.[695]

WHAT CONSIDERATIONS SHOULD I KEEP IN MIND?

Most *Dialogue & Exposure Therapies* directly engage the issues they aim to address: voices, memories of previous traumas, or intrusive thoughts. Many accept and dignify the individual's experience without judgment, no matter how odd the experience seems. There is good reason: these experiences are closely entwined with the individual; dismissing the experience is effectively dismissing the individual. Most therapists agree that recovery is more assured when we start from someone's own reality instead of imposing one.

Many *Dialogue & Exposure Therapies* walk a fine line, temporarily increasing individuals' stress levels during direct engagement with their troubling experiences. But, when done in a controlled and sensitive way, this engagement can strike at the heart of the issue and decrease the power of these experiences, giving the patient increasing control over them, and in some cases, eliminating them.

Dialogue Therapies (which focus on psychosis) and *Exposure Therapies* (which focus on trauma) are grouped together because studies show that a majority of people with psychosis report having experienced either moderate or severe trauma (most typically emotional trauma).[696] It appears that trauma is a contributing factor to psychosis.[697, 698, 699, 700] Nearly three-quarters of voice-hearers report that their initial onset of audio verbal hallucinations occurred after a traumatic or strongly emotional event in their lives, including illness, change in a personal relationships, pregnancy, divorce, or accident.[658]

With this tie between trauma and psychosis, it is perhaps not surprising that some therapies that address these conditions are similar. For example, both *Virtual Reality Exposure Therapy* for trauma and *Avatar Therapy* for psychosis use a computer to portray a disturbing mental construct that is persistent in the individual's experience, intending to decrease the anxiety and impact of these experiences through exposure and gradual direct confrontation. Both are designed to be progressive and relatively short-term, ending when the individual can experience the mental construct with a "normal" reaction.

Although trauma and psychosis are linked, we shouldn't cast a universal accusing eye at parents, assuming they are a source of trauma in their children suffering with psychosis. However, some researchers have stressed that it is "clinically imperative" to routinely assess for possible traumatic experiences in cases of psychosis.[701, 702, 703]

In addition to helping with trauma, *Exposure Therapy* is also helpful in addressing phobias such as fear of heights and fear of flying.

While considering *Dialogue Therapy* as a way to engage voices directly, it is also important for voice hearers to think about more immediate coping routines that can be used simultaneously. Strategies such as humming, reading aloud, opening the mouth, listening to music or white noise, moderating social engagement and wearing an ear plug can limit the intensity and frequency of the voices. Having strategies identified and practiced in advance can reduce stress, which may help minimize auditory hallucinations.

Although the skill takes up to six weeks or longer to develop, lucid dreaming is also "virtual" and can reconstitute and re-experience traumatic memories to lessen or eliminate their impact.

VRET is especially helpful for military veterans. See also *Emotional Freedom Technique* (p. 161), an additional trauma therapy.

REAL-WORLD EXPERIENCE

Practitioner's Story 5 – Talking to people about their voices

Mark Ragins is a psychiatrist who went to medical school in the days when the experts warned students about inviting patients to talk about their auditory hallucinations, with the explanation that talking about them would "feed into them and make them worse."

"I was taught that the psychoanalysts wasted a lot of time trying to connect to people with psychosis and find meaning in their psychosis," he said. "I was taught that there is no meaning. All we needed to know was enough to prescribe medications and assess if the meds worked."

But, during his career, he began listening to reports of several promising developments for the treatment of psychosis: Cognitive Behavioral Therapy for psychosis, dialogic therapy, and voice hearers. But he knew that none of them were used often.

"Why?" he asks rhetorically. "I think one reason is that we'd have to actually talk to people in depth about their individual psychotic experiences, and we're unable, or simply refuse, to do that. Think about it for a minute. How can we help people develop more positive ways of thinking about and interacting with their voices without talking in detail about how they think about and relate to their voices now?"[704]

Bottom Line: *Dr. Ragins thinks it is counterproductive to label someone's compelling reality meaningless. The better we understand and accept a voice hearer's reality, the more we can eliminate the barriers, so those patients can get help. To judge their experience as meaningless can be stigmatizing and disempowering, and may close a path to recovery.*

Case Study 49 – Working with Voices (Schizophrenia)

Lana was diagnosed with schizophrenia after reporting she was hearing voices. After consulting with practitioners, she decided to ignore the voices in her head. "I asked them to leave me alone," she recalled. "In my ignorance, I handled this in a totally wrong way. You can't just put aside something that exists and manifests itself in you in such a strong way. The voices would lose their right to exist because of a lack of attention and energy, and of course this was not what they wanted."

Until she made her request to the voices, they had been "polite and friendly," but that immediately changed; their tone reversed. "It was a full-blown civil war," Lana admitted, "but I continued to ignore everything. I kept myself busy. My house had never been cleaner, and my garden was never taken care of better. My life became more peaceful, but in a constrained way; I almost couldn't relax anymore."[658]

Bottom Line: *Each report of experiences with voices is different. Hearers must find coping strategies that work for them.*

Case Study 50 – Voice Dialoguing (Schizophrenia)

Jacob heard only one voice, an extremely destructive voice that repeatedly demanded that he take his own life.

When the Voice Dialoguing facilitator spoke with the voice, it was extremely hostile and expressed anger and frustration toward Jacob. The facilitator asked the voice if it was hard to carry all this anger. The voice said it was. The voice also confirmed that it wanted Jacob to become stronger, and that its efforts to move Jacob in that direction weren't working. The facilitator asked the voice if it wanted help finding better ways to support Jacob. The voice appeared to be intrigued and agreed. [645]

From that time on, the voice began to evolve from a destructive bully to a supportive companion who tried to help Jacob express what he needed.

Bottom Line: *Voices are often very real to those who experience them. Directly working with that reality can be a way to help change it.*

Case Study 51 – Hearing Voices Network (Schizophrenia)

Eleanor Longden started hearing voices that became progressively worse, even menacing. Her life became a living nightmare as the voices became not only her tormentors, but her only companions.

She was hospitalized for three months and prescribed psychotropics, but they did little good. She felt "discarded by the mental health system" that didn't know how to help her. She also began to self-harm, became suicidal, and was hospitalized.

A breakthrough came when she worked with a new psychiatrist who suggested Hearing Voices Network (HVN), a form of group therapy. Together, the members searched for meaning in their voices. Eventually she regarded the voices as entities tied to abuse she suffered as a child.

She found this supportive group format helpful. She started treating the voices with respect and viewing their messages as metaphorical. This allowed her to set boundaries for them and gain significant control over them. Over three years, she was able to reduce, then eliminate, medication.

She regained her life, earned an advanced degree, and become employed. The voices occasionally return, but she remains in control. She has shared her experience on a TED Talk (https://goo.gl/pwJZ5u).[705]

Bottom Line*: Regardless of your beliefs about voices, treating them with respect as if they were real may dramatically decrease their impact.*

Case Study 52 – Hearing Voices Network (Schizophrenia)

Rachel hears thirteen different voices, some angry and violent, some scared, others mischievous. After joining a Hearing Voices Network group, she found ways to cope with the voices and no longer feels terrorized by them. Now she chooses whether she listens to them and how she responds..

Some of the voices are now much more helpful, serving as a window into her feelings, letting her know what problems need to be addressed.[706]

Bottom Line*: No matter your view on voices, talking with them sometimes helps. Do what works.*

Case Study 53 – EMDR (PTSD)

John was a combat medic for the United Kingdom's army. While serving overseas, his buddy stepped on a land mine. John gave him first aid and climbed into the chopper that flew him to a field hospital. His friend died en route.

John continually relived the moment, suffered from nightmares, and believed he could still smell his buddy's stomach contents. "I should have done more" was his constant refrain. He was diagnosed with post-traumatic stress disorder.

When he was given EMDR daily for four days, his anxiety and intrusive thoughts markedly decreased. The therapist made John visualize the experience over and over until he had no disturbance.

After two review sessions during the next month, his symptoms continued to fade. He volunteered to return to the front line. A one-year check-up found he had no abnormal residual disturbance from the event.[707]

Bottom Line*: To extract a trauma by its roots often requires going to its core and stripping it of its power.*

Case Study 54 – Virtual Reality Exposure Therapy (PTSD)

Bo, 30, fought in Iraq. When he returned home, nightmares became common. He avoided crowds and public places and had an exaggerated startle reflex. He was diagnosed with post-traumatic stress disorder.

During eleven sessions of Virtual Reality Exposure Therapy (p. 152), he watched a video screen as IEDs exploded in very realistic views of Iraq. He was highly engaged emotionally.

After his sessions, Bo allowed his tears to flow, the first time he had cried for the losses he had suffered. By the end of the therapy, Bo was able to socialize in groups in public places, and his nightmares became rare. His anxiety decreased whenever he experienced cues of the war. Although he still had some PTSD symptoms, he made substantial progress, so that it didn't interfere with his life any longer.[708]

Bottom Line*: The many therapies for PTSD nearly all call for controlled re-exposure to the trauma.*

Case Study 55 – Guided Self-Determination (Schizophrenia)

John had a 35-year history of paranoid schizophrenia. He felt he was being controlled by aliens. His delusions persisted, despite the use of psychotropics, therapy, psychoeducation, and Cognitive Behavior Therapy.

His condition was worsening at the time he was given Guided Self-Determination Therapy (GSD). GSD helped John feel that his experience was accepted and important. He began to drop his resistance to his doctors and their ideas.

Over time, John changed his perception, recognizing his delusions as unreal. He moved from resistance to receptiveness and from doubt to a new system of thinking. This change was facilitated by John's conviction that he had become in charge of what was happening in his life.[709]

Bottom Line*: When practitioners and supporters accept odd thoughts without judgement, people can relax and feel respected. This sense of self-worth can help motivate individuals to begin the process of self-change.*

Case Study 56 – Avatar Therapy (Schizophrenia)

Ed was a business executive who heard a woman's voice all day long discussing his business and conversing with subordinates. He was convinced the voice was real.

Using Avatar Therapy, Ed created a computer likeness of the woman, with her voice and face as he experienced it. The program allowed the therapist (in a separate room) to respond as the avatar in real-time so that the therapist's words were on the lips of the avatar.

Ed guided the dialogue with the avatar, asserting that she should no longer bother him. The therapist gave Ed increasing control over the avatar in various ways. After two thirty-minute sessions, Ed told the voice to stop, and it did. The woman's voice disappeared and didn't return.[666]

Bottom Line*: Success was found after respecting and directly engaging Ed's reality, giving him a way and the power to overcome it – not by convincing him it wasn't real or dismissing it.*

Case Study 57 – Exposure Therapy (OCD)

"Treating my OCD involved a lot of counseling," one former patient explained. *"I would endure exposure therapy, where I would be deliberately exposed to things that would spark my anxiety, the theory being that once exposed, I would be able to face my fears. The idea was to refrain from performing compulsions in these situations."*

His counselor asked him to turn a stove on and only check once to make certain it was turned off. *"I wanted to double check, but couldn't,"* he said. *"The counselor had me touch door knobs and money, then refrain from washing my hands."*

He described Exposure Therapy as *"grueling,"* but, he admitted, *"the more I faced my fears, the easier the battles became. Also, I learned how to cope with OCD: recognizing the worry, doubt, or anxiety as exaggerated and unlikely. [I learned] I could develop the courage to accept anything that I feared."*[532(d)]

Bottom Line: *Exposure therapies are hard work but can deliver a lifetime of reduced anxiety.*

WHAT ARE ADDITIONAL RESOURCES?

- Voice Dialoguing. http://goo.gl/fJ9ovd.
- Voice Coping Strategies. https://goo.gl/rfFHyq.
- Avatar Therapy. http://goo.gl/rdxYpH.
- Open Dialogism. www.dialogicpractice.net.
- Soteria. www.moshersoteria.com.
- Diabasis House – medication-free treatment. http://goo.gl/iF8j8J.
- Hearing Voices Network. www.Intervoiceonline.org.
- Guided Self-Determination. https://goo.gl/JpL8gM.
- Additional Psychosis, Schizophrenia and Voices tools (p. 342).

Energy Therapy

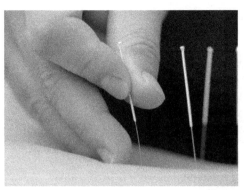

WHAT IS THE ESSENCE?

The broad and divergent collection of therapies clustered under the heading *Energy Therapy* accept the existence of non-biomedical energies and innate healing capacities that influence the body and mind.

The evidence supporting *Energy Therapy* is scant but growing. A small set of RCTs and many case studies support their effectiveness for mental health recovery.

Views on *Energy Therapy* vary. Some people find it consistent with their personal experience, belief system, or willingness to explore new possibilities. If you find it implausible, you can focus on the many other non-drug options for recovery. If you are open to considering these approaches, a belief in this energy isn't required to gain clinical benefit from *Energy Therapy*—just as you don't need to believe in aspirin to get pain relief.

One set of *Energy Therapy*ies is based in Eastern traditions and the concept of Qi (also chi), a "vital energy" that flows in the body. Qi approaches such as *acupuncture, acupressure, Reiki, Healing Touch,* and *Emotional Freedom Technique* identify and work with meridians of the body (specific energy pathways associated with internal organs and structures). The traditional practice of *Mind-Body Disciplines* (p. 111), like *T'ai Chi Chuan* and *Yoga,* are also based in *chi* (called *prana* in yoga).

WHAT EVIDENCE SHOWS THIS IS EFFECTIVE?

Acupuncture and Acupressure. Acupuncture is an ancient Chinese form of medicine that stimulates specific points on the body, based on the idea that stagnation, blockage, imbalance, or deficiency of *chi* can cause disease—including mental illnesses. There are many varieties:[710] *standard acupuncture* using thin needles; *electro-acupuncture*, which uses low-level electrical current on acupuncture needles; *laser acupuncture*; and *auricular acupuncture*, which positions needles in the ears. In acupressure, a close variant of acupuncture, pressure is applied by hand or an object to acupuncture points.

Evidence for acupuncture is growing. The National Institute of Health concludes that available research is promising. In most Eastern countries, acupuncture is well-accepted standard care validated by centuries of use.

- For *depression*. Acupuncture has proven as effective as antidepressants in treating moderate depression,[711] and it has been effective as a stand-alone therapy for major depression.[712]
- For *schizophrenia*. Both electro-acupuncture[713] and ear acupuncture[714] may reduce hallucinations. In China, eleven studies show that acupuncture yields symptom improvement, better than antipsychotic therapy alone. It is regarded as an additive benefit when used with antipsychotics.[715] These studies have not, however, been duplicated in Western settings. Other studies resulted in significant symptom improvement[716] when using laser acupuncture to reduce auditory hallucinations[717] for patients who were not taking antipsychotics. (See Case Study 59, p. 163.)
- For *PTSD*. A study found that service people given twice-weekly acupuncture in addition to normal PTSD care, had significantly improved symptoms as compared to those receiving normal PTSD care alone.[718] (See Case Study 60 and Case Study 61, p. 163.)
- For *anxiety*. Studies have shown that acupuncture can cause a significant drop in resting heart rate,[719] improve the immune response,[720] and increase central nervous system hormones associated with mental health.[721]
- For *insomnia*. Acupuncture has consistently proven effective in treating insomnia, both historically[722] and in a large meta-analysis,[723] including being of benefit for those with schizophrenia.[724] Acupuncture increases the secretion of the sleep enhancing hormone, *Melatonin* (p. 202).[725]
- For *alcohol and substance abuse*. In one study, the rate of alcohol abstinence rose dramatically in patients given auricular acupuncture on three specific points identified for substance abuse, as compared to a control group given acupuncture on sham points.[726] Another found cocaine-dependent patients on methadone receiving acupuncture more likely to provide cocaine-negative urine samples.[727] However, overall, the results are mixed; little conclusive supporting evidence exists.[728]
- *Acceptance*. 43% of conventional doctors refer patients for acupuncture.[729]

Reiki. Reiki is a Japanese technique where practitioners are purported to activate the natural healing processes of the patient's body and restore wellbeing by channeling energy into the patient by "laying on of hands."

Patients being treated for mild depression and stress who received six weeks of Reiki treatment showed both immediate and long-term improvements (up to a year) for depression, stress, and hopelessness.[730] In a study of nurses with "burn-out syndrome," biological indicators showed a significant relaxation response as a result of Reiki treatment.[731] Reiki is increasingly offered in hospitals, hospice care, and private practice settings, applied to a variety of illnesses and conditions.[732] In animal studies, Reiki treatment produced clear signs of reduced stress, indicated by changes in autonomic biological measurements such as heart rate.[733]

Healing Touch. In Healing Touch (HT), a practitioner uses their hands and intent to promote healing through very light or near-body touch. HT is purported to influence the energy field that penetrates and surrounds the body. In one study, people in active duty military with PTSD given both HT and *Guided Imagery* (p. 79) had significant reductions in PTSD symptoms and depression, and significant improvements in overall mental quality of life.[734]

Emotional Freedom Technique (EFT). Emotional Freedom Technique (EFT, not to be confused with Emotion-Focused Therapy) combines cognitive and behavioral techniques with physically tapping of the acupuncture meridians. EFT is based on **Thought Field Therapy (TFT)**, which uses acupoint stimulation to relieve traumatic memories. EFT is recognized by the American Psychological Association as a leading therapy for trauma.

EFT appears to significantly reduce psychological distress,[735] with results equal to that of *Eye Movement Desensitization and Reprocessing*[736] (p. 152).

- For *PTSD*. Small studies of veterans with PTSD found that 90%-100% no longer met PTSD criteria after 6-10 sessions of EFT[735] with many showing lower inflammation.[737] A study of 188 children orphaned by the Rwanda genocide found that 94% no longer had PTSD after a single TFT session – and remained that way for one year.[738] (See Case Study 58, p. 163.)
- *More broadly.* A meta-analysis of 18 RCTs using EFT/TTF found significant improvements with large effect sizes after a relatively few sessions.[739] People receiving a single 1-hour EFT session had reduced anxiety and depression as well as lower levels of cortisol (a stress hormone) as compared to controls.[740] It isn't clear why EFT/TTF works.[741]

Homeopathy. Homeopathy is based on a set of three concepts: the *Law of Similars* (a medicine that causes symptoms in a well person can cure a sick person with the same symptoms)—for which there is some biomedical support;[742] the *Law of Minimum Dose* (the more dilute a medicine, the more effective; vigorous shaking between dilutions increases potency); and the *Law of Cures* (symptom relief follows a certain progression).

Homeopathy is one of the most popular alternative treatments in the world, especially in the United Kingdom, where more than 40% of physicians refer patients to homeopaths;[743] 26% of the doctors in industrialized countries view homeopathy as legitimate and refer patients to homeopaths or prescribe homeopathic remedies themselves.[729] Patients typically report high satisfaction (65% to 75%) with homeopathy and experience only mild side effects, if any.

- For *anxiety*. One study of people with anxiety found significant improvement in both the homeopathy and the placebo groups, with no difference in the degree of improvement.[744] Most homeopathy literature for anxiety consists of case reports or uncontrolled studies.
- For *depression*. Evidence is limited.[16] The most commonly treated conditions in homeopathy are depression and anxiety, with positive outcomes seen 63% and 61% of the time, respectively.[745] The components of the treatment most responsible for the outcomes is unclear.

- From a *broader perspective*. Research on homeopathy is very limited.[16] The Faculty of Homeopathy, an international practitioner organization, notes that 104 RCTs on homeopathy exist with 54% showing inconclusive results and 5% negative results.[746] They note that tentative positive evidence exists for only one mental health disorder: insomnia. The active principle of homeopathy is unclear. Treatments typically contain no molecules of the original substance since they are so highly diluted.

Spiritist Therapy. Spiritist Therapy (or Spiritism) is a philosophy developed in the 19th century by Hippolyte Leon Denizard Rivail, whose pen name was Allan Kardec. Spiritism operates independently from any formal religion, medical, or governmental agency. There are more than 12,000 Spiritist centers in Brazil (offering free service to over 40 million people[747]) and in many countries outside of Brazil.[757] Key aspects of Spiritism include:

- **Integrative Mental Health Orientation.** Spiritist psychiatric hospitals often combine Western psychiatric protocols (including psychotropics and psychosocial therapies), *Wellness Basics*, select CAM therapies, and spiritual treatments that are individualized to the patient.[748]
- **Spiritual Energy Source.** Spiritism maintains that energy can influence mental states, and this energy can be viewed as an aspect of the individual's personality or as a distinct nonphysical being.
- **Disobsession.** Spiritist healers accept and confront the spiritual energy to remove its negative expression from the individual. It may work on the same principles as *Exposure Therapies* (p. 151).
- **Medical Intuitives.** Trained individuals called medical intuitives, believe they can sense and work directly with this spiritual energy.

Although there are no clinical trials testing Spiritist Therapy, a review of 181 cases[749] showed improvements of symptoms in nearly all cases, significantly in cases of schizophrenia, autism, cognitive impairment, panic attacks, OCD, and others. (See Case Study 62, p. 164.)

Holotropic Breathwork. Holotropic Breathwork, developed by Stanislav and Christina Grof, combines accelerated breathing with evocative music and other integration practices to help individuals enter a non-ordinary state of consciousness. It is a supportive approach to process intense emotions and activate our innate human healing ability. In a small study, it has been shown to increase self-awareness (a tipping-point insight needed in the awareness stage of recovery, p. 32) and decrease interpersonal mental distress.[750]

WHAT CONSIDERATIONS SHOULD I KEEP IN MIND?

Some studies and numerous case studies support the effectiveness of acupuncture and Reiki, though they lack a strong evidence base.

EFT and TFT show promise for trauma, although the benefit may result from *Affirmation* (p. 88) and *Cognitive Restructuring* (p. 89), not the tapping of acupoints.[751] The National Institute for Integrative Healthcare, a nonprofit research institution, offers EFT to returning vets for little or no cost.[752]

Spiritist therapy uses a variety of approaches, so mental health improvement is difficult to attribute to any specific therapy. Chinese and Western psychiatry differ substantially, so most studies of *Energy Therapies* have been done in China. Although reasonable studies exist here, many are small and poorly designed. Those noted above are among the most convincing and offer suggestive clinical evidence of effectiveness. Since these therapies have a cultural and historic validity, they are commonly accepted in the East.

REAL-WORLD EXPERIENCE

Case Study 58 – Emotional Freedom Technique (PTSD)

Sid was in one of the Twin Towers during the catastrophic 9/11 attack. He survived but developed a prolonged case of post-traumatic stress disorder. During several years of self-imposed seclusion, he was unable to work. Eventually, he tried Emotional Freedom Technique.

After a single session of EFT, he no longer had clinically significant symptoms. Sid also had reductions in four of seven measures of psychopathology. He took twelve EFT treatment sessions over eight weeks. At the end, he had a nearly complete elimination of symptoms and returned to work. A sixty-day follow-up assessment found that he had elevated results in only one of seven measures of psychopathology.[753]

Bottom Line*: EFT may seem very odd, but some have found it life-changing. We should keep an open mind about all therapies.*

Case Study 59 – Acupuncture (Schizophrenia)

Joyce was diagnosed with chronic schizophrenia and persistent hallucinations. She even felt physical pain from a bird that she thought was continually pecking at her back.

An acupuncturist gave her twelve weekly treatments, and Joyce found an immediate improvement in sleep and daily functioning. The hallucinations didn't go away, but they changed; she was less disturbed by them. Even the pain in her back from the imagined bird decreased. Her positive and negative symptoms, as well as depression, improved after three months of treatment.[754]

Bottom Line: *Dismissing energy therapies as implausible may close the door to an effective avenue of symptom relief and recovery.*

Case Study 60 – Acupuncture (PTSD)

Raul Rojas served two tours of combat in Vietnam, and the experience transformed his life.

"I'm 100% disabled because of PTSD," he said. "When I first started coming to the Acupuncturists Without Borders (AWB) clinic in

Albuquerque, I had spent years suffering from high anxiety…Because of the acupuncture, I have become calmer and my anxiety has drastically come down. I don't want the new vets to suffer for years like I did. Acupuncture is helping me get my life back."[755]

Bottom Line: *Acupuncturists Without Borders offers acupuncture to help heal the wounds of war in community acupuncture clinics.*

Case Study 61 – Acupuncture (PTSD)

Antoine was a 60-year-old Vietnam vet diagnosed with PTSD. For six months, he was treated with auricular acupuncture, which provided relief to a variety of his symptoms: chronic fatigue, depression, grief, generalized anxiety, headaches, insomnia, nightmares, irritability, and panic attacks.

A follow-up was conducted seven months after treatment was complete. Most of the reported symptoms had some level of relief, and some symptoms were completely resolved.[756]

Bottom Line: *Check with your local Veterans Administration for access to acupuncture.*

Case Study 62 – Spiritist Therapy (Schizophrenia)

Marcel, a young Brazilian man, started having delusions and hearing voices. Periodically he also became aggressive. He was diagnosed with schizophrenia and placed on antipsychotics.

He was advised to seek care at a nearby Spiritist psychiatric hospital. He received antipsychotics, occupational therapy, and group therapy. He was also given "energy passes" weekly by a trained healer, who transmitted energy to him without touch, and he engaged in medical intuition sessions. He received disobsession treatments three times a week.

After several weeks, his aggression and delusions stopped, and his psychotropic dosages were reduced significantly. He himself began the medical intuitive training. Marcel is now a medical intuitive working to heal others.[757]

Bottom Line: *Therapies from different cultures are worthy of consideration since there are many case reports of success.*

WHAT ARE ADDITIONAL RESOURCES?

- Homeopathy. www.Homeopathyusa.org, https://goo.gl/p9GGby.
- Spiritism. https://goo.gl/aQPrfy.
- Holotropic Breathwork. www.Holotropic.com.

5- Biomedical Restorative Therapies

Biomedical

Nutrient Therapy
Endocrine Therapy
Food Allergy Therapy
Detoxification Therapy
Pathogen Therapy

Physical Focus

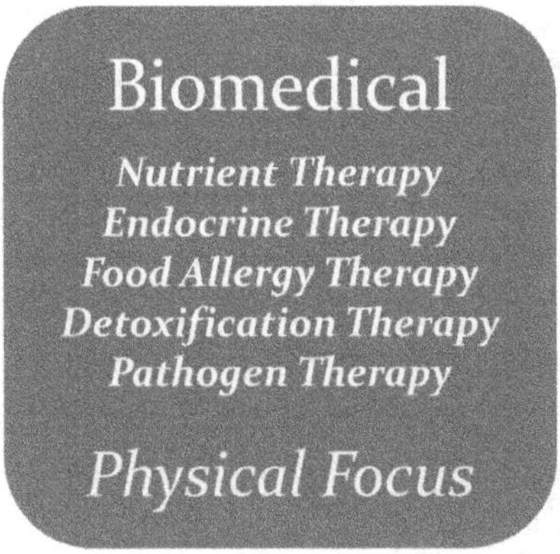

Figure 27 - Biomedical
Restorative Therapies

The second category of the *Wellness Continuum* (Figure 9, p. 47) offers *Restorative Therapies* that seek to address underlying causes and influencers of mental distress.

They are either *Psychosocial* (related to the mind) or *Biomedical* (related to the body); acknowledging that our physical health and mental health are deeply entwined. Helping one often helps the other.

Biomedical therapies (Figure 27) are grounded in a growing understanding of the mechanisms of the brain. (See *Brain Basics of Recovery*, p. 52.)

Ample research indicates that over 25% of mental health issues are directly linked to underlying physical issues.[61] The most prevalent of these are food allergies, nutrient imbalances, hypoglycemia, hypothyroidism, methylation irregularities, digestive disorders, inflammation, oxidative stress, environmental toxicity, and infections. These are relatively easy to detect, usually through standard blood and urine tests. If the conditions are addressed, mental health issues can often be significantly improved—and, in some cases, eliminated.

For instance, thyroid disorders are found in nearly 10% of the population. Anxiety, depression, poor memory, hallucinations, and delirium are all possible symptoms of thyroid disorders.[758] When thyroid issues are addressed, associated mental health issues often disappear rapidly.

Practitioners might be reluctant to run a thorough biomedical test protocol because of the costs-relative-to-benefit considerations. Their concerns are reasonable, but an extensive biomedical testing protocol should be considered mandatory to provide an accurate differential diagnosis. In the larger context, this is time and money extremely well spent. See the *Biomedical Test Panels* (p. 323) and the *Integrative Biomedical Practitioner Finder* (p. 320) to help identify the specific tests and the practitioners who value them.

Many *Biochemical Restorative Therapies* are based on pioneering concepts of Orthomolecular Psychiatry defined in the mid-20th century. One such concept is *Biochemical Individuality,* predicated on the fact that each person's body chemistry is unique. Testing protocols help identify individual characteristics. Knowing your unique body chemistry can be critical to recovery.

For instance, although most people with depression have low serotonin and respond well to SSRI antidepressants, 30% of those with depression have elevated serotonin. For them, SSRIs could be ineffective or even harmful.[19] (See Case Study 63, p. 190, as a dramatic example.) Although one orthomolecular therapy (the broad use of niacin for schizophrenia) was later shown to have less universal applicability than originally thought,[759] hundreds of gold standard trials confirm the value of nutrient therapy at the center of orthomolecular psychiatric care.

Biomedical Restorative Therapy spans a wide spectrum:

- *Nutrient Therapy* balances vitamins, nutrients, and vital bodily substances.
- *Endocrine Therapy* addresses malfunctions of glands.
- *Digestive Therapy* optimizes gut bacterial flora and nutrient absorption.
- *Food Allergy Therapy* addresses gluten, dairy, and other intolerances.
- *Detoxification Therapy* removes heavy metals and toxins from the body.
- *Pathogen Therapy* addresses infections from bacteria and viruses.

Nutrient Therapy

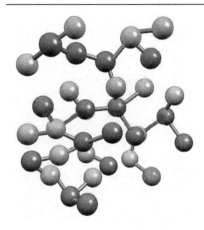

WHAT IS THE ESSENCE?

Nutrient Therapy aims to restore the optimum nutrient environment in the body by correcting imbalances or deficiencies in individual biochemistry. This therapy relies on substances natural to the body, such as vitamins, minerals, amino acids, trace elements, and fatty acids. Both nutrient overload and deficiencies can create mental health issues.

Much research shows that dietary choices and nutrient imbalances may cause or exacerbate mental health issues since they directly affect vital brain processes, including neurotransmitter synthesis, antioxidant recycling, epigenetic gene regulation and methylation (see *Brain Basics of Recovery,* p. 52). They also influence broader mechanisms that impact brain functioning, including the inflammation response to infection.

Nutrient Therapy is grounded in the original approaches of *Orthomolecular Psychiatry,* but it has been extended and validated through numerous recent clinical trials. *Nutrient Therapy* complements psychotropics and generally is very well tolerated.

Dr. William J. Walsh, PhD (see Figure 28, p. 168) is a leading voice in the field of *Nutrient Therapy*. His research strongly validates *biochemical individuality*: the idea that we each have unique body chemistry that requires a unique nutrient response. In fact, his research has determined the most common variations (called biotypes) of body chemistry for each mental health diagnosis.

Many people with mental health issues who have followed Walsh's nutrient testing and treatment protocols have experienced impressive results.

However, experimentation with *Nutrient Therapy* should be guided by practitioners using appropriate lab testing. (See *Biomedical Test Panels,* p. 323.) These tests can help identify specific nutrient deficiencies and overloads, thereby determining a person's biotype and unique nutrient needs.

No one should self-diagnose or self-treat, since a nutrient can be helpful for one biotype and ineffective or negative for another. Testing helps differentiate between potentially beneficial and non-beneficial nutrients for each individual.

And an important point for those on psychotropics: psychotropics appear to be more effective after nutrient imbalances have been corrected.[19]

Dr. William Walsh and Walsh Institute

Dr. William J. Walsh, PhD, is an internationally recognized expert on biochemical imbalances.[760] His work is grounded in Orthomolecular Psychiatry but extends well beyond it.[19]

The Walsh Research Institute, which he founded in 2008, works to unravel the biochemistry of mental health issues through research and the training of integrative mental health practitioners.

The institute has amassed what is probably the world's largest database of mental health laboratory analyses: more than three million records from blood and urine samples of more than 30,000 people with mental health issues. This database shows that umbrella diagnoses (like depression or bipolar) are composed of multiple subtypes (called biotypes), with each biotype requiring a different nutrient response.

The institute's research reveals six primary nutrient imbalances that are most commonly found in people with mental health symptoms:

- *Copper overload*
- *Vitamin B6 deficiency*
- *Zinc deficiency*
- *Methyl/folate imbalance*
- *Oxidative stress*
- *Amino Acid imbalance*

Nutrient Therapy based on biotypes has produced impressive results.[761]* *After six months of targeted nutrient therapy, 70% of patients with behavior issues, attention-deficit hyperactivity disorder, and depression reported feeling fine without psychotropic medication. The remaining 30% needed some psychotropics to avoid symptoms, but at lower doses than previously.*

The results for schizophrenia and bipolar also offer hope: 5% reported the ability to withdraw completely from psychotropics after Nutrient Therapy, and many others indicated that a combination of nutrient therapy and greatly reduced psychotropics eliminated their psychosis and allowed them to return to independent living.[19] Three-quarters of those with schizophrenia were able to reduce their medication when they combined it with Nutrient Therapy.

Dr. Walsh is a strong advocate for robust biomedical testing to guide Nutrient Therapy. His book, Nutrient Power,[19] *introduces his research.*

Figure 28 – Walsh Institute

Nutrient Therapy relies upon substances that occur naturally in the body, while *Herbal Therapy* (p. 223) uses plant-based remedies. Both have biochemical influences on bodily processes. Both typically have few if any side effects, although they affect individuals differently, based on their biochemical individuality. Although we have put them in different therapy groupings – *Nutrient Therapy* in *Biomedical Restorative* and *Herbal Therapy* in *Symptom Relief* – both have restorative features, and both offer relief from symptoms.

This section contains four subsections: *vitamins, minerals, amino acids, and other nutrients.* The evidence presented is dense and comprehensive, incorporating results from many clinical trials across a broad array of nutrients. As a result, *the best way to use this section is as an encyclopedic reference.* Skim it for evidence related to a diagnosis that interests you or use it to see how a particular nutrient influences a variety of diagnoses.

WHAT EVIDENCE SHOWS THIS IS EFFECTIVE?

Vitamins

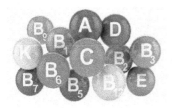

Vitamins are essential organic nutrients primarily obtained through food. They are micronutrients, as opposed to macronutrients like proteins, carbohydrates, and fats.

Vitamin A. Found in many foods, Vitamin A is important for vision, the immune system, and reproduction.

- For *alcohol abuse*. The consumption of excess alcohol is associated with declines in Vitamin A, which can result in vision problems or even blindness.[762]

Vitamin B1 (Thiamine).[763] Vitamin B1 is important in oxygen and energy metabolism; a deficiency of B1 can cause anxiety, depression, obsession thinking, defective memory, and time distortion. A chronic B1 deficiency (Wernicke-Korsakoff Syndrome) can cause brain damage.

- For *alcohol abuse*. One of the most dangerous side effects of alcoholism is that it often causes a B1 deficiency. Patients experiencing alcohol withdrawal typically have a more substantial deficiency.[764] Numerous studies show that B1 can help neurological issues of chronic alcoholism.[15] In one study, patients with alcohol-related psychosis were given thiamine. All but one had substantial improvements.[765]
- For *dementia*. Taking between three and eight grams of Thiamine each day may decrease the severity of mild to moderate dementia. [18a]

Vitamin B2 (Riboflavin). In addition to producing energy for the body, riboflavin is an antioxidant, fighting damaging free radicals.

- For *postpartum depression (PPD)*. When women consume insufficient amounts of Vitamin B2 during pregnancy, the risk of PPD increases.[766]

Vitamin B3 (Niacin, Nicotinic acid, Niacinamide). Niacin is a reuptake promoter.[767] It also reduces LDL cholesterol, much the same as statins, but without statin side effects.

- For *schizophrenia*. Although there are conflicting studies,[768] B3 trials have shown a recovery rate double the norm, a 50% reduction in hospitalization rates, and a significant reduction in suicides.[769] These patients also took Vitamins C and B6. During these trials, B3 mega-dosages proved nontoxic.[770] Dietary B3 may also protect against age-related mental decline.[771]

- For *alcohol abuse*. One study found that niacin supplementation helped wean patients from alcohol.[772]

- For *anxiety*. A case study found that 2,500 mg of niacinamide (nicotinamide) per day significantly improved severe anxiety.[773]

- For *dementia*. Oral niacinamide improves mental function in people with Alzheimer's Disease.[774]

- *Safety*. Niacin is generally safe, even in large doses. Some gastric upset and flushing may occur, but not with the use of niacinamide.

Vitamin B6 (pyridoxine, pyridoxal, and pyridoxamine). B6 is vital to mental health and its levels in the brain are about 100 times higher than levels in the blood. B6 is required for the efficient synthesis of three neurotransmitters: serotonin, dopamine, and GABA. People with a B6 deficiency can have abnormally low levels of any or all three.[19] B6 is also essential for recharging glutathione, an antioxidant in the brain. B6 deficiencies can usually be detected by an inexpensive urine test, when pyrroles are elevated. (See *Glossary*, p. 337, and Case Study 74, p. 193.) Vitamin B6 deficiency is one of the top six nutrient imbalances in people with mental health issues. (See Figure 28, p. 168.)

- For *depression*. A meta-analysis suggests that supplementing a healthy diet with between 100 and 200 mg of Vitamin B6 every day significantly improves premenstrual depression.[775] Low dietary and plasma B6 increases the risk and severity of depression in geriatric patients.

- For *schizophrenia*. 50mg B6 taken three times a day for between eight and twelve weeks in addition to medication significantly improved symptoms. Patients experienced a better sense of well-being, increased motivation, and greater interest in interactions.[776] A case study reported that using B6 dramatically reduced psychotropic side effects as well psychotic symptoms.[777] Two trials showed significant improvement in psychotic symptoms when B6 was taken with B3 and psychotropics.[778]

- For *alcohol abuse*. Metadoxine, a chemical relative of B6, has been effective in helping maintain abstinence, decrease alcohol cravings, and improve short-term memory.[778]

- For *dementia*. Low B6 is common in patients with Alzheimer's Disease (AD),[779] so B6 supplements and other nutrients improve AD symptoms.[780]

- *More broadly.* Deficiencies in B6 can contribute to depressed levels of dopamine and symptoms of ADHD, depression, anxiety, and sleep disorders.[19]

Vitamin B7 (Biotin).

- For *postpartum depression (PPD).* Even slight biotin deficiencies in pregnant women can produce metabolic problems that can lead to PPD.[781]

Vitamin B8 (Inositol).[782] Our brains have significant concentrations of inositol, which is found in beans, grains, nuts, and many fruits. In studies, doses ranging from 12,000 to 20,000 mg per day[783] have been effective in treating the same disorders aided by SSRI antidepressants.

- For *depression.* Inositol can reduce depression, hostility, tension, and fatigue, in some cases significantly.[784]
- For *bipolar.* One trial investigating the benefits of inositol studied a population of people with bipolar who were taking psychotropics. The patients given inositol reported at least a 50% reduction in depressive symptoms versus those in the placebo group.[782]
- For *panic and anxiety.* A trial comparing Prozac and inositol showed a greater reduction in the number of panic attacks during the first week when patients took inositol; the results were similar throughout the nine-week course.[785] Twelve grams of inositol per day can significantly reduce the severity and frequency of panic attacks.[786]
- For *obsessive-compulsive disorder.* Two studies found significant improvements in symptoms when individuals took inositol as compared to a placebo, with a level of improvement similar to psychotropics.[787, 788]
- *More broadly.* Inositol is believed to be ineffective for *schizophrenia, dementia, ADHD, and autism.*[789]
- *Safety.* Gastrointestinal side effects may be a problem, but inositol is generally well tolerated.[24]

Vitamin B9 (folate, folic acid, methylfolate). Folate plays an essential role in serotonin synthesis and serves as a *serotonin reuptake enhancer.*[19] It reduces the synaptic activity at serotonin, dopamine, and norepinephrine receptors,[767] and may provide neuroprotection. Folate in our bodies can be compromised by smoking, alcohol, poor diet, mood-stabilizers, and statins. Taking high doses of folate when the body has no folate deficiency may be harmful and mask a B12 deficiency.[18a]

- For *schizophrenia.* Because Vitamin B9 is often low in people with schizophrenia,[790] B9 supplements may significantly improve negative symptoms,[791] social recovery, and clinical symptoms.[792] Symptoms of folic acid deficiency are similar to those of schizophrenia, which can result in a misdiagnosis.[778]

- For *depression*. The relapse rate for patients with low B9 levels was more than ten times greater than the relapse rate for those with normal B9 levels.[793] L-methylfolate is a form of folate that more easily enters the brain, so it is the most effective form of B9 for depression. Adding 15 mg per day to psychotropics resulted in significant improvement in clinical and social symptoms,[794] and may be an effective, safe, and relatively well tolerated treatment for major depressive disorders when patients have little or no response to SSRIs.[795] Adding 5 mg per day may benefit female patients with depressive episodes who are taking fluoxetine.[796] (See Case Study 77, p. 194.)

- *For bipolar*. Mania is associated with abnormally low levels of folate in the body. In one study, 45 hospitalized patients with acute mania had significantly lower red blood cell folate than the control group, but there was no significant difference in serum folate levels.[797] Another study found that folic acid increases the effectiveness of lithium to control depressive symptoms.[798] Undermethylated bipolar patients cannot tolerate folic acid.[767]

- For *dementia*. Scientists have found a clear link between decreased folic acid and cognitive impairment in the elderly.[799] When the amount of folic acid is increased in their diet, the risk of Alzheimer's Disease decreases.[800]

- *For smoking cessation and alcohol abuse*. Many smokers and alcoholics have a high risk of Vitamin B9 deficiency. Former smokers who consume a high dose of dietary B9 reduce their risk of lung cancer.[801]

- *More broadly*. Abnormal folate levels are common in those with schizophrenia, bipolar, anxiety, and depression.[802] A gene mutation correlated with B9 occurs frequently in psychiatric populations, which indicates that B9 has potential as a treatment for schizophrenia, depression, and bipolar.[803] Methylfolate may be more effective than folic acid, since it is more easily absorbed, especially in people with a genetic error called MTHFR polymorphism.

- *Safety*. Vitamin B9 is generally quite safe. Taking folic acid may mask anemia caused by a Vitamin B12 deficiency, so practitioners should check serum B12 levels before recommending B9 for their patients. (See *Methylation*, p. 54.)

Vitamin B12 (Cobalamin). B12 is only synthesized by certain bacteria and humans obtain it typically from meat, dairy, eggs, and fish. Psychiatric symptoms may be the first manifestation of B12 deficiency; in that case, Vitamin B12 replacement therapy may resolve these symptoms. Checking serum B12 in any psychiatric disorder is recommended.[804] Although the normal reference range for B12 is 200-1100 pg/ml, about 10% of the people with values up to 350 or 400 may have B12 deficiency and experience neuropsychiatric issues.[805] Some doctors treat psychiatric patients using B12 supplementation with levels less than 500. [809] Vitamin B12 may be taken three ways: as a subcutaneous injection, nasal spray, or tablet under the tongue. Taking B12 in the form of a B12 complex is often recommended to ensure absorption.

- For *depression*. When individuals with low B12 supplement their antidepressants with Vitamin B12 supplements, they report significantly improved depressive symptoms.[806]
- For *schizophrenia*. B12 (methylcobalamin) levels in people with schizophrenia can be 3-fold lower than the general population[807] and this deficiency can cause symptoms similar to schizophrenia. B12 supplementation appears to improve negative symptoms[808] and there are cases where it has fully eliminate psychosis.[778] (See Case Study 75, p. 193.)
- For *obsessive-compulsive disorder*. Clinical experience shows that some patients with OCD have a dramatic decrease in symptoms with B12 treatment alone.[809]
- For *dementia*. Taking 1mg each week may reduce the rate of normal cognitive decline in the elderly and improve cognition in moderately demented individuals.[18a]
- For *bipolar*. If a B12 deficiency is detected, injections of B12 may reduce the risk of recurring manic episodes.[810] (See Case Study 76, p. 194.)
- For *insomnia*. Vitamin B12 influences the secretion of melatonin, which assists sleep. B12 can help maintain appropriate wake-sleep cycles[811] and can help avoid *Sleep phase insomnia* (p. 309).[812] Even when serum B12 levels are within normal bounds, patients can have B12 deficiencies that influence insomnia.[813]

Vitamin B Complex.

- For *depression*. Higher intake of B6/B12 for up to twelve years can mean less risk of depression in the elderly–the greater the B6/B12 dosage, the fewer depressive symptoms.[814] B vitamin therapy has proven helpful to address under-methylation, a condition often associated with mood and behavior disorders.[180]
- For *schizophrenia*. A meta-analysis found that high-dose B vitamins (B6, B8, B12) are consistently effective for reducing symptoms, but lower doses are not. The greatest benefit was for those early in their psychosis experience.[815]

Vitamin C. Vitamin C is a powerful natural antioxidant.

- For *major depression*. Patients who were treated with fluoxetine and Vitamin C for six months showed a significant drop in depressive symptoms, as compared to those who took fluoxetine plus a placebo.[816]
- For *schizophrenia*. Patients who were given Vitamin C with atypical antipsychotics showed a significant positive improvement in oxidative stress and symptoms.[817] Vitamin C is especially helpful when combined with Vitamin E[778] and this combination (with added essential fatty acids) has been shown to reduce psychotic symptoms during use and for four months afterwards.[818] Vitamin C also works well with antipsychotics; 77% of the people on antipsychotics who were given Vitamin C had fewer hallucinations and disorganized thoughts.[819]

- For *bipolar*. Vitamin C helps clear vanadium from the system; vanadium is a mineral that can aggravate moods and it is often abnormally high in patients with bipolar.[820] Both manic and depressive symptoms may improve significantly after a one-time three-gram dose of vitamin C.[821]

Vitamin D. Vitamin D is a hormone produced by the body when our skin is exposed to sunlight. It has many functions including activating genes that regulate the immune system and release neurotransmitters that influence brain function. Vitamin D deficiency is common, especially in people with dark skin, the elderly, and women: 61% of women of color have a vitamin D deficiency as do 35% of other women.[822]

- For *schizophrenia*. Sub-optimal levels of Vitamin D have been found in 97% of the population with schizophrenia.[823] In a study of 18,411 women, researchers discovered that those in the highest quartile of Vitamin D consumption had a 37% lower risk of psychotic-like behavior than women in the lowest quartile.[824] Suitable levels of Vitamin D during a boy's first year of life are associated with a reduced risk of schizophrenia later in life.[825] In addition, people with high Vitamin D levels and markers for *Inflammation* (p. 52) – a condition often associated with mental health issues – have a significantly decreased risk of a schizophrenia diagnosis.[826]
- For *Seasonal Affective Disorder (SAD)*. SAD, a depressive disorder, often occurs when there is little sunshine, coinciding with a drop in vitamin D levels in the body. Several studies suggest that SAD may be caused by changing vitamin D3 levels, which may affect serotonin levels in the brain.[827]
- For *depression*. When overweight subjects who suffer from depression are given Vitamin D supplements, they report a significant improvement in depressive symptoms.[828] Treating inadequate vitamin D levels in people with depression and other mental disorders appears to be a cost-effective therapy, improving long-term outcomes and quality of life.[829]
- For *Alzheimer's*. Low Vitamin D levels are a causal risk for Alzheimer's. Very low levels increase the risk of Alzheimer's by as much as 25%.[830]
- *More broadly*. 85% of psychiatric patients have suboptimal Vitamin D levels.[831] Historically, 25-hydroxy-vitamin D levels of 20 ng/mL were considered normal. During the past decade many researchers have argued that a blood level of at least 30 ng/mL is optimal; some advise even higher goals – 40-50 ng/mL.[832] One leading integrative psychiatrist prefers to see higher levels – 50-75 ng/mL – and recommends supplementation of 2,000-10,000 IU for deficiencies.[833] Vitamin D supplementation should be monitored by blood testing every few months.

Vitamin E (α-tocopherol). Vitamin E is an antioxidant and anti-inflammatory.
- For *depression*. Patients suffering with major depression had significantly lower serum vitamin E concentrations than their healthy counterparts.[834]

- For *dementia*. A two-year study found that patients with Alzheimer's Disease who took Vitamin E improved their symptoms and lived longer.[835]
- For *schizophrenia*. Vitamin E reduces the movement disorder side effects that are associated with antipsychotics.[836]

Choline. Choline is an essential nutrient often grouped with B-vitamins; it comes in a variety of forms. CDP Choline has been used to treat disorders that affect the blood in the brain, including strokes. A meta-analysis found evidence that CDP Choline is effective as a neuroprotectant.[837]

- For *bipolar*. A small, open-label study of six bipolar patients with treatment-resistant rapid cycling who were stabilized on lithium found that adding free choline in doses between 2,000 and 7,200 mg per day saw manic symptoms improve.[838] Phosphatidylcholine (15 to 30 g/d) may reduce the severity of mania and depressed mood in bipolar patients. According to several case reports, choline bitartrate reduced mania in patients on lithium with rapid-cycling; however, the impact on depression was mixed.[838]
- For *dementia*. A nine-month study of 349 subjects confirmed that CDP Choline is an effective treatment for mild vascular dementia.[839] A meta-analysis by Cochrane Stroke Review Group found, "There is some evidence that the CDP choline has positive effects on memory and behavior in the short- to medium-term in cerebral disorders in the elderly."[24]
- *For substance abuse*. Limited research indicates that citicoline appears to decrease cravings; in fact, high doses of citicoline is associated with a successful reduction in cocaine use by patients with both bipolar disorder and cocaine dependence. Citicoline may also hold promise for those who are dependent on alcohol and cannabis, as well as for those interested in reducing food consumption.[840]
- *Safety*. There are no reported side effects or drug interactions with CDP Choline,[24] and toxicology tests have shown it to be safe.[841]

Multi-Vitamins. Multi-vitamins can be a good source of nutrients. However, more personalized nutrient therapy can be given when preceded by suitable *biomedical testing* (p. 323).

- For *mood disorders*. One study compared a multi-vitamin containing ten times the adult requirements of Vitamins B1, B2, B6, B12, C, E, folate, biotin, and nicotinamide for a year in comparison to placebo. Those who were in the multi-vitamin group—both sexes—showed statistically significant improvements in mood, and women experienced a significant improvement in both mental health and sleep. Vitamins B1, B2, and B6 were found to be important for improving mood.[842]
- For *anxiety*. One study offered young men twelve times the adult daily requirements of B1, B2, niacin, pantothenic acid, B6, biotin, folic acid, B12, C, calcium, magnesium, and zinc. In one month, the multi-vitamin group had

significantly lower anxiety levels and significantly lower perceived stress than the control group.[843] Similar results are found with older men.[844]

- For *schizophrenia*. One trial found that those who stayed on mega-vitamin therapy after release from the hospital had a 50% lower rate of return hospitalization than those who stopped mega-vitamin therapy.[845]
- For *insomnia and fatigue*. Abnormally low serum levels of vitamins B1, C, E, pantothenic acid, folic acid, and B12 may increase daytime fatigue.[16]
- For *substance abuse*. Because of the many nutrient deficiencies associated with substance abuse, multivitamins and mineral supplements are commonly required after detoxification.[846] In one study involving recovering cocaine addicts, multivitamins worked as well as standard drug-withdrawal meds.[847]
- *Safety*. There are no reports of serious side effects from the use of multivitamins, even in the dosages well above daily minimum standards.[16]

Minerals

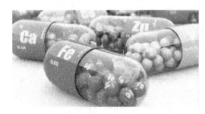

Minerals are inorganic nutrients that play a key role in ensuring health and well-being. Minerals include the trace elements copper, iodine, iron, manganese, selenium, and zinc, together with the macro elements calcium, magnesium, potassium, and sodium. Like vitamins, minerals are found in small quantities in the body and are obtained from a wide variety of foods.

Chromium/ Chromium Picolinate. Chromium is an essential micronutrient.

- For *depression*. Chromium is a good stand-alone therapy for depression and other mood disorders, and it can be effective as an add-on therapy with conventional antidepressants.[16]
- For *atypical depression*. One study found that 60% of those taking chromium picolinate (600µg/day) experienced a loss of their depressive symptoms.[848] It also appears to reduce carbohydrate craving in depressed patients.[849]
- *Safety*. Multiple studies have reported no toxic effects from chromium in dosages up to 1 mg/day, although people using insulin should monitor their insulin levels. Chromium may cause higher HDL cholesterol levels and increases in blood pressure. Given the risk of bipolar cycling, people who have (or may develop) bipolar disorder should be cautious about using chromium.[24]

Copper. Copper plays an important role in the synthesis of neurotransmitters.[850] An overload of copper tends to lower dopamine and increase norepinephrine; it can also signal Wilson's Disease. Copper imbalance is often associated with paranoid schizophrenia, depression, and autism,[851] as well as bipolar and ADHD.[19] In animal studies, diets very low in copper caused massive changes in the levels of neurotransmitters.[852] Most people with excess copper also have low zinc levels (zinc blocks absorption of copper in the intestines) and excessive oxidative stress. Copper overload is one of the top six nutrient imbalances in people with mental health issues. (See Figure 28, p. 168.) Nutrient therapy, which is inexpensive and relatively free of side effects, can correct copper imbalances.[19] (See Case Study 73, p. 193.)

Iron. Iron carries oxygen from the lungs to the body's tissues and is necessary for neurotransmitter synthesis. Throughout the world, iron is the most common nutrient deficiency; it can cause anemia, a lack of adequate healthy red blood cells.

- For *depression*. Iron deficiency anemia is associated with apathy, depression, and fatigue.[853] A lack of iron can aggravate the symptoms of *postpartum depression*,[854] so treating iron-deficient mothers with iron supplements improves mood.[855]

- *More broadly*. Iron deficiency increases the risk of mood disorders, autism spectrum disorder, attention-deficit hyperactivity disorder, and developmental disorders in children.[856]

Lithium. Lithium is a naturally occurring salt available as lithium carbonate (a prescription drug prescribed at near toxic levels) and lithium orotate (available OTC). Adequate lithium levels appear strongly associated with mental health. [857] It reduces inflammation (associated with mental ill-health), increases GABA (which reduces anxiety) and increases BDNF (which is correlated with better mood).[858] Ground water levels of lithium seem to be inversely linked to suicide, but some analysis suggests this link is uncertain.[859] Frequent blood tests for those on prescription lithium are needed to check if toxicity is causing kidney damage. (See Case Study 72, p. 192.) Low dose lithium is seldom used and appears to be an overlooked therapy choice for mental health.

- For *bipolar*. Considerable evidence shows that even very small doses may be beneficial in preventing suicides, dementia, and bipolar.[860] A small open study found that patients with bipolar responded to low doses (50 μg/meal) of a vegetable-based lithium compound.[861] Lithium treatment is also associated with greater brain gray matter volume in those with bipolar.[862]

- For *alcoholism*. In one study, 42 alcoholics were prescribed Lithium orotate and a low carbohydrate diet. Ten had no relapse for between three and ten years, thirteen didn't relapse for one to three years, and the remaining twelve relapsed between six and twelve months. Lithium orotate was found to be safe, and its adverse side effects are minor.[863]

- For *drug abuse*. A study of former drug users found that 400μg /day of lithium improved mood and energy.[864]

- For *autism*. Autistic children and their mothers have lithium levels significantly lower than normal.[865] One theory is that when pregnant women drank highly purified water to avoid toxic chemicals rather than tap water (in which trace lithium is found), the child was deprived of the trace lithium needed for normal brain growth.[866]

- For *dementia*. Five of seven epidemiological studies found an association between standard-dose lithium and low dementia rates.[867] Lithium appears to interfere with the production of plaque in the brain, so may help prevent Alzheimer's Disease, especially in younger patients with an inherited form of Alzheimer's.[868] Long-term use (301-365 days) in older adults with bipolar resulted in 23% decrease in dementia risk.[869] One study showed that 5% of people with bipolar on lithium develop dementia, but 33% of a comparable group from the general population develop dementia.[870]

- *Safety*. Prescription lithium is potentially toxic and can cause kidney and thyroid damage. Little clinical testing has been done on lithium orotate. It should be taken under the guidance of a trained practitioner.

Magnesium. Magnesium is the fourth most abundant mineral in the body; it contributes to more than 300 enzymatic reactions and can be found inside cells (particularly in the heart and brain) in high concentrations. Magnesium is also one of the first nutrients to disappear from food when it is processed, and one of the first nutrients to leave the body when it is stressed.[984a] For a variety of reasons (e.g. soil depletion and food processing), the average daily intake of magnesium has plummeted from about 500mg/day in 1900 to about 200mg today. Overall, the population is deficient in magnesium.[871]

Although it is difficult to assess magnesium levels through blood tests, its deficiency can lead to neurological (especially neuromuscular and "restless legs") disorders.[872] Common symptoms of magnesium deficiency are digestive issues, irritability, anxiety, insomnia, constipation, and calcium deficiency. Magnesium supplements are often prescribed for two or three times per day. Magnesium can also be absorbed through the skin by spending fifteen or twenty minutes soaking in hot water in which between one and two cups of magnesium sulfate crystals (Epsom salts) have been dissolved.[778]

- For *depression*. A meta-analysis shows that higher dietary magnesium is associated with lower levels of depression.[873] Conversely, a magnesium deficiency is linked to depression and other psychiatric disorders.[874] Patients with an undermethylated depressive biotype often thrive on magnesium.[19]

- For *bipolar*. Preliminary evidence suggests that in cases of acute mania or rapid cycling, magnesium is helpful as an additive to mood stabilizers.[875] In one study, magnesium and verapamil were much more effective than verapamil alone for acute mania.[876] In a case series, several patients remained stable on reduced psychotropics while undergoing magnesium therapy.[877]

- For *anxiety*. An early 20th-century trial found that magnesium worked effectively as a sedative for agitated patients and was helpful as an aid for sleep.[878] This was supported in a modern study that proved that a reduced anesthetic is needed when it is combined with magnesium sulphate.[879]

- For *ADHD*. When magnesium was deficient in children diagnosed with ADHD and they were given magnesium supplements for six months, the result was a significant decrease in hyperactivity (and an increase in magnesium, zinc, and calcium, which were often low). Hyperactivity increased in other children with ADHD who served as the control group; they were deficient in magnesium, but were not given magnesium supplementation.[893] Chronic deficits in magnesium in children with normal IQs are characterized by fidgeting, learning difficulties, anxiety, restlessness, and psychomotor instability.[880] (See *Broad Spectrum Minerals,* p. 180.)

- For *alcohol abuse.* Alcohol consumption is one of the major causes of magnesium loss; serum magnesium tends to decrease while urinary magnesium increases two- or three-fold.[881] Intravenous magnesium sulfate can relieve alcohol-associated headaches.[882]
- For *substance abuse.* Many people with substance abuse issues, especially alcohol, suffer from a magnesium deficiency. When eighteen methadone-maintained patients suffering with cocaine and opiate addictions were given magnesium supplements, they reported a significant reduction in craving and better abstinence rates.[883]
- For *insomnia.* The muscle relaxant properties of magnesium can help relieve Restless Legs Syndrome, which can cause insomnia.[884]
- *Safety.* High dosages may slow heart rate and cause dizziness. Magnesium is a mild sedative, so it should be taken at bedtime.
- *More Broadly.* 125-300 mg of magnesium glycinate (a form gentle on the digestive tract) at meals and a bedtime (four times daily) produces clinically significant mood improvement. 200-300 mg of magnesium glycinate or citrate before bed supports sleep onset and duration through the night.[871]

Manganese. Manganese decreases dopamine neurotransmission,[885] as does the class of psychotropic medications known as SSRIs.

Selenium. Selenium is an essential antioxidant found in foods in varying quantities, depending on the selenium content of the soil where they are grown.

- For *depression.* Five studies have reported that a low selenium intake was associated with poorer mood.[886] Pregnant women who took daily selenium had significantly less postpartum depressive symptoms than a placebo control group.[887] For selenium-deficient patients, 100µg/day significantly improved depression and anxiety.[888]
- For *schizophrenia.* U.S. states with low-selenium levels record a high incidence of schizophrenia. Schizophrenia levels in Finland decreased after selenium was added to fertilizers and animal feed.[889]

Zinc. Zinc combats free radicals and helps control oxidative stress that can kill brain cells.[19] Zinc deficiency is the most common chemical imbalance in people with mental health issues (see Figure 28, p. 168); more than 90% of those diagnosed with depression, schizophrenia, ADHD, and autism have low blood zinc levels.[19] Zinc deficiencies can cause copper overload, which can alter neurotransmitter levels.

- For *depression*. A meta-analysis suggests that zinc supplements have potential benefits as a stand-alone intervention or when used in conventional antidepressant drug therapy. Research shows that zinc significantly lowered depressive symptoms.[890] (See Case Study 71, p. 192.)
- For *schizophrenia*. Zinc is effective in reducing the amount of copper in the body, and excess copper has been associated with schizophrenia.[891]
- *More broadly*. Zinc should be taken with the evening meal; if taken in the morning it can cause nausea. Zinc deficiencies, which are common in vegetarian diets, can usually be corrected in two months.

Broad Spectrum minerals. In early trials, broad-spectrum micronutrient supplements appear to be as effective as psychotropics—but with fewer adverse effects—when treating mood disorders, ADHD, aggressive behavior, and misconduct. Broad-spectrum treatments may also improve stress responses, cognition, and a sense of well-being in healthy adults.[892]

- For *ADHD*. Hyperactive children have a much greater incidence of magnesium, copper, zinc, calcium, and iron deficiencies than healthy children, and magnesium deficiency is the most frequent.[893]

Amino Acids

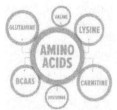

Amino acids are organic compounds that are vital for neurotransmitter synthesis. There are three major types: *essential* (not made by the human body), *non-essential* (made by the human body) and *conditional* (those needed occasionally, as in times of stress). Digestive enzymes are responsible for producing amino acids; the enzymes are activated by hydrochloric acid in the stomach.[894] Amino Acid imbalance is one of the top six nutrient issues in people with mental health issues. (See Figure 28, p. 168.)

D-alanine. When D-alanine is added to antipsychotics, there is significant improvement in the treatment of schizophrenia.[895]

D-Amino Oxidase Inhibitors (DAAO). DAAO is an enzyme that oxidizes D-amino acids. It can be useful in reducing the dose of D-serine needed to improve psychosis. Using DAAO with D-serine can remove some side effects associated with high doses of D-serine.[896]

D-cycloserine. D-cycloserine is a colorless amino acid produced by some bacteria. It is sometimes used as an antibiotic.

- For *anxiety*. Patients suffering from anxiety report significantly less social anxiety when they combine D-cycloserine with exposure therapy, as compared to patients working with exposure therapy alone. [897]

D-serine. D-serine is an amino acid used in the synthesis of proteins.

- For *schizophrenia*. Patients with treatment-refractory schizophrenia reported significant improvements in negative, positive, cognitive, and depression symptoms when D-serine was used with risperidone (an antipsychotic).[898]

DL-phenylalanine (DLPA). DLPA contains two forms of the amino acid Phenylalanine. The "L" form, thought to improve mood, is a natural substance found in protein-rich foods. The "D" form is made synthetically.

* For *depression*. DLPA reduced depression in 31 of 40 people participating in a preliminary trial.[899] Some physicians suggest a daily dose of three or four grams for people with depression, while others suggest that a much lower dose, between 75 and 200 mg per day, was effective.[900] In one trial, people with depression who were given between 150 and 200 mg of DLPA per day had symptom relief comparable to the relief offered by antidepressants.[901]

GABA (gamma-aminobutyric acid). GABA is both an amino acid and neurotransmitter. When levels of GABA are low, people often suffer from anxiety, depression, and psychosis.[19] GABA can be taken as a food supplement; it increases alpha brain waves (associated with relaxed, effortless alertness) significantly, while decreasing beta brain waves (associated with high stress).[902]

Glutathione (GSH). Glutathione is an antioxidant that helps prevent cellular damage caused by free radicals, heavy metals and other sources, making it critical to the body's detoxification. It is formed from three amino acids - cysteine, glycine, and glutamate – and can be found in virtually every cell of the body. Research[903] suggests that the GSH levels are significantly reduced in patients with schizophrenia,[904] bipolar, and major depression, suggesting that GSH supplementation may aid recovery. (See Case Study 65, p. 190.)

Glycine. Glycine is the simplest naturally occurring amino acid. It is a constituent of most proteins.

* For *schizophrenia*. In one study, researchers found glycine levels significantly lower in patients with schizophrenia than in controls.[905] Patients on psychotropics had even lower levels of glycine. High doses of glycine may significantly reduce positive[906] and negative[907] symptoms, and high doses rarely worsen psychosis. Many studies indicate that glycine reduces the symptoms of schizophrenia in people unresponsive to drug therapy.[778]

Homocysteine. Homocysteine is an amino acid derived from ingested methionine found in cheeses, eggs, fish, meat, and poultry. It is toxic to neurons and blood vessels and can induce DNA strand breakage and oxidative stress. Excessive homocysteine is often associated with a deficiency in vitamin B12.[908]

* For *schizophrenia*. Homocysteine levels are higher in people with schizophrenia (65% higher in men and 25% higher in women controls), so researchers suggest homocysteine may contribute to chizophrenia.[905] Symptoms also occur during a genetic disorder (homocysteinuria), where the levels of homocysteine are not adequately controlled.[19]

L-Carnitine and Acetyl-L-Carnitine (ALCAR). Acetyl-L-carnitine is a synthesized form of L-carnitine, a derivative of the amino acid lysine. Our bodies manufacture L-carnitine, which is used in the brain. Both L-carnitine and ALCAR are antioxidants that act as neuroprotectants.

- For *depression*. When ALCAR is prescribed as a supplement for elderly patients with chronic depression, its antidepressive qualities are as effective as fluoxetine.[909]
- For *dementia*. ALCAR may slow the rate of cognitive impairment in the normal aging process, as well as early dementia.[18a] ALCAR may be enhanced if it is taken with Coenzyme Q10 or omega-3 fatty acids.
- For *alcohol abuse*. Two grams taken daily may improve memory in abstinent alocholics.[18b]

L-Carnosine. L-Carnosine is a protein-building block found in the heart and brain and concentrated in muscles when they are working.
- For *schizophrenia*. When patients were given L-carnosine, they performed significantly faster on certain cognitive tests, although reaction times and errors were not significantly different between treatments.[910]

L-Glutamine. L-glutamine is the most abundant amino acid in the bloodstream, responsible for 30%-35% of the amino acid nitrogen in blood.
- For *alcohol abuse*. One study found that when alcoholics were given L-glutamine daily in divided portions with meals, they had less desire to drink; L-glutamine can also reduce anxiety.[911]

L-Lysine. L-lysine is an essential amino acid that supports growth and overall health. It is available in many food sources.
- For *schizophrenia*. In chronic schizophrenia, L-lysine can improve negative and general psychopathology symptoms.[912]
- For *anxiety*. A week-long oral treatment with lysine and arginine significantly reduced chronic anxiety.[913]

L-Theanine. The amino acid L-Theanine, which is an extract from green tea, has been widely used to treat anxiety and depression, particularly in Asian countries. It can stimulate GABA synthesis, thereby increasing dopamine, reducing serotonin, and creating feelings of calm and well-being.[16]
- For *anxiety*. L-theanine is effective for moderate to severe anxiety without causing drowsiness. A calming effect is usually found within thirty or forty minutes after taking a dose ranging from 50 to 200 mg, and the benefit lasts as long as ten hours. Improvement for moderate anxiety is often seen with 200 mg doses taken once or twice a day. More severe anxiety may require 600 or 800 mg taken in smaller doses through the day.[16]
- For *schizophrenia*. L-theanine can reduce anxiety in patients with schizophrenia spectrum diagnoses better than a placebo.[914]

L-Tyrosine. L-Tyrosine is a building block amino acid for neurotransmitters and thyroid hormones, both of which can have a dramatic impact on mental health. L-tyrosine helps combat stress. Although it is sold as a supplement, it occurs naturally in chicken, turkey, fish, milk products, peanuts, and a variety of seeds and nuts. The evidence supporting L-tyrosine is limited.

- *For mood disorders.* One study found that people exposed to a stressful environment, including cold and reduced oxygen levels, significantly increased their physical performance and mood when taking L-tyrosine.[915]
- *For depression.* L-tyrosine levels in the blood are much lower in depressed patients than in normal populations, one study showed. The L-tyrosine levels rebounded once patients recovered from their depression.[916] A single case study yielded impressive results. (See Case Study 78, p. 195.)

5-HTP (5-hydroxytryptophan/ L-Tryptophan/L-5-HTP). L-Tryptophan becomes 5-HTP in the body and converts quickly to serotonin. In 1989, L-Tryptophan was taken off the market and replaced by 5-HTP because of contamination from a single vendor, but 5-HTP is generally preferred over L-tryptophan because it crosses the blood-brain barrier more easily and requires smaller doses.

- For *depression.* 5-HTP has shown strong benefits in dealing with depression; some researchers support its use as additive to psychotropics. A meta-analysis of thirteen small studies found between 29% and 69% of subjects responded favorably to 5-HTP.[917] In one study of people with long-term refractory depression, 43 of 99 experienced complete recovery and eight improved significantly.[918] Two separate studies showed that patients with depression who were given L-5-HTP showed a significant reduction in depressive symptoms—in fact, the reduction was equal to what psychotropics can accomplish. The first study showed that L-5-HTP was as effective as fluoxetine for people with first-episode depression;[919] people with all degrees of depression experienced benefits within two weeks of treatment. The second study showed efficacy equal to a decarboxylase inhibitor,[920] and concluded that taking between 50 and 3,000 mg daily for between two and four weeks might improve symptoms of depression.[921]
- For *bipolar.* An acute depletion of L-tryptophan in the diets of patients with bipolar results in depression.[922] Daily 5-HTP supplements can have anti-depressant effects.[923] One study found that use of L-tryptophan at between 6 and 12 grams per day resulted in a significant reduction in mania.[924] Another found that taking three grams three times per day with lithium was superior to taking lithium alone.[925] However, some studies show no benefit.[16]
- For *anxiety.* In one study, people with panic disorder found that taking 5-HTP inhibits panic.[926]
- For *schizophrenia.* Several studies found lower concentration of tryptophan in the serum of schizophrenia patients.[927] As compared to a placebo, L-tryptophan benefitted the memory functions of patients with schizophrenia, although it had no effect on the patients' psychotic state or on the side effects of medications.[928]
- For *insomnia.* According to one study, tryptophan supplementation was 100% effective in promoting sleep for people who wake between three and six times a night.[929]

- For *smoking cessation*. Daily tryptophan supplementation with a high-carbohydrate diet can lessen smokers' withdrawal symptoms; it also substantially improves their success rates.[930]
- *Safety*. 5-HTP is reasonably well tolerated, with no serious side effects. However, it can cause nausea and sedation, which diminish with continued treatment.[16] Use with MAOIs (an early class of antidepressants) is not recommended.

Methionine. Methionine, along with SAM-e, has the greatest positive effect on people with depression of the undermethylated biotype.[19]

N-acetylcysteine (NAC). NAC is produced by the amino acid L-cysteine and is a precursor to glutathione, the most important antioxidant in the brain. NAC has been used to treat a variety of inflammatory disorders;[26] NAC appears to increase glutathione levels. Oxidative stress and imbalanced glutathione have been associated with bipolar and depression.

- For *schizophrenia*. NAC reduces the core symptoms of schizophrenia, eliminating apathy and improving social interaction and motivation.[931] It appears that these benefits are the result of NAC's anti-inflammatory qualities.[149]
- For *bipolar*. One trial of patients on mood stabilizers found that those who were given N-acetylcysteine (2 gm/day) showed a significant improvement in depression, mania, quality of life, and social and occupational functioning, as compared with patients taking a placebo.[932] A broader review found it helpful for bipolar depression.[933] Another study confirmed the additive benefit of NAC (one gram twice daily) to mood stabilizers for depressive symptoms, but found no significant benefits for mania.[934]
- For *addictions*. Evidence suggests that NAC reduces cravings in people suffering from cocaine,[935] cannabis, and cigarette addictions.[931]
- *Safety*. NAC appears to be well tolerated. Response to NAC usually does not occur for at least eight weeks.

Phosphatidylserine (PS). PS is derived from the amino acid serine, which is important in cognition. PS is found in high concentrations in fish.

- For *depression*. Women given PS for thirty days experienced a 70% reduction in the severity of their depressive symptoms.[936]
- For *dementia*. One study on PS showed improvements in depression, memory, and behavior.[937] Another found that memory dysfunction associated with aging improved after twelve weeks of daily PS supplementation.[938]

Sarcosine. Sarcosine (N-methylglycine), is an amino acid associated with glycine synthesis and degradation.

- *For schizophrenia*. According to one study, sarcosine improved general psychiatric symptoms and depression, with possible benefits for such negative schizophrenic symptoms as blunted affect.[939] Another study found sarcosine superior to a placebo in four separate measurements of symptoms, including both positive and negative symptoms.[940] Yet another found that six months of sarcosine supplements may reverse damage to the brain's glutamate system and improve both the negative and cognitive symptoms.[941] In reviewing recent studies, [942] the European Psychiatric Association notes that two grams per day of sarcosine in addition to antipsychotics may improve both positive and negative symptoms.[943] One study of people who had never taken psychotropics found a 20% improvement in both positive and negative symptoms when taking 1-2 g/day over six weeks.[944]

- *Safety.* Sarcosine has been tolerated well, with no notable side effects.

Taurine and Acamprosate. Acamprosate is a medication derived from taurine, an amino acid and antioxidant.

- For *alcohol abuse.* Taruine (1 gm three times a day) reduces the level of a toxic alcohol byproduct and may decrease the severity of withdrawal.[18b]

Branched-chain Amino Acid drink. Drinking a mixture of amino acids (leucine, isoleucine, and valine) specifically excluding the amino acids tyrosine and phenylalanine (a precursor to tyrosine) can depress the mood.[945]

- For *bipolar.* This drink may benefit patients with acute mania. One study of 25 patients found that those who drank it had a significant reduction in manic symptoms within six hours of treatment, and they sustained the improvements for a week after the study.[946]

Other Nutrients

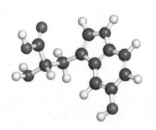

In addition to vitamins, minerals and amino acids, other substances that occur in the body are helpful for mental health.

EMPowerplus is a custom mix of minerals, vitamins, amino acids, and antioxidants available over the counter.

- For *bipolar.* A review of 358 people with bipolar using EMPowerplus showed a significant decrease in symptoms at three months, and the improvement was sustained for six months; the average rate of symptom reduction was 45%.[947] A small study found symptom reduction in as little as two weeks, with enough symptom reduction at six months to justify lowering the doses of psychotropics.[948] An observational study of 22 subjects found that 19 responded positively to treatment (10 significantly, 7 moderately, 2 slightly). Of the 15 subjects on psychotropics prior to the study, 11 were symptom-free without psychotropics over the six to nine-month follow-up period. In a similar study of 19 subjects, 15 improved (12 significantly, 3 moderately, 1 slightly).[16] (See Case Study 70, p. 192.)

- *Safety.* Some people reported occasional gastrointestinal discomfort. Also, a micronutrient formula may increase the power of mood stabilizers, thereby allowing a gradual reduction of mood stabilizers while on EMPowerplus.

Vitamins and Fatty Acids. MRIs show that people with elevated vitamins B, C, D, E, and Omega-3 function better cognitively—and actually, their brains increase in size.[192] Micronutrient treatment for ADHD patients have shown robust improvements in symptoms, depression, and global functioning—with no adverse effects.[949]

Cholesterol. Cholesterol is a vital building block of many hormones that influence mood. Cholesterol is also important in minimizing *Inflammation and Oxidative Stress* (p. 52), both closely associated with mental health issues. Evidence is substantial that changes in cholesterol level or an intrinsically low level may result in variations in mental state or personality.[950]

- For *depression.* For both men[951] and women,[952] cholesterol levels are consistently lower in more severely depressed patients.[953]

- In terms of *suicide.* People whose serum is within the lowest quartile of cholesterol concentration are more than six times likelier to commit suicide than those in the highest quartile.[954] In addition, case studies indicate an association between low cholesterol and marijuana craving.[984(a)]

Coenzyme Q10 (Q10). Q10 is a nutrient and naturally occurring antioxidant and anti-inflammatory found in the body and in many foods.

- For *bipolar depression.* 200mg/day Q10 improves depression after 8-weeks with a large effect-size (large improvement) compared to placebo with minimal adverse effects.[955] This confirms smaller studies using 800-1200mg/day dosages.[956]

Creatine Monohydrate. A nitrogenous organic acid that occurs naturally in vertebrates, creatine helps supply energy to all the body's cells, especially muscle cells, so it increases muscle mass.

- For *depression.* A small open study suggests that creatine augmentation is beneficial in unipolar depression, but it may possibly precipitate a manic switch in bipolar depression.[957]

Folinic Acid. Folinic acid (5-formyltetrahydrofolate) is a vitamer for folic acid (Vitamin B9) and has the full vitamin activity of B9. It is on the World Health Organization's List of Essential Medicines.

- For *treatment-resistant depression.* A small study found that high-dose folinic acid improved symptoms for treatment-resistant depressive patients with low cerebral spinal fluid folate.[1512] (See Case Study 79, p. 195.)

Idebenone. Idebenone is a semi-synthetic antioxidant closely related to coenzyme Q10 (a molecule that plays a central role in bodily energy production); in fact, it may be more potent than Q10.[18a]

- For *dementia.* Elderly patients who received Idebenone (120 mg/day for 6 months) with Alzheimer's-type dementia saw significant improvement in mild and moderate dementia.[958] Further improvement continues into the second year of use.[959]

Indole-3-acetic acid (IPA). The subject of extensive studies, IPA is the most common naturally-occurring plant hormone of the auxin class.

- For *insomnia*. A small study of people with moderate insomnia found that total sleep time, duration of stage-two sleep, and total non-REM were significantly increased when they took IPA.[960]

Lipoic Acid (alpha-lipoic acid). Lipoic acid is a vitamin-like antioxidant substance found in yeast, liver, kidney, spinach, broccoli, and potatoes. It is also manufactured in the laboratory.

- For *dementia*. Lipoic acid acts as a neuroprotectant and can improve cognition in people suffering with dementia.[961]

Omega-3 Fatty Acids. Omega-3 fatty acids are important in cellular metabolism, having anti-inflammatory properties (see *Inflammation*, p. 52) that can improve brain function. There are three types: EPA (ethyl eicosapentaenoic acid), DHA (docosahexaenoic acid), and ALA (alpha-linolenic acid). EPA and DHA are found in fish and shellfish, while ALA is plant-based and found in flaxseed oil. A deficiency of DHA can lead to depression, ADHD, bipolar, schizophrenia, and dementia.[19] Interestingly, Omega-3 supplementation with higher EPA concentrations appears to help depression while lower EPA concentrations (and higher DHA/ALA) appears to help anxiety.

- For *bipolar depression*. A meta-analysis found that adding omega-3 fatty acids to mood stabilizers improves depression, but there is little evidence it can improve mania.[962] These fatty acids help depression in both unipolar depression and bipolar.[963] One study showed that EPA (1-2 g/day) improved depression.[964] Another found that additive omega-3 helped people remain in remission significantly longer than placebo.[965] EPA appears to be more beneficial than DHA for bipolar depression.

- For *anxiety*. A 19 trial meta-analysis found that people with anxiety who took Omega-3s ($\geq$ 2,000 milligrams a day with < 60% EPA) saw a modest reduction in anxiety. Those having more severe anxiety benefited the most.[966]

- For *depression*. The findings are inconclusive, but some studies show promise. The ratio of EPA/DHA appears to be important. Adding EPA Omega-3 to antidepressants for treatment-resistant severely depressed patients led to dramatic and sustained improvement within one month in all the symptoms of depression, including unremitting and severe suicidal thoughts.[967] EPA may have a therapeutic effect equal to Prozac.[968]

- For *phobias*. Symptoms of social phobia improved dramatically.[967]

- For *schizophrenia*. Preliminary information suggests that when certain omega-3 fatty acids are ingested by those not using antipsychotics, they have sustained improvements in positive and negative symptoms.[16] Trials show omega-3 fatty acids (EPA) may prevent first-episode psychosis.[969]

Additionally, patients taking EPA require lower antipsychotic doses.[970] In a study of 81youths with signs of early schizophrenia, 5% of those who took fish oil later developed schizophrenia, as compared to 28% who took a placebo.[971] Patients receiving a polyunsaturated fatty acid had a marked reduction in symptoms during a two-month follow-up; at six months, few symptoms remained.[972]

- For *substance abuse*. A small study showed fish oil decreased anxiety in substance abusers.[973]
- *Safety*. Fatty acids should be taken with food for best absorption into the body. They may alter glucose metabolism in diabetics.[16]

Resveratrol. Resveratrol is derived from plants; the highest levels are found in red wine and the skins of red grapes. It has anti-oxidant, anti-inflammatory, and anti-carcinogenic properties.

- For *dementia*. Resveratrol is neuroprotective for Parkinson's disease and Alzheimer's that can slow cognitive decline.[974] It also improved learning and memory ability in an experiment using rats with vascular dementia.[975]

SAM-e (S-Adenosyl Methionine). SAM-e is a naturally occurring and essential substance concentrated in the liver and brain. It plays an important part in regulating serotonin and dopamine,[976, 977] and is an uptake inhibitor for serotonin, dopamine, and norepinephrine.[19] It has been called a "first-line CAM treatment" for mild, moderate, or even severe depression.

- For *depression*. A meta-analysis supports its use in treating mild-to-moderate depression, with 8 of 14 studies showing positive results,[978] and one study showing that SAM-e was as effective as antidepressants, but tolerated significantly better.[979] Another suggests that SAM-e can improve memory-related cognitive symptoms in depressed patients.[980] Analysis of extensive clinical experience[19] indicates that people suffering from depression with the undermethylated biotype (sometimes associated with OCD tendencies) "thrive" on SAM-e.
- *For substance abuse*. Preliminary studies suggest that SAM-e may help treat chronic liver disease caused by medications or alcoholism.[981] It also significantly improved anxiety, depression, fatigue, anorexia, insomnia, and nausea, while helping alcoholics remain abstinent.[982]
- *More broadly*. It is vital to use the finest SAM-e. It must be carefully manufactured and packaged. Because it rapidly oxidizes, it must be properly processed and coated. There are inferior sources of SAM-e; check to make sure it is packaged in foil blister packs to maintain potency.

WHAT CONSIDERATIONS SHOULD I KEEP IN MIND?

Nutrient Therapy is one of the most promising mental health therapies, and it can help all diagnoses. It should be approached with the guidance of a practitioner who will prescribe nutrients based on lab test results and clinical exams. We should avoid self-diagnosis and self-treatment and work with practitioners who use robust *Biomedical Test Panels* (p. 323) that can identify possible disorders that span all *Biomedical Restorative Therapies* (p. 165).

Based on test results, you and your practitioners can design a personalized nutrient response to deal with your own relevant issues: diet, vitamin deficiencies or overload, allergies, toxins, and others. Each of us has a *biochemical individuality*, which means that nutrients should not be considered "one size fits all". For instance, some people with depression will thrive on folate, while it may be ineffective or detrimental to others.

In addition, remember that all interventions carry some risk, including *Nutrient Therapy*. For instance, excess zinc supplementation can lead to copper deficiency; SAM-e supplementation may lead to bipolar switching; and excessive Vitamin D supplementation can cause kidney stones. This should not lead you to avoid the significant value of *Nutrient Therapy* but encourage you to seek the best-available guidance and support from practitioners well-grounded in its science. The risks of *Nutrient Therapy* are often considered negligible compared to psychotropics.

The compelling benefit of *Nutrient Therapy* is the potential to reduce—and, if possible, eliminate—mental health symptoms. When symptoms are reduced, the optimal dosages[983] of psychotropics can often be reduced.

Compared to psychotropics, the time required for the body to respond to nutrient therapy is considerably longer. Pyrrole disorders can see improvement in as little as a week, zinc deficiencies in two months, methylation issues in two to four months, and copper overload in up to a year. People with type A blood, substance abusers, and people who do not absorb nutrients from food well (malabsorption) respond more slowly to nutrient therapy.[19]

The timing for ingesting certain nutrients is important. For instance, zinc is best taken with the evening meal, and B6 in the morning. Compounding prescribed nutrients can be helpful, considerably reducing the number of capsules (by as much as 80%), which makes compliance easier. This helps, because *Nutrient Therapy* often requires many individual tablets or capsules. Also, blending necessary nutrients into a daily smoothie can be helpful. Work with your practitioners on approaches that can make *Nutrient Therapy* easier.

A proper diet is critically important. (See *Diet & Digestion*, p. 61.) Eating nutritious foods can reduce the need for *Nutrient Therapy*. As evidence, countries where fish (rich in omega-3 fatty acids) is a mainstay in the diet have significantly lower rates of depression.

Nutrient Safety. Nutrient therapy is relatively safe; however, there are potential side effects and it is important to get high quality nutrients. Some patients are sensitive to nutrients that are deficient in their system. Transitional side effects are also possible, as nutrient levels move to more desirable levels. If this happens, dosages can be reduced.

Countless people have recovered by using nutrient approaches.[984]

REAL-WORLD EXPERIENCE

Case Study 63 – Importance of Knowing Your Biotype (Depression)

Pete developed suicidal depression at mid-life, so his doctors prescribed lab tests to find the root of the problem. While he waited for the results, he saw a psychiatrist who put him on an SSRI antidepressant.

The depression became sharply worse. The psychiatrist doubled the SSRI dosages. Six days later, Pete committed suicide. When the lab results came back, they showed that Pete had a low folate biotype associated with intolerance to SSRIs.

__Bottom Line__: Biomedical lab tests help determine the best therapeutic response and can help prevent harmful therapies.[24]

Case Study 64 – Amino Acid Therapy (Depression)

Marsha, a 36-year-old entrepreneur, ate well, exercised, and pursued a healthy life style. But she became increasingly depressed and unable to sleep.

Routine blood work showed that thyroid and iron levels were normal. She was given Lexapro. Then Abilify was added. And Ativan. Within eight weeks, her doctor prescribed Wellbutrin and Lamictal. They didn't help her problems.

Marsha went to an integrative practitioner who did initial testing of iron and vitamins B12 and D, followed by many other tests covered by Marsha's insurance. Nothing significant was found, so an amino acid screen was run. Results showed that Marsha's system had low levels of all essential amino acids. The practitioner quickly started her on an amino acid powder plus a digestive enzyme with hydrochloric acid (HCl).

Marsha lost all symptoms after four weeks of treatment.[6]

__Bottom Line__: Exhaustive biomedical testing may uncover an easily treatable disorder that otherwise might cause a lifetime of misery.

Case Study 65 – Glutathione (Schizophrenia)

Mrs. J abruptly began hearing voices. It was so severe that she could not feed herself and she soon became catatonic. She continued in this state for seven months until a doctor ran detailed lab tests which uncovered a significant deficiency of glutathione, a major antioxidant.

Intravenous glutathione was administered along with calcium, magnesium, N-acetylcysteine and B12. Within 48 hours Mrs. J saw a dramatic turnaround. Her full recovery took six weeks. During this time her response varied, and her nutrient levels were adjusted to accordingly. She has fully recovered and shows no trace of her former mental state.[985]

__Bottom Line__. There is strong evidence that oxidative stress is linked to mental health issues. Maintaining needed antioxidant levels is therefore vital.

Case Study 66 – Pellagra (Dementia)

At the age of 45, James was admitted to the hospital because of disorderly behavior and symptoms of dementia. He was diagnosed with psychosis.

A biomedical test identified pellagra, a niacin deficiency. After James was placed on nutritional therapy focused on niacin supplements, he made a complete recovery within six months.[986]

Bottom Line*: We have known for over fifty years that pellagra can cause mental health issues. Often, contemporary psychiatry doesn't run the test to check for it.*

Case Study 67 – Broad Nutrient Therapy (ADHD)

Free lab tests and nutrient therapy were provided to 33 special education children in a poverty-ridden section of Chicago who had been diagnosed with attention-deficit hyperactive disorder or behavioral disorders.

After the children were given nutrient therapy based on their individual test results, 71% of those with ADHD showed significant improvement in their academics. Some improvements were stunning: 13 of 16 children with behavioral problems improved, and several children who had a history of serious assaultive behavior completely stopped all negative behaviors. Parents were thrilled and amazed with the improvement in their children.

The tests cost $300 per child.[19]

Bottom Line*: Inexpensive lab tests and simple nutrient therapy can make a significant difference in the lives of at-risk children, their parents, and their communities.*

Case Study 68 – SAM-e (Depression)

Jim, a business consultant, was 50 years old when he suffered his fourth bout with depression. Overnight, it seemed to his family, he turned from his normal self-confident, outgoing, dynamic self to someone with significant insecurity, worry, and indecisiveness. He couldn't sleep.

Zoloft had worked for him in the past, but he didn't want to go back on it because it caused extreme sexual dysfunction. Instead, he started a trial of SAM-e at 400 mg in the morning. When his practitioner suggested he increase the dosage to 800 mg twice a day, all his depressive symptoms disappeared. After being symptom-free for three months, he lowered the dosage to a maintenance level of 400 mg twice a day and experienced no side effects.[15]

Bottom Line*: Get a full biomedical lab test. Those with undermethylated biotype often thrive on SAM-e with no side effects.*

Case Study 69 – Cholesterol Supplementation (ADHD)

Fred was an aggressive and unhappy young man. At the age of 16, he was diagnosed with attention-deficit hyperactivity disorder. A biomedical test panel revealed that his cholesterol level was low.

His practitioner prescribed cholesterol supplements. As his cholesterol levels slowly increased, there was a significant drop in aggression.[984a]

Bottom Line*: We often think of cholesterol as something we should seek to reduce. However, it is vital to many bodily functions. Inadequate levels can cause mental health issues.*

Case Study 70 – EMPowerplus (Bipolar)

At the age of 18, Josh's world started to unravel. He began having severe manic episodes, delusions, and rage. The diagnosis was bipolar.

During a month in the hospital, doctors prescribed lithium and antipsychotics. Josh remained relatively stable for two years, but he felt groggy, sedated, and unhappy. He also felt weak and complained of a tightening in his chest. He told friends he didn't feel like the person he had been before.

Because Josh couldn't tolerate the side effects any longer, he stopped taking lithium. He then felt his world spiral out of control. His moods started to cycle rapidly, and his friends and family members worried about suicide.

A psychiatrist formerly associated with the Mayo Clinic suggested EMPowerplus. They tried it, and Josh began to improve. Change was significant within five weeks. Josh returned to the person he had been before his bipolar diagnosis.

Bottom Line*: See www.truehope.com. EMPowerplus can be taken as a powder mixed into smoothies.*

Case Study 71 – Zinc Supplementation (Depression)

Amy, 34, took good care of herself with exercise, a healthy diet, and yoga. But she still suffered from depression.

A broad biomedical exam indicated that she had a low serum zinc level. Her practitioner suggested nutrient therapy, with a primary focus on zinc supplements, starting at 90 mg/day and tapering to 60 mg/day.

Amy noticed a significant improvement in mood.[984a]

Bottom Line*: Zinc deficiency is one of the six major nutrient imbalances that can cause mental health issues.*

Case Study 72 – Lithium Orotate (Bipolar)

By the time Glenda turned 60, she had a thirty-year history of bipolar. Lithium helped significantly, but after twenty-five years on prescription lithium carbonate, she was taken off the medication because she was suffering renal failure. She became homebound for five years.

A biomedical exam pointed to many nutrient deficiencies. They were corrected, but without major improvement. However, when lithium orotate was prescribed, her mood improved substantially.

By experimentation, Glenda determined that she could maintain this improvement with as little as 5 mg of lithium orotate every four days without any kidney issues.

Bottom Line*: Some research suggests that lithium orotate much more readily passes the blood/brain barrier than lithium carbonate.[984a]*

Case Study 73 – Copper Overload (Suicidal Depression)

Kathleen developed suicidal depression after the birth of her third child. Two years of therapy and psychotropics did little to help her. Finally, a biochemical evaluation revealed that she had copper overload.

Initially, she was treated with zinc, slowly increasing the dosage to 75 mg/day. She was also given vitamins B3, B6, C, and E, as well as manganese and omega-3 fatty acids.

During the initial ramp of zinc, Kathleen's anxiety increased, but after six months of nutrient therapy, her copper levels returned to normal ranges. Her depression disappeared.[19]

Bottom Line*: Copper overload is one of the six major nutrient imbalances that can cause mental health issues.*

Case Study 74 – Pyrrole Disorder (Schizophrenia)

Mary was a successful businesswoman, but at the age of 29, she had a severe mental breakdown after her mother died in an automobile accident. She was diagnosed with schizophrenia. After many different psychotropics, she became suicidal, with daily episodes of hysteria.

A biomedical exam revealed that she had signs of a pyrrole disorder. Doctors immediately prescribed large doses of zinc and B6, among other nutrients. She responded quickly and made substantial improvement within a month. At her three-month check-up, all psychiatric symptoms were gone, and she was off all psychotropics.

Mary had two serious relapses over the next two years—when she temporarily stopped her nutrient therapy. At last check, she was maintaining the nutrient therapy and had remained healthy for six years.[19]

Bottom Line*: The pioneering work of orthomolecular psychiatry found the association between pyrrole imbalances and mental health symptoms. Make sure your biomedical practitioner checks your pyrrole levels.*

Case Study 75 – Vitamin B12 (Schizophrenia)

When he was a college student, Ben become depressed, paranoid, and delusional. Blood tests revealed a severe B12 deficiency. Intramuscular injections of B12 resolved all his mental health symptoms.

Another example of B12 benefits is the story of Mark, an Iraq veteran who returned from war with chronic anxiety and fatigue, despite the fact that he ate well and exercised regularly. His B12 levels were low, but within conventional ranges, so his physician was not concerned. The doctor prescribed psychotropics. Mark suffered severe side effects. He then consulted an integrative psychiatrist who knew that some people in the lower band of acceptable ranges for B12 can develop mental health symptoms. Mark was given B12 injections, and within a month his symptoms disappeared. He reported that he felt better than ever.[6]

Bottom Line: *Always remember bio-individuality. Even though your B12 levels may be within typical ranges, your body may require a different level. Consider B12 therapy when B12 results are in the lower band.*

Case Study 76 – Vitamin B12 (Bipolar)

Mrs. A, 35, was admitted to the hospital after three weeks of manic episodes lasting several hours. Her symptoms included grandiosity and hyperactivity. She was diagnosed with bipolar and treated with valproic acid (an antiseizure med used for bipolar) for three weeks. There were no signs of improvement. Blood tests indicate her serum vitamin B12 level was very low.

Vitamin B12 (1000 µg/day) was administered intravenously for one week. After the third day, Mrs. A did not experience any new manic episodes. B12 injections were given weekly for one month, and neurologic symptoms improved. She continued the injections, this time monthly. One year after B12 vitamin replacement started, her mental status was still normal.[987]

Bottom Line: *Don't scrimp on biomedical testing. It may point to clear issues that can be readily addressed.*

Case Study 77 – Low Folate (ADD)

Marilyn, 36, had an IQ of 132, but she lacked motivation. She had been diagnosed with attention-deficit disorder as a child, and Ritalin was prescribed. As a young adult, she developed depression. Zoloft was prescribed, but her depression worsened. Several other SSRIs failed. She chose Klonapin, since it helped reduce anxiety.

Blood tests revealed a histamine level of 16 ng/ml. She was treated with high doses of folic acid, Vitamin B12, and niacinamide, followed by zinc, manganese, chromium, and vitamins B6, C, and E. She stayed on Klonapin for several months. At her follow-up appointment, Marilyn reported significant improvement. New lab tests fine-tuned her nutrient therapy.

Her Klonapin was discontinued by slowly reducing dosages. She continues nutrient therapies and says she is "95% better".[19]

Bottom Line: *Nutrient therapy is perhaps the best kept "secret" in psychiatry and should always be considered.*

Case Study 78 – L-tyrosine (Depression)

Alice suffered from chronic depression for many years. She tried an antidepressant, but it made her agitated. With Alice's consent, her doctor started her on a "crossover" trial, where she was given either L-tyrosine or a placebo at various times without her knowledge of which she was taking.

When she was taking on L-tyrosine, Alice improved dramatically, reporting that she felt "better than she had in years." Her energy, self-esteem, and ability to sleep improved dramatically. Within one week of switching to the placebo, all her depressive symptoms returned. When she switched back to L-tyrosine, her symptoms once again improved quickly. She had no side effects from the L-tyrosine.[988]

Bottom Line*: The crossover test that yielded dramatically different results between L-tyrosine and the placebo offers strong evidence that L-tyrosine works for her. Consider crossover approaches with your practitioners as you plan non-drug treatments.*

Case Study 79 – Folinic Acid (Refractory Depression)

Ben, an energetic middle-schooler, started to feel a sense of "nothingness" at age 13. These thoughts soon became overwhelming. Over the next year he was given a variety of drugs, electroconvulsive therapy and extensive inpatient care. Nothing worked to help is constant depression.

Ben's parents stumbled upon research that showed that some cases of treatment refractory depression were caused by issues in central nervous system metabolism. Ben was tested and found to be folate deficient. Within a month of starting high doses of folinic acid, "we felt like we had our Ben back," said his mother. Ben has been thriving ever since.[989]

Bottom Line*: Prevailing paradigm practitioners (see p. 20) rarely do robust biomedical testing. If you don't look for a problem, you can't find it. Assertive self-advocacy is vital. Robust testing helps leave no stone unturned.*

Case Study 80 – Intravenous Nutrients (Depression)

Kevin, 46, suffered from chronic depression and anxiety from childhood. Eight years of psychoanalysis provided little relief.

His doctor started him on weekly intravenous vitamins and nutrients (Myer's cocktail) providing almost complete symptom relief. Oral and intramuscular (IM) administration of the same nutrients were not effective. Through trial and error, the combination of nutrients was adjusted. After four years he was able to reduce the frequency of injections to once monthly or less.[990]

Bottom Line*. Intravenous administration of nutrients can achieve blood concentrations not obtainable with oral, or even IM, administration. Work only with trained and licensed practitioners.*

WHAT ARE ADDITIONAL RESOURCES?

- Nutrient Power by William Walsh. http://goo.gl/DxoIvQ.
- Nutrient Quality by Brand. www.ConsumerLab.com.
- Nutrient/Drug Interactions. www.NaturalDatabase.com.
- Mensah Medical. www.MensahMedical.com.
- Dr. James Greenblatt, MD. http://goo.gl/cPbpv5.
- Pfeiffer Medical Center. www.hriptc.org.
- Omega-3 Fatty Acids Detail. http://goo.gl/E69VrS.

Endocrine Therapy

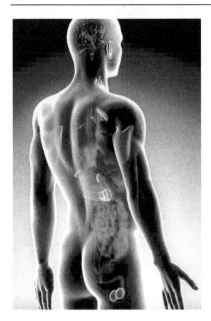

WHAT IS THE ESSENCE?

The endocrine system is the collection of glands that produce hormones regulating our metabolism, growth, sexual function, reproduction, sleep, and mood.

Endocrine therapy can restore hormonal balance by supporting one or more of the major glands, including the thyroid, adrenal, parathyroid, and pituitary.

Endocrine therapy is typically straightforward, and may significantly improve, even potentially eliminate, mental health symptoms.

The medical community has long known that hormones can have a profound effect on our mental health. Increased testosterone in men is associated with increased anger and hostility,[991] while women experience a continuous cycle of hormonal fluctuations from puberty through post menopause, and this cycle affects brain chemistry and mood.

Too much (disorders starting with "hyper") or too little (disorders starting with "hypo") of certain hormones can cause significant mental health issues. (See Figure 29, p. 198, for the more common endocrine disorders that can impact mental health. See also case studies of mental health recovery from these disorders, p. 205-208.)

Glands interact in complex ways, so multi-glandular coordinated therapies may be necessary when dysfunctions occur. For example, the thyroid works in concert with the adrenal. If one needs therapeutic support, the other often does, too.[992]

Endocrine disorders are relatively common, found in over 5% of the U.S. population,[993] while the frequency of borderline cases is greater (up to 15% for hypothyroidism[994]). Certain subgroups exhibit dramatic rates of disorders (for example, 20% of women over sixty years of age have borderline hypothyroidism[995]). People struggling with mental illnesses have even higher rates of endocrine disorders.

WHAT EVIDENCE SHOWS THIS IS EFFECTIVE?

The following table highlights the variety of ways endocrine issues can impact mental health. Each gland is examined in more detail.

Disorder/Imbalance	Gland	Potential Symptoms
Hypothyroidism	Thyroid	Depression, psychosis
Hyperthyroidism	Thyroid	Anxiety, depression, mania
Hypoparathyroidism	Parathyroid	Depression
Hyperparathyroidism	Parathyroid	Anxiety, mania, psychosis
Hyperglycemia (Diabetes)	Pancreas	Bipolar, depression, psychosis
Hypoglycemia	Pancreas	Depression
Addison's Disease	Adrenal	Depression
Cushing's Syndrome	Adrenal	Depression, psychosis
DHEA Imbalance	Adrenal	Depression
Pheochromocytoma	Adrenal	Anxiety, psychosis
Pituitary Tumor	Pituitary	Depression, psychosis
Oxytocin Imbalance	Pituitary	Poor social skills
Melatonin Imbalance	Pineal	Anxiety, insomnia, depression
Estrogen/Progesterone Imbalance	Ovaries	Schizophrenia
Polycystic Ovary Syndrome	Ovaries	Depression
Low Estrogen	Ovaries	Depression
Irregular Menstrual cycle	Ovaries	Anxiety, ADHD
Testosterone Imbalance	Testes	Depression, anger

Figure 29 – Endocrine Disorders influencing Mental Health[996]

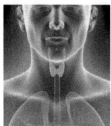

Thyroid. Located in the neck, the thyroid gland secretes hormones that influence metabolism and growth. Thyroid disorders are surprisingly common; 9.5% of the population has hyperthyroidism (overactive thyroid),[997] and 15% of the people admitted to psychiatric hospitals have mild or greater hypothyroidism (underactive thyroid). Both conditions can cause mental health issues,[998] triggering depression, bipolar, borderline personality disorder, and psychosis.[999]

Thyroid disorders are generally diagnosed through blood tests. When effective thyroid treatment is begun, the response is usually quite favorable.[1000] (See Case Study 81, p. 205 and Case Study 82, p. 205.)

- For *depression*. Hypothyroidism is strongly associated with depression. Even a borderline case can significantly alter mood.[1001] At least 15% of patients diagnosed with depression have a minimal thyroid insufficiency, with evidence of an autoimmune thyroid disease.[1002] A large trial showed that the thyroid hormone T3 is as effective as lithium in treating resistant depression.[1003] In depressed patients, small changes of thyroid hormones, even within normal ranges, have significant effects on the functioning of the brain.[1004]

- For *bipolar*. About 25% of people with bipolar have thyroid dysfunction.[1007] Studies of people with bipolar or unipolar depression found that thyroid supplements were effective with antidepressants, particularly in women. T3 hormone supplements resulted in remission for one-quarter of the patients with bioplar.[1005] Two-thirds of bipolar patients in depressive states have subclinical hypothyroidism; these individuals recover significantly more slowly than those with optimum thyroid profiles.[1006] Lithium (p. 177) is a natural salt used to treat bipolar disorder; it can cause hypothyroidism.

- *For schizophrenia.* Abnormal thyroid hormonal status was observed in 29% of patients with schizophrenia-spectrum disorders.[1007] Animal studies suggest antipsychotics can influence thyroid.[1008]

- *More broadly.* Treating an underlying thyroid problem (typically with drugs and/or surgery) often alleviates a variety of underlying psychiatric symptoms.[1009]

Adrenal.[1010] The adrenal gland is located over the kidneys and produces several

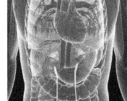

important hormones, including cortisol, aldosterone, DHEA, pregnenolone, and adrenaline.

Adrenaline stimulates our fight-or-flight response and provides energy in times of stress. Because stress is so closely tied to mental health issues, it isn't surprising that the adrenal gland influences our mental health.

Although adrenal issues are relatively rare, both the underproduction (Addison's Disease) and overproduction (Cushing's Syndrome) of adrenal hormones can cause mental health issues--which include shifts in mood, memory problems and even, in severe cases, psychosis.[1011] In addition, with continual stress, the adrenal can be overtaxed, leading to hypoglycemia.

Addison's Disease is potentially life-threatening. It destroys parts of the adrenal, thereby decreasing hormone secretions. Many different stressors can trigger an Addisonian crisis. One researcher found that 70% of the people with Addison's Disease experienced changes in their mental state, predominantly in moods and behavioral changes. (See Case Study 83, p. 206.)

Cushing's Syndrome is associated with high levels of the stress hormone cortisol (hypercortisolism) and reduced methylation[1012] (p. 54). Most cases of Cushing's Syndrome are caused by taking medicines or party drugs that add too much cortisol to the body. However, it can be caused by a tumor on the adrenal gland or pituitary gland (Cushing's Disease).[1013] (See Case Study 84, p. 206.)

A tumor on the adrenal gland can also cause pheochromocytoma, a situation where the adrenal causes persistent high blood pressure. Like other adrenal disorders, pheochromocytoma can produce a variety of psychiatric symptoms. It can be addressed effectively with adrenal therapy.

DHEA and 7-keto DHEA tend to decline as men and women age. Lower levels of DHEA are associated with depression; this can be reversed with DHEA supplements.

- For *depression*. In a three-week trial of DHEA involving patients with midlife onset depression, half of them improved significantly. In addition, DHEA was associated with better sexual functioning.[1014] A case study also suggests that DHEA may have antidepressant and pro-memory benefits.[1015] Others suggest that DHEA is effective in treating major depression.[1016] (See Case Study 90, p. 208.)
- For *schizophrenia*. When DHEA levels increase, negative symptoms improve in patients with schizophrenia, although no improvement occurred for depressive and anxiety symptoms.[1017]
- For *insomnia*. DHEA supplements significantly increase REM sleep during the first two hours.[1018]
- For *dementia*. People who took DHEA twice daily for six months improved their mental performance dramatically higher than those taking a placebo.[1019]
- *More broadly*. When patients with bipolar and PTSD had low DHEA-sulfate levels and received 7-keto DHEA treatment, their symptoms improved noticeably.[15]
- *Safety*. DHEA is typically well tolerated, but it may cause testosterone levels to rise, which can lead to new issues. 7-keto DHEA, however, does not convert to testosterone or other hormones, so it doesn't have the potential side effects of DHEA.

Pregnenolone is a precursor hormone made from cholesterol. It appears to have neuroprotective properties with positive effects on learning, memory, inflammation, and GABA neurotransmitter receptor response.[1020]

- For *schizophrenia*. When used in conjunction with antipsychotics, pregnenolone was found to significantly improve positive[1021] and negative[1022] symptoms.
- For *anxiety*. 400mg pregnenolone reduces self-reported anxiety.[1023] The mechanism at work is believed to be the neurosteroid allopregnanolone which has known ability to ease anxiety. Pregnenolone converts to allopregnanolone. Allopregnanolone fluctuations over the course of a woman's menstrual cycle impact mood.[1024]
- For *bipolar*. One study found that pregnenolone was associated with a significant improvement in depression, as compared to the placebo group. It also seemed to trend toward improvement in manic symptoms.[1025]

Pituitary and Hypothalamus. The pituitary and hypothalamus are located in 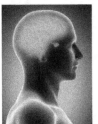 the base of the brain, the region that coordinates the autonomic nervous system—which, in turn, controls body temperature, thirst, hunger, sleep, and emotions. Among the major hormones produced in this region are oxytocin and protirelin.

Oxytocin strongly influences our social behavior and emotions. Associated closely with trust, relaxation, and psychological stability,[1026] oxytocin is released when people bond socially, regardless of whether the experience is positive or negative. Even playing with your dog can cause an oxytocin surge.[1027] Oxytocin also helps the female uterus contract and boosts milk production in the breasts.

- *For schizophrenia.* One study found that oxytocin improves psychotic symptoms.[1028].
- *For autism.* A small study of children with autism-spectrum disorders used brain scans to study oxytocin's impact. Researchers found that oxytocin temporarily normalized brain regions responsible for social deficits.[1029]
- *More broadly.* Oxytocin can be used to enhance interpersonal skills and individual wellbeing. In midlife men, it has even been shown to increase the positive emotions during meditation.[1030] It might also have more applications for neuropsychiatric disorders, especially the disorders characterized by persistent fear, repetitive behavior, reduced trust, and an avoidance of social interactions.[1031]

Protirelin (thyrotropin-releasing hormone, TRH), which is produced by the hypothalamus, promotes the secretion of thyroid-stimulating hormones from the pituitary gland. When a patient is given an intravenous injection of TRH, there is an immediate rise of thyroid-stimulating hormone (TSH) in the blood. Protirelin caused a prompt decrease in psychotic symptoms in 50% of those with schizophrenia. Patients then tended to experience a relapse slowly.[1032]

Thymus. The thymus gland, located behind the sternum, is only active until 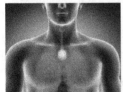 puberty. Afterwards, it starts to shrink slowly, replaced by fat. Thymalin is a polypeptide derived from the thymus gland. Synthetic Thymalin is composed of several amino acid constituents. Thymalin was combined with psychotropic drugs in treating 36 patients with schizophrenia who were therapeutically resistant. Thymalin users showed considerable improvement; psychic disorders were eliminated, and neuroleptic complications were reduced.[1033]

Parathyroid. The parathyroid is a gland located next to the thyroid that secretes
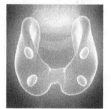
a hormone responsible for regulating the body's supply of calcium. Parathyroid problems can cause calcium imbalances, which may result in psychiatric symptoms, such as severe depression and poor memory.

Hyperparathyroidism (hormonal overproduction) is often caused by a tumor on the parathyroid that can be removed by surgery. The *Biomedical Test Panels* (p. 323) your practitioners use should include a serum electrolyte and calcium concentration test that are markers for potential parathyroid issues.[1034] (See Case Study 85, p. 206.)

Pineal. The pineal is a pea-sized gland in the brain that produces the hormone
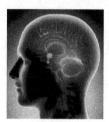
melatonin (available in synthetic form as N-acetyl-5-methoxytryptamine). A powerful antioxidant, anti-inflammatory, and sleep aid, melatonin is released in a daily (circadian) rhythm, with peak levels occurring at night. (See also *Chronotherapy,* p. 240, and Case Study 89, p. 208.)

• For *insomnia*. Studies suggest that melatonin may help people with disrupted circadian rhythms and those with low melatonin levels (e.g. seniors and people with schizophrenia) sleep better. Melatonin supplements may help prevent jet lag, particularly in people who cross 5 or more time zones. A meta-analysis found that melatonin decreases the time to fall asleep and increases overall sleep time.[1035]

• For *schizophrenia*. Studies suggest that melatonin is helpful with the side effects of tardive dyskinesia and weight gain.[1036] Drug-free patients with schizophrenia have a lower nighttime secretion of melatonin; this did not improve following anti-psychotic drug treatment, which may explain why many people with schizophrenia suffer with insomnia.[1037]

• For *major depression.* One study found that melatonin had no effect on depressive symptoms,[1038] while another found substantial improvement.[1039]

• For *substance abuse withdrawal.* Melatonin can significantly reduce acute nicotine withdrawal symptoms, including anxiety, restlessness, tension, irritability, anger, depression, impatience, and cigarette cravings.[1040] It also reduces benzodiazepine withdrawal symptoms.[1041]

• *Safety.* Melatonin, as a hormone, should be taken under practitioner guidance. It is best to begin with very low doses, close to the amount that our bodies normally produce (< 0.3 mg per day).[1042] Melatonin supplements often come in dosages much higher. High doses can lead to a "hangover" effect that leaves users groggy. A meta-analysis found that high doses of melatonin are ineffective; "After a few days, it stops working," when the brain's melatonin receptors are exposed to too much of the hormone, they become unresponsive.[1043]

Pancreas. The pancreas is a large gland organ located behind the stomach. As a 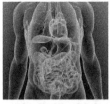 part of the digestive system, the pancreas produces important enzymes and hormones that break down foods. It releases insulin, to control blood sugar (glucose) levels.

Of all the tissues in the body, the brain is most dependent on the moment-by-moment supply of blood glucose to function properly.[1044] If glucose is too low,[1045] a condition called hypoglycemia occurs, and with it a smorgasbord of mental health symptoms: anxiety, phobias, irritability, depressions, obsessive behavior, mood swings, psychosis, forgetfulness, and anti-social behavior.[1046] A defining symptom of diabetes, hyperglycemia occurs when glucose is too high. Hyperglycemia can also occur without diabetes. For example, insulinoma, a tumor of the pancreas, can produce excessive insulin and low blood sugar; insulinoma is often misdiagnosed as a psychiatric disorder.[1047]

Paradoxically, eating excess sugar can result in low blood sugar. Classic signs of hypoglycemia are low blood pressure and lowered body temperature. (To determine whether hypoglycemia is an issue, see *Biomedical Test Panels,* p. 323.) Hypoglycemia is less common in non-diabetic persons. The most common forms of hypoglycemia occur as a complication of diabetes treatment.[1048] If the patient is on insulin, the insulin dosage may need to be reduced. Low blood sugar can also cause other endocrine issues as glands work overtime to regulate blood sugar. As a result, hypoglycemia may create the need for more expansive endocrine therapy.

The good news is that hypoglycemia is often fully reversible. Those with hypoglycemia or periodic low blood glucose levels and mental health issues should consider a *hypoglycemic diet*: eliminating sugar, white flour, alcohol, caffeine, and tobacco consumption, and eating six small daily meals rather than three large meals.[1049] Fish, seafood, and starchy roots provide a healthy source of energy and could reduce the prevalence of depression.

- For *depression.* Research indicates that a diet high in added sugar reduces the production of Brain-Derived Neurotrophic Factor (BDNF),[1050] a brain chemical that plays an important role in forming new synapses. Low BDNF levels have been linked to depression.[1051] Levels of BDNF are particularly low in people with an impaired glucose metabolism – diabetics and pre-diabetics. As the amount of BDNF decreases, sugar metabolism worsens.[1052]

- For *bipolar.* As many as 53% of the people with bipolar have a metabolic disorder of pre-diabetes or diabetes.[1053]

- For *schizophrenia.* Results from four out of five placebo-controlled studies confirm that excessive sugar and saturated fats worsen the long-term outcome of schizophrenia. A diet with high saturated fat, high glycemic load, and low omega-3 PUFA may also increase the schizophrenia symptoms.[1054]

- *More broadly.* **Research indicates that diets containing high amounts of refined sugar are correlated with worsening symptoms of schizophrenia**

and a higher rate of depression. Research recommends limiting sugar consumption to 10% of total energy (or calorie) intake.[1055]

Ovaries. The ovaries produce a variety of hormones. *Estrogen*, the primary female hormone, maintains the body's female characteristics. In the brain, it boosts the synthesis of neurotransmitters that affect sleep, mood, memory, libido, and cognition. *Progesterone* ensures the development and function of the breasts and female reproductive tract. In the brain, it exerts a calming effect and improves sleep. Polycystic ovary syndrome (PCOS) is one of the most common endocrine disorders that affects 5-10% of women of childbearing age and is characterized by abnormal hormone levels.

- For *depression*. An analysis of over 1 million women over 14 years found that the use of hormonal contraception, especially among adolescents, was associated with later depression, suggesting depression as a possible side effect of hormonal contraceptives.[1056] In addition, there is a high prevalence of depression among women with PCOS.[1057]
- For *schizophrenia*. Overall, trials testing estrogen on women with schizophrenia have produced mixed results.[1058] However, some studies have found combining estrogen and antipsychotics yields a significant decrease in positive and negative symptoms,[1059] and appears to have anti-inflammatory value.[149]
- For *postpartum depression*. One study found that transdermal estrogen (absorbed through the skin) offered a rapid improvement of mood.[1060]
- *Safety.* **Estrogen therapy is associated with increased risk of breast cancer**, and women with schizophrenia have a lower incidence rate of breast cancer than the general population.[1061]

Menstrual Cycle. Since the dawn of time, women have known about the strong tie between hormonal changes during the menstrual cycle and mental health symptoms.[1062] Women with irregular cycles have more than twice the chance of being diagnosed with anxiety disorders; 65% of women with bipolar have dramatic mood changes during their menstrual cycles; and 59% of women with bipolar have long cycles.[1063] Irregular cycles, late onset of menses, and the first year of menses are associated with depression, obsessive-compulsive disorder, and eating disorders.[1064]

Testes. Testosterone stimulates the development of male secondary sexual characteristics; this hormone is produced mainly in the testes, but also in the ovaries and adrenal.

- For *schizophrenia*. Men with schizophrenia who were treated with testosterone supplements and antipsychotics experienced a significant improvement of negative symptoms.[1065]
- For *depression*. Testosterone gel may produce antidepressant effects in depressed men with low testosterone levels.[1066]

WHAT CONSIDERATIONS SHOULD I KEEP IN MIND?

Hormonal disorders and imbalances are common in people with mental health issues. As a result, your practitioner (typically your primary care physician, integrative medicine practitioner, or a referred endocrinologist) should perform a thorough endocrine evaluation as part of your larger *Biomedical Test Panel* (p. 323). When you and your practitioner examine the test results, both out-of-range and borderline indicators should be considered, since even borderline conditions may cause or exacerbate mental health symptoms.[1067] Testing is especially important when depression has resisted treatment and when there is rapid bipolar cycling.[1068]

For women with mental health issues, biomedical psychiatric testing should include assessments for menstrual cycle and gynecologic problems, especially if symptom severity coincides with the menstrual cycle. Women who take psychotropics should have repeat menstrual screening tests, since drugs may impact the menstrual cycle.[1062]

Endocrine issues can be caused by ingesting endocrine disrupters, which are chemicals associated with heavy metals, plastics, metal food cans, detergents, flame retardants, cosmetics, pesticides, and pharmaceuticals. Antipsychotics are endocrine disrupters; they can cause insulin resistance.[1069]

Endocrine therapy can take many forms, including hormone supplements, detoxification from endocrine disrupters (See *Detoxification* Therapy, p. 212.), surgery, and radiation. Often, endocrine therapy is effective in correcting the underlying hormonal condition and may relieve mental health symptoms significantly. Discuss possible side effects of endocrine therapy with your practitioners, because excess ovarian hormones, including estrogen, contribute to the development of breast cancer.[1070]

REAL-WORLD EXPERIENCE

Case Study 81 – Hyperthyroidism (Anxiety)

Without warning, Audrey started having daily anxiety attacks. Her doctor prescribed psychotropics and urged her to start breathing techniques, which she did. Audrey improved, but was still edgy and preoccupied. Gradually, she became very fatigued, slept erratically, and felt "in a fog".

Her practitioner ordered a thyroid blood test. The diagnosis: hyperthyroidism. Audrey started thyroid therapy and felt better immediately. All psychiatric symptoms went away.[1071]

Bottom Line*. Thyroid disorders are the leading endocrine cause of mental health issues.*

Case Study 82 –Hypothyroidism (Schizophrenia)

Helen had monthly bouts of catatonia (physical immobility and odd behavior) over fourteen years. With these came hallucinations and delusions. She worsened to the extent that she was admitted to the hospital.

Brain scans were run, but nothing appeared abnormal. Doctors then tested her thyroid levels; two were within normal bounds and a third was "somewhat elevated", so no thyroid issue was immediately apparent. Helen remained in the hospital for seventeen months without improvement.

Finally, her doctors felt that a mild case of hypothyroidism may be influencing her symptoms. Within four weeks of beginning thyroid therapy, Helen improved dramatically and was released from the hospital. She had no recurring bouts of catatonic or psychosis symptoms for four years.[1072]

Bottom-line*. Even borderline endocrine disorders can have a dramatic impact on mental health.*

Case Study 83 – Addison's Disease (Schizophrenia)

Karen was undergoing thyroid therapy, and it was working—until one day, when she became agitated, aggressive, and delusional.

A biomedical exam revealed that her cortisol levels were undetectable. Further tests uncovered endocrine abnormalities. Karen was in an Addison's (adrenal) crisis.

She was placed on a regimen of hydrocortisone and fludrocortisone. Karen's electrolytes and other measures returned to normal within a week, though she continued to have subtle cognitive difficulties. However, after two months, she was completely well mentally and physically.[1010]

Case Study 84 – Cushing's Syndrome (Schizophrenia)

Paul, an otherwise healthy 23-year old, started having overwhelming psychosis resembling schizophrenia. A thorough endocrine exam revealed that he had Cushing's Syndrome. Initial treatment was radiation therapy of the pituitary, but that failed to make a significant improvement.

His medical team then surgically removed the adrenal gland, and Paul began adrenal replacement therapy. This resulted in complete remission of all physical and mental symptoms within six months.[1073]

Case Study 85 – Hyperparathyroidism (Schizophrenia)

Becky was admitted to the hospital in a delusional psychotic state. Blood tests revealed that her serum calcium level was 14.3 mg/DL. (The standard reference range is between 8.2 and 10.2 mg/DL.) This and other tests were consistent with hyper-parathyroidism. A benign tumor on the parathyroid gland was found and surgically removed.

Becky's calcium levels returned to normal and her psychosis ended.[1510]

Case Study 86 – Elevated Testosterone (Depression and Suicide)

Beth was a well-adjusted and talented child with a strong support system, but gradually she became depressed. At fifteen, she tried to injure herself. Her psychiatrist prescribed Prozac. A week later, Beth attempted suicide. Her psychiatrist switched her to Lexapro. Within days, she became homicidal. Her psychiatrist then hospitalized her and prescribed Abilify. But Abilify caused her to feel "blunted", so her prescription was changed yet again, to Risperdal. When members of her medical team didn't see progress, they added the generic Lamictal.

Beth was the pawn in a game of rapid-fire psychotropic roulette.

Finally, Beth's mother had enough. She insisted that Beth be evaluated for hormonal irregularities, pointing out that Beth had entered puberty at age eight and had irregular menses. Hormonal testing revealed Beth had an elevated testosterone level. She started taking birth control pills to establish a regular monthly cycle, and she became stable. After Beth decided to stop all psychotropics, she became free of all psychiatric symptoms.[1074]

Bottom Line*: Psychiatrists know psychotropics. But you know your child better than any psychiatrist ever will. Beth's mother trusted her knowledge of her daughter and demanded hormonal testing—and that proved to be Beth's gateway to recovery.*

Case Study 87 – Low Estrogen (Schizophrenia)

Since puberty, Ms. A had irregular menses, mood swings, anxiety, and a feeling of unreality. But, when she was prescribed oral contraceptives in her late teens, her symptoms improved significantly. Then she went to college. After a month of hallucinations and delusions, Ms. A. stopped her college studies and eventually admitted herself to the hospital. She was diagnosed with schizophrenia.

Seeing the potential of a hormonal imbalance, her doctors tested the young woman and found low estrogen levels. She was prescribed oral contraceptives that included estrogen and progesterone. Within one week, her psychotic symptoms improved significantly and in three weeks they disappeared. Antipsychotic medication was never needed.[1075]

Case Study 88 – Progesterone (Schizophrenia)

Ann was diagnosed with schizophrenia at age 14. She self-medicated with alcohol, and that helped her get through the day, but not surprisingly, she became addicted. She joined Alcoholics Anonymous, and at age 35, she was put on Zoloft. Zoloft caused her to become suicidal.

Her psychiatrist offered her no acceptable solution, so she conducted her own research. She found that her severe premenstrual symptoms might be relevant, so she started taking large doses of natural progesterone.

Ultimately, a two-year process of self-initiated experiments led her to wellness when she began using progesterone, amino acids, and vitamins.

Ann is now very high functioning and attributes her success to finding the right nutrients and hormone supplements through experimentation.[1076]

Bottom Line*: Own your recovery and interview practitioners until you find the best one for your needs and the best answer to your problems.*

Case Study 89 – Melatonin (Aggression)

For decades, George and his wife had enjoyed a loving relationship, with no physical aggression whatsoever. And then suddenly, when George was 79, he started punching his wife while they were in bed.

A psychotherapist suggested the violence was caused by latent subconscious anger. George was confused. His family was in an uproar.

George was treated with 3 mg rapid-onset melatonin and 6 mg slow-release melatonin at bedtime for a REM sleep disorder. The nighttime scuffles ended, and the couple slept peacefully thereafter.[15]

Case Study 90 – DHEA (Depression)

Elena suffered from severe depression most of her life. She tried almost every antidepressant and found that each one had difficult side effects. None seemed to help enough to make the side effects worth the effort.

Electroconvulsive therapy left her with persistent memory loss. She tried SAM-e and Rhodiola rosea, but neither helped much. She was diagnosed with breast cancer and underwent chemotherapy. Finally, her DHEA-sulfate levels were checked in her post-menopausal state, and they were found to be extremely low.

She took 50 mg/day of 7-keto DHEA while staying on an antidepressant. After one week, her mood, energy, and cognitive function improved. She increased the dosage of 7-keto DHEA to 75 mg/day. She slept better, and all depression disappeared.[15]

WHAT ARE ADDITIONAL RESOURCES?

- Integrative Hypothyroid Treatment. http://goo.gl/R00nAo.
- Glycemic index & glycemic load, http://goo.gl/hNuH3R.
- Endocrine Web. www.EndocrineWeb.com.

Food Allergy Therapy

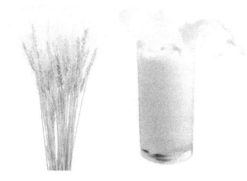

WHAT IS THE ESSENCE?

Foods can cause two negative reactions: *allergy* or *intolerance*. An *allergy* is when the body's immune system produces antibodies directed at the food. There are no medications for food allergies; sufferers can only diligently avoid certain foods. An *intolerance* is the body's inability to fully digest a food.

One test of patients with schizophrenia found that 92% reacted to one or more substances as follows: Wheat (64%), corn (51%), milk (50%), tobacco (75%, with 10% becoming psychotic), and hydrocarbons (30%).[1077] Gluten (a protein present in wheat, rye and barley) allergies appear to show the highest correlation to mental health issues, followed by dairy.

One mechanism by which a food allergy can threaten mental health is *Inflammation* (p. 52). People with food allergies are also more prone to react adversely to food dyes, aspirin, foods with salicylates, food additives, food preservatives, and the insecticides used to reduce food spoilage.

WHAT EVIDENCE SHOWS THIS IS EFFECTIVE?

Gluten. *Celiac Disease* (CD), which occurs in about 1% of the population, is an immune response to gluten. 35% of the people with CD have a history of mental health issues.[1078] Gluten sensitivity (GS) is estimated to be six times more common than Celiac Disease, but often both occur together, triggering a variety of neurologic and psychiatric disorders.[1079]

As many as 57% of the people with neurological dysfunctions will test positive for gluten sensitivity.[1080] The Mayo Clinic advises that the medical community may need to consider universal screening for CD,[1081] which is sometimes difficult to detect from gastrointestinal symptoms.[1082] Closely related to Celiac Disease and Gluten Sensitivity are allergies to wheat and other cereals.

- For *bipolar*. Individuals with bipolar have a much higher risk of having increased levels of IgG antibodies (a protein produced in response to bacterial and viral infections) to gluten, as compared to those without.[1083]
- For *depression*. A study reported that one-third of the individuals with Celiac Disease also suffer from depression.[1084]
- For *schizophrenia*. Of all mental health diagnoses, CD has the strongest tie to schizophrenia.[1085] Studies indicate that CD is between three[1086] and fifty[1087]

times more prevalent in people with schizophrenia than in the general population. Anti-gliadin antibodies (a marker for Gluten Sensitivity) occur in 23.4% of people with schizophrenia, as compared to 2.9% of the general population.[1088] When people with schizophrenia were hospitalized and put on a gluten-free, milk-free diet, they were released to an open ward considerably faster than those assigned a high-cereal diet.[1089] The patients on the gluten-free milk-free diet were also discharged more than twice as fast as those on a high cereal diet.[1090] An epidemiological study showed that the reduction in gluten rations during WWII significantly correlated to reduced schizophrenia rates in five countries.[1091] Studies have found that some people with schizophrenia improve markedly on a gluten-free, casein-free diet.[1092, 1093]

Dairy. Lactose (a sugar) and casein (a protein) are components of milk that can cause allergies or intolerances that have become prevalent, although they vary across population groups. It can affect more than 50% in African American, Hispanic, Asian, and American Indian populations.[1094] Lactose intolerance increases with age, and becomes quite common in the elderly.

- For *schizophrenia*. People being treated for mental health issues should be evaluated for dietary changes.[1095] Studies have shown that people with schizophrenia have increased levels of antibodies to bovine casein.
- For *depression*. Studies on 30 women suggest that lactose intolerance can cause or deepen depression.[1096]

Other Foods. A history of allergies is reported by 71% of people with depression.[1097] This is 3.5 times the rate of the general population.[1098] Also, as allergy scores increase, so do anxiety symptoms.[1099] Dietary changes can help tremendously; 70% of children with attention-deficit hyperactivity disorder (ADHD) who followed a "few foods" diet for five weeks showed significant improvements in behavior and no longer met ADHD criteria.[1100]

Schizophrenia was extremely rare in Pacific island populations who consumed no dairy and or grains. When these populations were introduced to grains, schizophrenia became common.[1101]

Food Allergy Tests. A variety of techniques determine food allergies. One of the easiest is an *elimination diet*: remove the food from your diet for between two and four weeks to determine if your symptoms improve, then later reintroduce the food to see if symptoms worsen. Blood and skin prick tests can give allergy markers. Perhaps the best test is an *oral food challenge*, conducted under the care of a skilled allergist at a medical facility. During a challenge, the allergist feeds you increasing doses of suspect foods. Following each dose, you are observed for any signs of a reaction.

WHAT CONSIDERATIONS SHOULD I KEEP IN MIND?

We are sometimes allergic to the foods we crave, particularly the foods we view as "comfort food". This may be because one of the body's stress responses to these foods is to release endorphins which can improve our mood.[1102] Also, we may be allergic to foods that produce anxiety after eating.[1103] Paradoxically, eating a food to which we are allergic can temporarily mask or inhibit an allergic response, offering short-term relief from our symptoms.

Start with lab screening for possible allergies (p. 210). Or we can try simple elimination diets ourselves. When we identify food sensitivities, we should reduce or eliminate those foods—while maintaining a wholesome diet.

While we are evaluating our responses to possible food allergies, we need to maintain a good mental health diet. (See *Diet & Digestion*, p. 62). Allergies run in families, so we should test first for allergies present in our families.

REAL-WORLD EXPERIENCE

Case Study 91 – Dairy Allergy (Anxiety)

Beth had symptoms of intense anxiety. After extensive biomedical testing, doctors discovered that she had elevated levels of casomorphin – a peptide derived from the digestion of the milk protein, casein.

When she was questioned, Beth admitted that she consumed a large amount of Coffeemate, a powdered cream alternative, in her coffee every day. Coffeemate contains very high levels of casein. When her physician recommended eliminating all dairy from her diet, she saw a modest improvement in the symptoms, but the removal of Coffeemate from her diet resulted in a very substantial improvement in her anxiety.[6]

Case Study 92 – Gluten Allergy (Schizophrenia)

Glenda, 33, claimed she had telepathic thoughts. She also had hallucinations. When she was diagnosed with schizophrenia and started medications, she developed severe diarrhea. A brain scan showed frontal cortex dysfunction. Blood testing revealed she had celiac disease.

When Glenda went on a gluten-free diet, a remarkable recovery began. In six months, all her psychiatric symptoms were gone, and her frontal cortex returned to normal. She was able to discontinue the use of antipsychotics and remained symptom-free at a one-year follow-up.[1104]

WHAT ARE ADDITIONAL RESOURCES?

- Gluten Sensitivity. www.glutenfreesociety.org.
- Celiac and bipolar. http://goo.gl/tZ4Mna.
- Celiac Disease Facts and Figures. http://goo.gl/HGKIQQ.
- Elimination diets. https://goo.gl/PybAjE, https://goo.gl/4UDdZE.

Detoxification Therapy

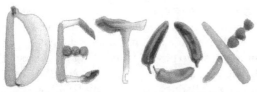

WHAT IS THE ESSENCE?

Certain classic neurotoxins, such as lead, mercury, and pesticides, are well known to cause mental health issues, but those are just the tip of the iceberg when it comes to toxic substances. It is perhaps not unexpected that the increasing occurrence of mental health symptoms in developed countries is associated with increasing exposure to toxic substances.

The techniques used to remove toxic substances from the body vary. In some cases, we just need to stop exposure to the offending substance or condition. In other cases, a strong intervention is required. For example, when heavy metals are detected, doctors turn to chelation: certain molecules bond with the metal ions and are then excreted.

WHAT EVIDENCE SHOWS THIS IS EFFECTIVE?

Heavy Metal Toxicity. Toxic levels of heavy metals that cause mental health issues[180] can often be detected using lab tests (typically, hair samples). Toxicity is most commonly caused by the following:

- **Aluminum.** Only a very small amount of orally ingested aluminum can be absorbed in the GI tract, and our kidneys effectively eliminate aluminum from the body. When the GI barrier is bypassed, however (particularly during intravenous infusions, dialysis, or advanced renal dysfunction), aluminum accumulates rapidly in the body.[1105] Aluminum levels in drinking water are correlated with Alzheimer's Disease rates in Britain.[1106]

- **Cadmium.** Cadmium is an extremely toxic metal commonly found in industrial workplaces. Acute exposure to cadmium fumes may cause "the cadmium blues." The concentration of cadmium is significantly higher in the hair samples of people with schizophrenia than those without the disorder.[1107]

- **Lead.** People are 3.4 times more likely to develop Alzheimer's if their jobs expose them to high levels of lead, either by breathing lead dust or from direct skin contact.[1108] One study showed a direct link between low-level long-term exposure to lead and both cognitive performance issues and childhood/adolescent behavior. Any lead content will affect the central nervous system.[1109]

- **Mercury.** In a group of 465 patients diagnosed as having chronic mercury toxicity (CMT), 32.3% reported severe fatigue, 88.8% had memory loss, and 27.5% suffered with depression.[1110] Mercury toxicity is associated with reduced neural uptake of norepinephrine and dopamine.[1111] Mercury can be ingested by eating some fish and shellfish (usually larger and older fish, see Figure 13, p. 65), breathing air from coal incinerators, or breathing vapors from burning fuels that contain mercury. Some dental and medical treatments can also lead to mercury toxicity.

Electromagnetic Fields (EMF). EMFs are produced by power, electrical, and wireless devices commonly found in the home, workplace, school, and community. EMFs affect the central nervous system, and there are reports of a link between EMFs and Alzheimer's Disease, insomnia, headaches, sexual dysfunction, chronic fatigue, learning, and memory issues and other neuropsychiatric problems.[1112] (See Case Study 94, p. 214. Also see *Earthing*, p. 255, as a potential approach to help address EMF exposure.)

- For *suicide and depression*. Higher rates of depressive symptoms and suicide have been associated with EMF exposure. Electrical utility workers have double the suicide rate of the general population, possibly because of melatonin depletion triggered by EMF exposure.[20] People living near power lines are more than twice as likely to suffer from depression.[1113]
- For *attention-deficit hyperactivity disorder*. Evidence suggests an association between EMF exposure and conduct problems in adolescents[1114] as well as a potential tie to ADD/ADHD.[1115]
- From a *broader perspective*, it shouldn't surprise us that our mental health can be influenced by Electromagnetic fields when we have an entire category of *Electromagnetic Therapies* (p. 244) that can strongly influence mental health.

Pesticides. The EPA banned the two most commonly used organophosphate (organic compounds containing phosphorus) pesticides from residential use in the year 2000. Pyrethroid pesticides are now the most commonly used pesticides for residential pest control; they appear to be much safer for humans.

- For *depression*. One study of 19,000 farm workers found that those exposed to high levels of organochlorine and fumigants pesticides were between 80% and 90% more likely to be diagnosed with depression.[1116]
- For *ADHD*. Boys who were exposed to pyrethroids were three times as likely to have ADHD. Hyperactivity and impulsivity increased as exposure to pyrethroids increased. The same does not seem to hold true for girls.[1117]
- *More broadly*. In tests using rats, pesticides altered their brain cells, neurotransmitters, and production of a protective acid.[1118]

Solvents.
- **Tetrachloroethylene (PCE)**. PCE is a neurotoxin and carcinogen that has been used to line water pipes in Massachusetts and as a dry-cleaning solvent. People with prenatal and early childhood exposure to PCE had elevated risks of bipolar and post-traumatic stress disorder, which increased among subjects with the highest exposures.[1119]

- **Carbon disulfide (CS2)**. CS2 is a volatile liquid used in insecticides, solvents, and other industrial applications. There is clear evidence that it can cause neurotoxic damage.[1120]
- **Hydrogen sulfide.** Both CS2 and hydrogen sulfide are neurotoxins that can affect moods and how we respond to stress. One study found that two neighborhoods experiencing ten times the state's suicide rate and 6.4 times the rate of brain cancers had a local asphalt plant emitting these neurotoxins into the atmosphere.[20]

WHAT CONSIDERATIONS SHOULD I KEEP IN MIND?

We all should take steps to minimize our exposure to toxins. Typically, the greatest exposure is at work or home. We should eliminate any lead paint or lead pipes in a safe and professional manner. We should also avoid aluminum cookware. Use organic lawn and garden products. Replace furnace air filters regularly. And keep a flow of fresh air through our homes. We should also avoid dry-cleaning services that use PCE.

If heavy metals are detected, chelation therapy is usually recommended. For milder situations, chelating agents such as garlic, Vitamin C, zinc, and amino acids are helpful.[1121] For more severe situations, ethylene diaminetetraacetic acid (EDTA) and other agents can be administered intravenously, intramuscularly, or orally.[1122]

Chelation agents bind with the heavy metals; both are then eliminated through urination. Chelation must be conducted by a specially trained medical professional, and only used in cases of known heavy-metal toxicity, since it contains inherent risks: allergic reactions, kidney damage, lowered levels of dietary elements, and in some cases, death. More than thirty deaths have been recorded with IV-administered EDTA since 1970.[1123] Over-the-counter chelation products are not approved for sale in the United States.

REAL-WORLD EXPERIENCE

Case Study 93 – Lead Toxicity (Depression)

John, at age 54, started fixing up an old house he had recently purchased. Not long after he began renovations, he developed severe depression, anger, and nausea. Psychotropics didn't help. A biochemical blood test revealed that the lead level in his blood was 80 times the normal level. He had been scraping lead-based paint from his home.

John was hospitalized and given chelation therapy to remove the lead. He was back to normal in a week. Doctors prescribed zinc, selenium, and Vitamin C to protect him from lead that might be slowly leaching from his bones.[19]

Case Study 94 – Electromagnetic Field Toxicity (Schizophrenia)

Denard, 17, had a three-year history of intrusive thoughts, as well as increasing depression. He became more and more aggressive toward his parents. Psychotropic medication failed to control the symptoms—in fact, they caused numerous side effects, which added to the family's misery.

Doctors finally determined that an extremely strong EMF was in his bedroom (>200 mGauss), caused by an electrical entry to the house that was right beside his bed. He changed bedrooms and all other sources of EMF exposure were minimized. Within twelve weeks, the intrusive thoughts abated considerably, the mood symptoms declined, the medication was stopped, and the parents reported that their son's behavior had completely turned around. He was friendly and motivated.

One episode of symptom aggravation occurred later, immediately after Denard spent four hours online in a high school computer lab. The symptoms subsided within 72 hours of deliberate EMF avoidance. All adverse symptoms completely cleared within six months, and he remained well over the next two years.[1112]

WHAT ARE ADDITIONAL RESOURCES?

- Toxic Metals and Mental Health. http://goo.gl/MMKjw5.
- Toxins. Multiple Chemical Sensitivity. http://goo.gl/yseS1z.
- Indoor pollutants. http://goo.gl/xYUz6E.

Pathogen Therapy

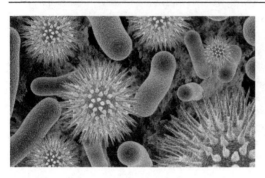

WHAT IS THE ESSENCE?

Living bacteria, viruses, parasites, and other infections appear to be able to cause mental health issues. While the psychiatric impact of infections is known, testing for infections is rarely a part of a mental health diagnostic process.

One of the greatest and most common bacterial threats is Strep; 15% to 40% of the cases of sore throats in children are caused by Strep.

WHAT EVIDENCE SHOWS THIS IS EFFECTIVE?

A variety of evidence suggests a tie between mental health and infections. One study of the medical records of over 3 million people found that those who had been hospitalized for an infection had a 62% increased risk of later developing a mood disorder.[1124] Schizophrenia is more common in those born in the winter months when infections or more prevalent.[1125] Additionally, one study found that 53% of patients in psychiatric hospitals had parasites.[1126]

Infections can activate the immune system and cause inflammation. A large body of research links autoimmune activity and inflammation with psychiatric symptoms. Although the list of possible infectious agents is endless, the following are some of the most common infections tied to mental health issues.

Algae Virus. Acanthocystis turfacea Chlorella virus 1 (ATCV-1) is an algae found commonly in streams and ponds. In one study, subjects with ATCV-1 had more difficulties with speed and accuracy in a test of visual processing.[1127]

Bartonella. Bartonella is a tick-born infection sometimes acquired from cat scratches. At least nine varieties have been discovered as human infections. Bartonella is well known to cause neurologic disorders, and researchers believe that it may also cause psychiatric disorders.[1128] The prevalence of Bartonella is not yet clear. (See Case Study 96, p. 219.)

Borna virus. The Borna virus infects a broad range of warm-blooded animals, from birds to primates. Infection causes movements and behavioral disturbances similar to some neuropsychiatric syndromes.[1129]

Candida Albicans. Candida, a yeast, is part of the normal human intestinal flora. However, studies have seen increased psychiatric symptoms in people with increased candida, including high rates of panic attacks, depression, and poor concentration.[1130] 26% of men with schizophrenia and bipolar (almost double the percentage of controls) had a current or previous candida infection.[1131] Common medical treatments, including antibiotics[1132] and anti-hyperchlorhydric agents, increase the risk of candida.[1133] Up to 75% of women experience at least one episode of vaginal candida in their lifetimes.[1134] (See Case Study 99, p. 219.)

Clostridia difficile. Clostridia difficile is a gut bacterium that can overgrow and release toxins that attack the intestinal lining. It is a major cause of infectious diarrhea in the United States. High levels of HPHPA (see p. 325) in the blood can be an indication of clostridia difficile, which also occurs with severe neurological and psychiatric disorders, including autism, severe depression, and schizophrenia.[1135] Psychotic individuals with high HPHPA have been successfully treated using Vancomycin (a bacterial antibiotic). Follow-up probiotics (e.g. Lactobacillus acidophilus) can prevent clostridia difficile from regaining a foothold. (See Case Study 97, p. 219.)

Fungus. Elevated serum creatine phosphokinase (CPK) MM level is often found in acute psychosis.[1136] Dr. Richard Jaeckle, a psychiatrist and allergist, finds that psychotic patients with elevated CPK, uric acid, and white cell counts may respond favorably to antifungal treatment.[1137]

Lupus. Individuals suffering from systemic lupus erythematosus (SLE) can develop several psychiatric conditions, including psychosis.[1138] Some medications prescribed to treat lupus—especially corticosteroids such as prednisone—can cause clinical depression.[1139] Lupus can affect the brain, and when that happens, one of the main symptoms is depression.[1140]

Lyme Disease.[1141] Lyme disease is an inflammatory disease characterized at first by a rash, headache, fever, and chills, and later by possible arthritis and neurological and cardiac disorders. It is caused by bacteria transmitted by ticks.

- For *depression*. Between 26% and 66% of patients with late Lyme disease exhibit depression.[1142]

- For *schizophrenia*. People suffering from psychosis are 2.6 times more likely to have Lyme in their system than the general population.[1143] The Western Blots Test can detect exposure to Borrelia burgdorferi (the bacteria that causes Lyme Disease). Doxycycline can relieve psychotic symptoms significantly.[1144] Lyme is difficult to diagnose, so consider a Lyme screening questionnaire.[1145] (See Case Study 98, p. 219.)

- *More broadly*. Lyme Disease is associated with several psychiatric conditions, including paranoia, dementia, schizophrenia, bipolar, panic attacks, depression, and obsessive-compulsive disorder. One study found deficits in memory and mental flexibility in people with Lyme disease.[1146]

Neurocysticercosis. The most common parasitic disease in the world, neurocysticercosis affects the central nervous system.[1147] It is found predominantly in Asia, Eastern Europe, and Latin America.

- *For depression*. One study in Brazil found that depressive symptoms are frequent in patients with neurocysticercosis.[1148]

- *Overall*, psychiatric issues are found in about 65% of neurocysticercosis cases, with depression and psychosis being the most common symptoms.[1148] (See Case Study 100, p. 220.)

Rickettsiae. A significant source of disease in the U.S., Rickettsiae (unrelated to the disease known as rickets) is a diverse collection of bacteria that can lie dormant in the body for months or even years. Rickettsiae is carried by lice, mites, and ticks, and is manifested in typhus, Rocky Mountain Spotted Fever, and other diseases.[1149] When properly identified, Rickettsiae can often be controlled with common antibiotics. Although headaches and rash are more common symptoms, depression, delusions, and hallucinations can occur in typhus strains of Rickettsiae. See (Case Study 101, p. 220.)

Strep (Streptococcus spp) Bacteria. Some children display obsessive-compulsive disorder behaviors after being infected with Strep.[1150] One animal study confirmed this tie by observing rat behaviors linked to antibodies in brain areas.[1151] This condition is sometimes called "pediatric autoimmune neuropsychiatric disorders associated with strep," or PANDAS.

Toxoplasma Gondii (T-gondii). About one-fifth of all people are infected with Toxoplasma gondii, a parasite transmitted in soil, uncooked meat, and feces. The research on T-gondii is mixed. One meta-analysis found that T-gondii infection is associated with schizophrenia, bipolar, and possibly addiction and OCD.[1152] Another estimates that as many as 20% of schizophrenia cases may be related to T-gondii,[1153] although that claim is repudiated by a third study that found no association between T-gondii and psychiatric symptoms.[1154]

WHAT CONSIDERATIONS SHOULD I KEEP IN MIND?

People living in or visiting areas with ticks and fleas should be alert to Lyme, Bartonella, and other sources of infection. Especially if you have recently visited foreign countries or tick-infested areas, have a complete evaluation for pathogens.

The course of the infection most relevant to psychiatry is a chronic, low-grade, persistent infection or an infection lying dormant. At a later point in time, some triggering event, like chronic stress, may activate the infectious agent.

Treatment for infections varies, but it often starts with antibiotics. One such antibiotic, Minocycline, penetrates the blood-brain barrier easily, and is often used to combat Lyme and Bartonella infections.[1144] Minocycline has been used to relieve symptoms for both schizophrenia[1155, 1156] and depression.[1157] If antibiotics are prescribed, restock gut flora with probiotics after antibiotic treatment.

Infections often lead to *Inflammation* (p. 52), a contributing factor to mental health symptoms. As a result, anti-inflammatory treatments including aspirin and *Cholesterol* (p. 53) may be helpful.

REAL-WORLD EXPERIENCE

Case Study 95 – Multiple infections (OCD, Depression)

John, 18, developed extreme compulsive behavior, mood swings, GI complaints and headaches. CBT and psychotropics helped little.

A practitioner grounded in Functional Medicine ran extensive tests and found five different pathogen infections including salmonella, Bartonella, and candida. John was given antibiotics, targeted nutrients and then probiotics to restore his gut microbiome. Within 12 weeks, all symptoms were gone.[1158]

Bottom Line: Look for pathogens as a part of normal psychiatric care.

Case Study 96 – Bartonella (Depression, Panic)

When three patients developed acute psychiatric disorders—dramatic personality changes, agitation, depression, and panic attacks — physicians found that each had been exposed to ticks or fleas. Physical symptoms indicated Bartonella, so they were given. All three significantly improved. Physical and mental health were restored once the Bartonella was cured.[1128]

Bottom Line: Ticks, lice, and fleas can carry pathogens. Exposure to areas known to harbor insects should alert us to the dangers of Bartonella.

Case Study 97 - Clostridia Difficile (OCD)

Jake was a young man who had significant obsessive-compulsive disorder symptoms. He was given multiple psychotropics and a variety of alternative treatments, including EMPowerplus, but nothing seemed to help. Then a blood test detected an elevated HPHPA marker that suggested the presence of Clostridia difficile, an unhelpful gut bacterium. Doctors started Jake on high doses of probiotics. He soon had a complete recovery of treatment-refractory OCD.[984a]

Bottom Line: The gut pumps out neurotransmitters used by the brain. Fixing simple gut issues may significantly help the brain.

Case Study 98 - Lyme Disease (Depression)

Three different people who had developed a psychiatric disorder for the first time after an infection of Lyme disease were interviewed. One reported major depression and panic disorder; the second suffered from depression and mania; the third had panic disorder.

Each of the three patients underwent antibiotic treatment for Lyme disease. The psychiatric symptoms for all three people disappeared.[1159]

Case Study 99 - Candida Albicans (Bipolar)

Kate, 24, had severe mood swings and was diagnosed with ADHC. She responded well to a micronutrient treatment, experiencing improvements in all her psychiatric symptoms.

She maintained the treatment and was stable for two years. However, her psychiatric symptoms worsened when she developed a candida infection.

Her candida was treated with olive-leaf extract, probiotics and micronutrients. In two months, Kate was free of psychiatric symptoms.[1134]

Bottom Line: The gut-brain axis is vital to mental health. Kate's axis was compromised by candida, which inhibited micronutrient absorption.

Case Study 100 - Neurocysticercosis (Schizophrenia)

Kumar lived in India. Over three months, he saw a gradual change in behavior, including delusions of persecution. He also suffered a seizure. Doctors diagnosed schizophrenia and gave him anti-seizure medication. They noticed several small movable nodules under his skin, but that did not influence the diagnosis.

When his psychosis did not improve, Kumar took a blood test and CT scan. They revealed markers for neurocysticercosis. He was placed on albendazole to target the parasite. Three months later, the nodules under his skin disappeared, and so did his delusions.[1160]

Bottom Line: *If you live in, or have traveled to, an area where neurocysicercosis is present, you should test for possible infection.*

Case Study 101 - Brill Zinsser Disease (Panic, Delusions)

Several times a year, Rachel's life unraveled—and this had been going on for decades. She experienced crippling bouts of fever, panic, paranoia, and delusions. She said she saw visions of her deceased parents.

Dozens of psychiatrists examined her over the years, all coming up with the same "obvious" diagnosis: depression and panic caused by traumas during her war-torn early life. They prescribed antidepressants and psychotherapy, but nothing stopped the attacks.

Her new psychiatrist looked deeper, however, and observed that as a child, she lived in an area where Rickettsiae was prevalent. He tested her for the parasite and found she had Brill Zinsser disease. Doses of common antibiotics ended Rachel's debilitating attacks for the rest of her life.[1161]

Bottom Line*: Seemingly irrelevant questions like, "Where did you live as a child?" may identify the solution to a lifetime of debilitating symptoms. Seek practitioners who think outside of the small box of psychotropics.*

WHAT ARE ADDITIONAL RESOURCES?

- PANDAS. www.pandasnetwork.org.

6 – Symptom Relief Therapies

The third category of the *Wellness Continuum* (Figure 9, p. 47) includes *Symptom Relief Therapies* (Figure 30). These approaches do not seek to cure; instead, they help minimize the presence, impact, and discomfort of mental health symptoms, thereby reducing stress, improving functioning, and gaining a greater sense of well-being.

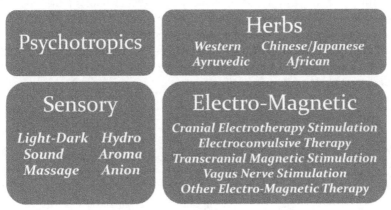

Figure 30 - Symptom Relief Therapies

Their relief is temporary, so recurring use is required to manage the symptoms.

Because everyone responds differently to drugs and *Symptom Relief* therapies, rarely will lab tests identify the optimum response. The therapies to consider include:

- **Psychotropics**. By far the most widely studied and widely prescribed *Symptom Relief* therapy, drugs offer benefits and limitations. (See *Changes in Treatment*, p. 24.) They can be essential for stabilizing patients in crisis, typically providing fast-acting symptom relief that may be complete but is more often partial. And their symptom relief comes at a cost: side effects. Physicians often prescribe more than one psychotropic at a time (*polypharmacy*), a practice that is sometimes appropriate, often overused, and rarely studied sufficiently to confirm the safety of such a practice. (See *Over-Care Avoidance*, p. 257.) Unfortunately, a comprehensive review of psychotropics would require a book many times the size and scope of this book.

- **Herbal Therapies** are plant-based remedies often grounded in traditional medical practices spanning Western, Ayurvedic (India), Chinese/Japanese, and African medicinal practices. Most have small but growing evidence of their efficacy, but they do have a measure of historical validity from sustained use over centuries. They have far fewer and milder side effects than psychotropics.

- **Sensory Therapies** seek calming relief by stimulating or quieting one of the five senses to reduce stress and promote relaxation.

- **Electromagnetic Therapies** apply electricity or magnetism to the central nervous system. With one exception, they use low-amplitude energy: *Electroconvulsive Therapy* can use up to 500 volts, sufficient to induce convulsions and cause persistent memory loss—which makes it the most controversial therapy in mental health. The low-amplitude therapies have little or no side effects. We lack a good understanding on why Electromagnetic therapies work, but it appears that some regions of the brain can steer the brain into a variety of states very easily when stimulated, while other regions have less effect.[1162]

Herbal Therapy

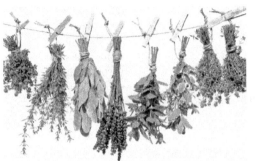

WHAT IS THE ESSENCE?

Herbal Therapy is based on the use of plant-based substances for symptom relief, while *Nutrient Therapy* (p. 167) uses substances that occur naturally in the body.

Both influence bodily processes biochemically. Both have mild (if any) side effects, and their efficacy varies from person to person, based on the individual's biochemical individuality. Although we have put *Nutrient Therapy* in **Biomedical Restorative** and *Herbal Therapy* in **Symptom Relief,** both can have restorative and relief characteristics.

Psychiatric research on herbs is limited, but rapidly growing. The primary reason for this is economic: research funding is much lower for herbs than for psychotropics, since the profit potential from herbal sales is much lower. However, available clinical evidence shows that many herbs are a viable alternative for symptom relief, as many cultures attest.

Leading Integrative Mental Health doctors believe that the safety factor for herbals weighs heavily in favor of experimenting with them, despite limited scientific research.[15] **However, herbs can have psychotropic properties that may interact with prescription medication.** Therefore, always work with certified and skilled practitioners trained in the specific school of medicine that uses a particular herb and investigate the latest research for safety and effectiveness. Also, take herbs in minimal effective dosages, starting low.

This section contains four subsections, each with herbs from different geographic origins: **Western, Chinese/Japanese/Kampo, Ayurvedic (India), and African.** The evidence is dense and comprehensive, incorporating results from clinical trials across a broad array of herbs. As a result, *the best way to use this section is as an encyclopedic reference.* Skim it for evidence related to a diagnosis that interests you or use it to see how a particular herb influences a variety of diagnoses.

Western Herbs

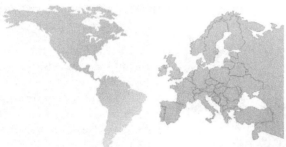

Western herbs are grown and used most commonly in the Americas and Europe. Some species are variable, depending on where they are grown.

American Skullcap (Scutellaria lateriflora). Skullcap can refer to two herbs: American skullcap and Chinese skullcap (Scutellaria baicalensis). Both forms are used to treat different conditions and are not interchangeable. American skullcap is native to North America, but is now widely cultivated in Europe and other areas of the world. It has been used for more than 200 years as a mild relaxant and as a therapy for anxiety, nervous tension, and convulsions.

- For *anxiety*, a placebo-controlled trial found that skullcap reduced generalized anxiety and tension in healthy volunteers.[1163]

Anthocyanin. Anthocyanins are water-soluble pigments belonging to a class of molecules called flavonoids. They occur in all tissues of higher plants; blueberries, raspberries, and red cabbage are especially rich in anthocyanins, which have antioxidant and neuroprotective properties.

- For *alcohol abuse.* Anthocyanin decreases the negative effect of alcohol in rats; no substantive research is available to date involving humans.[1164]
- For *cognitive decline.* Ample research indicates that *Oxidative Stress* (p. 52) is responsible for age-related cognitive decline. A study on rats suggests that the antioxidant properties of anthocyanin may reverse certain neurological and behavioral aging.[1165]

Borage. A dried flower extract of Echium amoenum (Boraginaceae), borage has been used for centuries to reduce anxiety, improve mood, and reduce inflammation. It originated in Iran and some Mediterranean countries, but is found throughout the world. All borage trials indicated below were led by the same researcher.

- For *depression.* Borage shows significant superiority over the placebo in reducing depressive symptoms and anxiety.[1166]
- For *obsessive-compulsive disorder.* Borage significantly reduced OCD and anxiety symptoms over the placebo.[1167]
- For *anxiety.* When added to an SSRI (a common antidepressant), borage significantly reduced anxiety without side effects,[1168] as compared to SSRI plus placebo.

California Poppy (Eschscholzia californica). A flowering plant native to the United States and Mexico, the California poppy has sedative properties so mild that children can take it, so it is a component in a variety of herbal remedies. Although it is in the same family as the potent Oriental poppy, its active ingredients are alkaloids, not opioids. It is often consumed as a tea, with one-quarter ounce of dried extract added to six or eight ounces of boiling water.

- For *anxiety*. One randomized controlled trial determined that a combination of California poppy, calcium, and hawthorn reduced anxiety significantly more than the placebo.[1169]

Cannabidiol. Cannabidiol (CBD) is a non-psychoactive constituent of cannabis (marijuana) that offers anti-inflammatory properties. CBD is distinct from other cannabis constituents including tetrahydrocannabinol (THC) that can make you "high", and cannabinol. The legal status of CBD varies.

- For *schizophrenia*. A clinical trial found that CBD can reduce psychotic symptoms significantly and in a way similar to antipsychotics, but the side effects are much less.[1170] Although the evidence is not extensive, most studies of people with and without schizophrenia suggest that CBD has antipsychotic properties. (See Case Study 103, p. 237.)
- For *anxiety*. A number of animal studies confirm CBD's ability to reduce anxiety and interfere with the memory of traumatic events akin to post-traumatic stress disorder.[1171] Other studies suggest that CBD inhibits anxiety and psychotic symptoms.[1172]
- For *depression*. Although there are no human studies of the effects of CBD on depression, studies on rats suggest it may be effective.[1171]
- *Safety*. One analysis reviewed more than 130 papers assessing the impact of CBD on humans and animals and found, although more research is needed, "Several studies suggest that CBD is well tolerated and safe in humans at high doses and with chronic use."[1173]

Chamomile. Chamomile is the common name for several daisy-like plants of the family Asteraceae. It is most often used as tea to calm an upset stomach or to help with sleep.

- For *depression*. One small well-designed study found depressive symptoms were significantly reduced in those taking chamomile as compared to the placebo.[1174]
- For *anxiety*. Chamomile significantly reduces anxiety compared to the placebo at the end of eight weeks of treatment.[1175]

Corydalis (Corydalis favela). A plant native to the northern hemisphere and Africa, corydalis can influence the nervous system, providing pain relief and promoting relaxation.

- For *insomnia*. Preliminary evidence shows that people were able to fall sleep more easily after taking 100 or 200 mg/day of a corydalis extract (cdl-tetrahydropalmatine) without drug hangover symptoms such as dizziness or vertigo.[1176]

Damiana (Turnera diffusa). Damiana is a small shrub with aromatic leaves found on dry, sunny, rocky hillsides in Texas, Southern California and Latin America. It belongs to the family Passifloraceae. The native people of Mexico have used it as a general tonic for wellness, and to help cure asthma, depression, impotence, and menstrual problems.

- For *anxiety*. Mother tinctures (85% ethanol extracts) of Damiana have shown significant anti-anxiety potential.[1177]

Echinacea (Purple Cone Flower). Echinacea is an herb in the daisy family. The Great Plains Indian tribes used it for at least four centuries and Germans use it to heal urinary tract infections. It has also been prescribed as a natural cancer treatment, to boost the immune system, alleviate pain (toothaches, headaches, measles) and respiratory issues, and as a laxative and anti-inflammatory.

- For *anxiety*. Three varieties of Echinacea have reduced three different measures of anxiety with consistent results.[1178]
- *Safety*. Echinacea has an excellent safety profile.

Galanthus (snowdrop). An herb in the Amaryllis family that grows in Europe, the Middle East, and North America from bulbs, Galanthus produces a bell-like white flower without petals. Galantamine is an extract used in the treatment of mild to moderate Alzheimer's Disease and various other memory impairments, in particular those of vascular origin.

- For *dementia*. In a meta-analysis of more than 2,000 people with Alzheimer's, those receiving galantamine had statistically significant improvements in hallucinations, anxiety, apathy, and aberrant motor behaviors.[1179]

Galphimia glauca. Widely used for mental and emotional issues, Galphimia glauca is extracted from a small evergreen shrub found in Mexico and Central America.

- For *generalized anxiety disorder*. In comparison to lorazepam (a psychotropic), Galphimia showed greater effectiveness and high percentages of therapeutic tolerability and safety.[1180]

Ginseng. Ginseng is a slow-growing perennial in the genus Panax that has been credited with improving cognition and energy. Several species are components in Eastern and Western medicine. When taken regularly, it has cumulative strengthening effects as a psychotherapeutic agent.[1181]

- For *insomnia*. Various forms of ginseng are widely used for insomnia, daytime fatigue, and sleepiness. Doses of between 200 and 600 mg/day seem to be effective at enhancing daytime wakefulness. A 40-mg dose significantly improves daytime wakefulness and sleep quality in healthy adults.[1182]

- For *schizophrenia*. Ginseng significantly improves working memory.[1183] American ginseng has antipsychotic-like properties that may benefit negative and cognitive symptoms of schizophrenia.[1184]
- For *dementia*. A Mayo Clinic study found that ginseng has a protective quality against Alzheimer's Disease, due to its antioxidant properties.[1185]
- *Safety*. Ginseng is usually well-tolerated,[16] but can produce restlessness, nervousness, insomnia, or agitation.[1186] Short-term use of ginseng at recommended doses appears to be safe for most people,[1187] but should not be used with MAOIs (a class of tranquilizers) or caffeinated products.[16]

Hops (Humulus lupulus). A mild sedative, hops grows in the northern hemisphere. This plant is used most notably in the manufacture of beer.
- For *insomnia*. One study found that hop compounds increased the ketamine-induced sleeping time and reduced body temperature, confirming its sedating effect for insomnia.[1188]

Kava kava (Piper methysticum or Kava). Originating in Polynesia, the mild narcotic and hypnotic known as kava is of great cultural significance to Pacific Islanders, who still drink it as a relaxing non-alcoholic beverage; they trace its use back to antiquity.
- For *anxiety*. In more than a dozen Randomized Controlled Trials (RCT), kava has been shown to be effective for treating generalized—but not severe—anxiety.[24] A Cochrane Review of eleven studies found that kava was better than a placebo for short-term treatment of generalized anxiety, and its effectiveness compares favorably with benzodiazepines and other anti-anxiety drugs—but with fewer side effects.[16] In a 25-week RCT, WS 1490 (a kava extract) was significantly superior to the placebo, starting from the eighth week of use. Adverse effects are rare.[1189]
- *Safety*. Kava is generally considered safe for short-term use. It is estimated that 250 million daily doses of kava were prescribed in the 1990s, with only two cases of hepatoxicity.[1190] However, in rare cases, it may cause severe liver damage and interact with alcohol and other drugs. It should only be used with practitioner supervision and *never with an MAOI inhibitor (a tranquilizer)*. Some countries have banned kava, but a growing number of them have reversed that ban.

Lavender. Lavender is a fragrant flowering plant in the mint family. English lavender is the most common species, although there are many others.
- For *depression*. Lavender tincture (1:5 in 50% alcohol) taken as 60 drops/day improved symptoms when used with an antidepressant.[1191]
- For *insomnia*. Lavender is useful in aiding sleep, when applied as aromatherapy.[1192]

Lemon Balm (Melissa Officinalis). Lemon balm is a perennial herb from the mint family whose leaves have a mild lemon aroma. It was used alone or in multi-herb combinations as far back as the Middle Ages to reduce stress and anxiety, promote sleep, improve appetite, and ease pain and discomfort from indigestion. It is sometimes combined with valerian, hops, and chamomile.

- For *stress and anxiety*. In one RCT, lemon balm was found to significantly improve calmness.[1193]
- *Safety*. No serious side effects have been identified.[15]

Milk Thistle (Silybum marianum). Milk thistle has been used medicinally for over 2,000 years, particularly in Iran, most commonly for the treatment of liver, kidney, and gallbladder disorders.

- For *obsessive-compulsive disorder*. One RCT found that 600 mg daily of milk thistle was as effective as Prozac.[1194]
- For *alcohol abuse*. Numerous RCTs confirm it can successfully treat alcohol-induced liver damage.[778]
- *Safety*. In clinical trials, milk thistle appears to be well tolerated.[1195]

Nicotine patch. A patch impregnated with nicotine can be worn on the skin to deliver a continuous nicotine dose that can help smokers quit.

- For *major depression*. Nicotine patches can produce short-term improvement in depression, with only minor side effects for non-smokers.[1196]

Periwinkle (Vinca minor). A low-growing flowering plant native to Europe, Asia, and Turkey, periwinkle has been used to reduce swelling, treat toothaches, improve concentration and blood pressure, and for a drying effect on injured tissues. Vinpocetine is a chemical made from vincamine, which is an extract of periwinkle.

- For *dementia*. One sixteen-week study found that vinpocetine helped improve cognitive performance, quality of life, and depression,[1197] while another found that it can improve cognition and memory in people with dementia who have hardening of the arteries in the brain.

Psilocybin. Psilocybin is a hallucinogenic found in some toadstools.

- For *obsessive-compulsive disorder*. Psilocybin was safely used and several subjects had acute reductions in core OCD symptoms.[1198]

Rhodiola Rosea. Rhodiola rosea (a.k.a. "golden root" or "arctic root") is a perennial flowering plant that grows in cold regions. Eurasian traditional medicine used it as a natural tonic to improve mental and physical performance under stress.[15]

- For *anxiety*. A small pilot study found that 340 mg/day for ten weeks resulted in a significant decrease in generalized anxiety disorder symptoms.[1199]
- For *PTSD*. In people with PTSD, a rhodiola rosea extract can protect brain cells from an overabundance of glutamate (a neurotransmitter), which causes over-excitement and anxiety.[1200]
- *More generally*. An RCT shows it may significantly improve depression, insomnia, and emotional instability.[1201]

St. John's Wort (Hypericum perforatum). One of the most well-researched herbs, St. John's Wort is a flowering perennial plant found in the United States, Europe, and Asia.

- For *mild-to-moderate depression.* Twenty-three randomized controlled trials focused on mild or moderately severe depressive disorders were conducted with St. John's Wort and a placebo. Compared to the placebo, the St. John's Wort groups showed significantly superior results, similar to those of standard antidepressants.[1202]

- For *moderate to major depression.* Studies are inconclusive but appear to be leaning toward endorsing its effectiveness. Two studies, later criticized, found St. John's Wort ineffective.[1203] A more recent study found major improvement in treating depression,[1204] with one showing better symptom relief than psychotropics.[1205] The proprietary Schwabe St. John's Wort formula appears to be effective for major depression.[24]

- For *bipolar.* One study suggests that St. John's Wort may cause mania or psychosis in some people with bipolar disorder, although a cause/effect relationship has not been established.[1206]

- For *obsessive-compulsive disorder.* One study found it can provide significant improvement,[1207] but a contradictory study found little benefit.[1208]

- For *insomnia.* It may provide significantly better sleep quality for depressed patients.[16]

- For *alcohol abuse.* St. John's Wort can reduce voluntary alcohol intake[1209] and alcohol withdrawal symptoms in rats.[1210]

- *Safety.* St. John's Wort is generally well tolerated, but can decrease the effectiveness of certain drugs (including antidepressants and birth control pills).[1211] It can also induce mania or hypomania in susceptible individuals and result in a photosensitive rash for those exposed to prolonged sunlight.[16] Side effects tend to ramp with dosages. *It is recommended that St. John's Wort not be used with MAOIs* (an early class of antidepressants). (See *Passion Flower*, p. 232.)

Valerian (Valeriana officinalis). Valerian is a perennial flowering plant with sweetly scented pink or white flowers. A botanical medicine popular with Europeans, it has mild sedative and tranquilizing properties.

- For *insomnia.* A review of sixteen RCTs found that six showed improved sleep with valerian, while nine did not.[1212] One meta-analysis concluded that a dose of 600 to 900 mg at bedtime improved sleep quality with few side effects.[1213] The German Commission E recommends a dosage of 2 to 3 grams of the dried root one or more times a day for "restlessness and nervous disturbance of sleep."[1214]

- *Safety.* In humans, valerian is thought to be fairly safe, although side effects may occur: headache, dizziness, stomach problems, or sleeplessness.[1215]

Chinese/Japanese Herbs

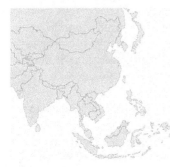

Various closely-related medical systems have developed in Asia, with *Traditional Chinese Medicine* (TCM) being the most prevalent. *Kampo Medicine* is a variant of TCM, adapted to the Japanese culture. Often Chinese and Japanese remedies are made with multiple herbs, so it is difficult to determine the impact of individual herbs. *TCM/Kampo herbs should be used under the guidance of a practitioner well-trained in the appropriate traditional medicine.*

Aralia elata. Aralia elata is a component within traditional Chinese herbal formulas. Oleanolic acid (OLA) is derived from roots and leaves of aralia elata.

- For *alcohol abuse*. Aralia elata can decrease acute alcohol intoxication, possibly by reducing alcohol absorption in the gut. It also appears to reverse alcohol-related liver damage in rats.[1216]

Betel Nut (areca catechu). The areca nut is the seed of the areca palm, which grows in the tropical Pacific, Asia, and parts of east Africa. Commonly referred to as betel nut, it is often chewed while wrapped in betel leaves.

- For *schizophrenia*. Chewing a betel nut is associated with lowering positive[1217] and negative symptoms.[1218]

Centella asiatica (gotu kola). A perennial common in Asia, Centella asiatica has been used to treat many conditions for thousands of years in India, China, and Indonesia, both individually and in a compound known as *Madhya Ramayana*. It is not to be confused with kola nut (Cola nitida), which contains caffeine and should be avoided in cases of anxiety.

- For *anxiety*. An open trial[1219] and a double-blind randomized trial[1220] found Centella asiatica effective to reduce anxiety symptoms, including the startle response to loud noises.
- *More broadly*. It can significantly help anxiety-related disorders by reducing stress and associated depression.[1221]

Chaihu-Shugan-San. CSS is a well-known Chinese herbal preparation used for conditions involving depression.

- For *depression*. Meta-analyses based on six Randomized Controlled Trials indicated that CSS in combination with various SSRIs was more effective than antidepressant drugs alone.[1222, 1223]

Chaihu Xiaoyao (CXM). CXM is a traditional Chinese medicine compound.

- For *major depression*. Combining CXM and an antidepressant (paroxetine) is more effective than using the antidepressant alone, and CXM can enhance the drug's effectiveness with greater safety.[1224]

  Chotosan. Chotosan is an eleven-herb compound of TCM.
- For *dementia*. Chotosan is effective in treating vascular dementia, and has been associated with global improvement in psychiatric symptoms.[1225]

  Free and Easy Wanderer Plus (FEWP). Free & Easy Wanderer (Xiao Yao San, Xiao Yao Wan, XYS) and Free & Easy Wander Plus (FEWP, Jia Wei Xiao Yao San) are two of the most widely prescribed herbal extracts in American TCM clinics. XYS typically contains eight herbs: Bupleurum root, Chinese angelica root, white peony root, poria, bighead atractylodes rhizome, roasted ginger, prepared licorice root, menthol and peppermint.
- For *depression*. A meta-analysis found that XYS appears to be effective for depression.[1226] One trial showed significant improvement with FEWP, equal to that of antidepressants.[1227]
- For *bipolar*. When FEWP was given to 50 patients with bipolar, 26 showed marked improvement, 17 had some improvement, and 7 patients showed no improvement.[1228]
- For *PTSD*. Earthquake survivors with PTSD given XYS with additional herbs had significantly better symptom relief for depression, anxiety, hostility and obsessive-compulsive behavior than a placebo group.[1229]

  Ginkgo biloba. Ginkgo biloba is considered to be the oldest living tree species. Ginkgo leaf extracts are widely prescribed in Europe and are among the bestselling herbs in the United States. More than 400 studies have evaluated ginkgo, most of them originating in Germany. It appears to have antioxidant, anti-inflammatory, and neuroprotective characteristics. An anticoagulant, gingko may influence insulin, sugar, and blood pressure.
- For *anxiety*. A four-week RCT using between 240 mg and 480 mg of ginkgo extract (EGb761) found it reduced anxiety significantly.[1230]
- For *schizophrenia*. A meta-analysis found that when used with antipsychotics, it can improve cognitive function and positive (but not negative) symptoms. Using gingko may mean lower dosages of antipsychotics could be effective.[1231]
- For *insomnia*. A dosage of 240 mg/day when used with conventional antidepressants in depressed people may improve sleep quality and reduce their nighttime awakenings.[1232]
- For *dementia*. Meta-analyses have shown ginkgo provides significant benefit for symptoms of cognitive deficiencies[1233] and major neuroprotective factors for treating memory problems.[24] A trial found that Alzheimer's patients taking ginkgo scored significantly higher on cognitive tests than the control group after one year of treatment.[1234] Although some trials suggest ginkgo

can't prevent Alzheimer's disease, Mental Health America indicates ginkgo may be considered as an evidence-based treatment for mild and possibly early dementia, with limited benefit in delaying or avoiding some of the symptoms of Alzheimer's Disease.[24]

- *Safety*. The toxicity of ginkgo is very low,[1181] although it may have an anticoagulant effect, so caution should be used when treating patients with clotting disorders.[24] In addition, mild gastrointestinal upset, dizziness, irregular heartbeat, and allergic skin reactions may occur.[16] Commonly available ginkgo products may be different than the preparations used in clinical studies. *EGb 761 is the only preparation of ginkgo that should be used.[1235]*

Huperzine-A (Huperzia serrata or *qiang ceng ta*). A Chinese moss produces Huperzine-A. Its derivative, ZT-1, is being developed as a new drug for dementia.

- For *schizophrenia*. A pilot trial found that Huperzine-A had beneficial effects in treating cognitive and negative symptoms of schizophrenia.[1236]
- For *dementia*. Huperzine-A may positively influence general cognitive function, behavioral disturbance, and functional performance, with no obvious adverse effects in patients with Alzheimer's Disease.[1237]

Kudzu (Pueraria lobata and Pueraria flos). Pueraria lobate (root-based) and Pueraria flos (flower-based) are extracts from the herb Kudzu, which enhances alcohol removal from the body. This is a traditional hangover remedy.[1238]

- For *alcohol abuse*. The kudzu extract reduced alcohol (beer) consumption.[1239] However, it did not appear to affect cravings or abstinence.[1240]

Passionflower (Passiflora incarnata). Passionflower is a name for approximately 400 species of the genus Passiflora, which are primarily vines, some of them with showy flowers, others with edible fruit. Passionflower is used as a mild sedative, often in combination with other herbs.

- For *anxiety*. A four-week RCT using 45 drops of passionflower extract found it as effective as oxazepam (an anti-anxiety psychotropic) in reducing anxiety, but with fewer side effects.[1241] Another RCT using 500 mg of passionflower concluded that it reduced pre-surgery anxiety much better than a placebo.[1242] A third trial found that patients receiving a six-extract formula (Passiflora, Crataegus, Ballota, Valeriana, Cola, and Paullinia) showed improved anxiety symptoms over the placebo.[1243]
- For *depression*. Passionflower can significantly enhance the potency of St. John's Wort, which is used to treat depression.[1244]
- For *substance abuse*. When used with clonidine (a drug that lowers blood pressure and reduces heart rate), it significantly decreased the psychological symptoms of withdrawal from opioid dependence.[1245]

Saffron (Crocus sativus). Saffron is a spice derived from the flowering plant commonly known as the "saffron crocus".

- For *depression*. Four trials found saffron stigma extract to be more effective than a placebo and equivalent to psychotropics in effectiveness, while two studies found saffron petal extract significantly more effective than a placebo and the equivalent to fluoxetine when taken with saffron stigma extract.[1246, 1463] Saffron can improve mild to moderate depression.[1247]

Schisandria Chinensis Bail. Of Chinese origin, Schisandria Chinensis Bail is also used extensively in Russia as a tonic reputed to have a variety of health benefits.

- For *schizophrenia*. Its benefits may be similar to those of an antipsychotic.[1248]

Yoku-kan-san-ka-chimpi-hange (Yokukansan, yi-gan san, YGS). YGS is a seven-herb remedy widely used in traditional Japanese herbal medicine for over 500 years, to help restlessness in children.

- For *insomnia*. YGS is used to increase the duration and quality of sleep.[16] One study found markedly increased sleep time and efficiency in stage-two sleep, while decreasing the time it took to fall asleep.[1249]
- For *dementia*. It might be effective for dementia associated with Alzheimer's Disease, Lewy Body Disease, Parkinson's Disease with dementia, frontotemporal dementia, and vascular dementia.[1250]
- For *schizophrenia*. YGS has been shown to improve hostility symptoms,[1251] decrease psychosis in late-onset cases,[1252] and reduce both positive and negative symptoms in those with psychosis.[1253]

Other Chinese/Eastern herbal compounds for depression. A variety of Chinese and other traditional herbal medicines have shown efficacy for depression. This includes *Danzhi Xiaoyao Powder* (for symptom improvement of depression),[1254] *Ganmai Dazao* (to reduce side effects and enhance efficacy of antidepressants),[1255] *Jieyu Pil* (as effective as an antidepressant, but with less adverse reaction),[1256] *Xiong-gui-tiao-xue-yin* (shows significant benefit for postpartum depression),[1257] and many others.

Ayurvedic Herbs

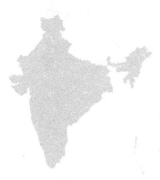

Ayurvedic herbs are a component of broader Ayurvedic medicine, India's ancient health and healing system, which is based on the integration of body, mind, and spirit; three *doshas*, or bioenergic principles must be in balance to promote healing, according to practitioners.

In Ayurvedic medicine, a person's doshas define his or her unique "constitution," including strengths and vulnerabilities. This concept is similar to *Biochemical Individuality* (p. 166) found in much of *Nutrient Therapy*.

Ayurvedic therapies encompass dietary changes, herbal remedies, oil massage, aromatherapy, sound therapy, color therapy, yoga, and breathing exercises. *Ayurvedic herbs should be used under the guidance of a trained Ayurvedic practitioner. It is important to note that one-fifth of U.S.-manufactured and Indian-manufactured Ayurvedic products bought on the Internet contained detectable lead, mercury, or arsenic.*[1258]

Brahmi (Bacopa monnieri or Aindri). Grown throughout India, Bacopa monnieri is a small creeping herb with antioxidant properties. The principle ingredient in the compounded herbal formula Mentat, since antiquity, Bacopa monnieri has been used as a sedative and relaxant for neuropsychiatric diagnoses, epilepsy, and insomnia.

- For *anxiety*. In an open clinical trial, subjects showed significant reduction in anxiety after between two and four weeks of treatment.[1259] A well-designed trial in Australia found a significant drop in anxiety after twelve weeks using Brahmi.[1260]
- *More broadly*. This well-tolerated herb is effective in treating depression and as an aid for cognitive functioning.[1261]

Brahmyadiyoga. Brahmyadiyoga is an herbal compound containing Brahmi (above) and other Ayurvedic drugs, including Rauwolfia serpentina (below, which is a known antipsychotic[1262]).

- For *schizophrenia*. Several studies of Brahmyadiyoga show positive outcomes, although it has only been tested in small trials.[1263]

Curcumin (turmeric). One of the most prevalent nutritional and medicinal compounds in India, curcumin is anti-inflammatory and anti-oxidant.

- For *major depression*. Curcumin may be used as an effective and safe treatment for depression.[1264]
- For *dementia*. Curcumin can inhibit the formation of plaque found in the brains of Alzheimer's Disease (AD) patients. Curcumin supplements "may correct immune defects of AD patients and provide a previously uncharacterized approach to AD immunotherapy."[1265]

Geriforte. Geriforte is an Ayurvedic medicine whose primary ingredient is chyawanprash, an ancient tonic for delaying aging and boosting immunity. It is often prescribed for those dealing with stress, anxiety, and fatigue.

- For *anxiety*. Evidence suggests that geriforte may reduce generalized anxiety symptoms.[1266]

Mentat (BR-16A). A widely used compounded Ayurvedic herbal formula, Mentat includes the herb Shankhapushpi, which appears to have neuroprotective and beneficial antioxidant properties.

- For *depression*. A small study found that Mentat improved self-confidence and depression without side effects.[1267]
- For *schizophrenia*. A small study of patients who agreed to a three-week wash-out of antipsychotics saw significant improvement in both positive and negative symptoms.[1268]
- For *alcohol abuse*. Mentat shows promise in reducing relapse for abstinent alcoholics.[1269]

Rauwolfia serpentina (Indian snakeroot or sarpagandha). Rauwolfia serpentina is a flowering perennial shrub native to India and East Asia. Its roots are a traditional Ayurvedic treatment for insomnia, anxiety, and schizophrenia.[1270] Reserpine, an extract of this plant, is used as an Ayurvedic tranquilizer and was the first medication found to be effective for treating psychosis. Reserpine was widely used for schizophrenia before tranquilizing psychotropics were introduced in the mid-1950's.[1271]

- For *schizophrenia and psychosis*. Reserpine has been used to calm psychosis. Seven of eight double-blind studies from the 1950s found Resperine was associated with clinical improvement in most patients, with four of these studies showing significant improvement.[1272] Studies suggest that dosages of 7mg/day may be needed for significant improvement.
- For *bipolar*. In a small case set, bipolar patients who were acutely manic and had not responded to lithium and antipsychotics improved dramatically when their antipsychotic was replaced with Rauwolfia serpentine.[1273] Reserpine does show promise in the management of manic episodes resistant to lithium and typical antipsychotics.[1274]
- *Safety*. Reserpine may worsen depressive moods, so *Reserpine should not be used by people with depression*.[16] Trials from the 1950s suggest that a gradual increase of Reserpine from 5mg/day to 8-12 mg/day reduces some side effects. A more recent review of earlier studies advised that Reserpine should be considered only after reasonable alternatives have failed.[1272]

Withania somnifera (Ashwagandha, Indian ginseng, poison gooseberry, or winter cherry). Withania somnifera is a plant in the nightshade family. It is frequently used alone for insomnia, agitation, and anxiety, thanks to its sedative-hypnotic and mood-stabilizing properties.

- For *bipolar*. Preliminary studies indicate that withania somnifera improves auditory-verbal working memory, reaction time, and social cognition.[1275]
- For *anxiety*. A meta-analysis of five studies found that Withania somnifera improved anxiety or stress symptoms better than placebo, with significant improvement in most cases.[1276]

   Additional Ayurvedic Compounds. Ayurvedic herbs are often combined in a wide variety of compounds.

- For *depression*. Kushmanda Ghrita,[1277] Mucuna pruriens, Acorus calamus, Convolvulus pluricaulis, and Celastrus panniculatus have all shown positive results in depression trials. Generally, Ayurvedic herbs are used in combination for depression.

African Herbs

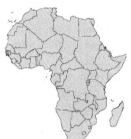

Alstonine. Alstonine is a plant-based extract used by traditional psychiatrists in Nigeria.

- For *schizophrenia*. Alstonine has antipsychotic effects, according to anecdotal evidence.[1278]

   Crassocephalum bauchiense leaf. This traditional Cameroon medicine has been used to treat epilepsy, insomnia, dementia, and psychotic disorders.

- For *schizophrenia*. A study of its use in rats found antipsychotic and sedative properties.[1279]

   Jobelyn. Used in Nigeria for a variety of medicinal purposes, jobelyn is an herb derived from sorghum bicolour.

- For *schizophrenia*. It exhibits antipsychotic-like activity without antipsychotic side effects, and may reduce psychotic symptoms.[1280]

   Yohimbine. Yohimbine comes from the bark of the Pausinystalia yohimbe tree in Central Africa.

- For *narcolepsy*. At 8 mg/day, it may be effective for daytime drowsiness.[1281]
- *Safety*. It has been known to cause diarrhea, insomnia, gastrointestinal issues, and flushing.

WHAT CONSIDERATIONS SHOULD I KEEP IN MIND?

   Herbs generally have less robust evidence than other therapies, but lengthy historical evidence indicates they are relatively effective and safe. Herbs typically have few and mild side effects—especially when compared to psychotropics.[16] As with any therapy, work with trained practitioners skilled in the use of herbs. Aromatherapy (p. 241) can be considered a form of herbal therapy since it uses essential oils from herbs and other plants.

Finding quality sources is vital, to ensure potency, consistency, and the absence of contaminants. The FDA has established quality standards for herbs and supplements, but herbs receive much less scrutiny and far fewer assurances of safety. [16] For sources of quality herbal compounds, see below.

REAL-WORLD EXPERIENCE

Case Study 102– Valerian (Insomnia)

Twenty people receiving mental health services at a large urban hospital all agreed to participate in a sleep-related study. All complained of insufficient sleep.

They were asked to try a popular national brand of valerian ("Nature's Way", 470 mg valerian root). They took 1 capsule each night before bed and were allowed to increase their dose to 3 capsules after Week 1.

On a 5-point scale with 1=no effect and 5=extremely helpful, 15 of the 20 described their response as either a 4 or 5.[1282]

Case Study 103 – Cannabidiol (Schizophrenia)

Diagnosed with schizophrenia, Ladova, 19, was given a typical regime of antipsychotics, but she experienced severe reactions to the drugs. Her doctors then prescribed oral doses of Cannabidiol (CBD) for four weeks.

Ladova experienced a significant improvement in all aspects of the psychiatric rating scale. Doctors concluded that the results of the CBD treatments were similar in effectiveness to psychotropics for patients with schizophrenia. During treatment, Ladova had no side effects. However, when she was taken off CBD, her psychotic symptoms worsened.[1283]

Bottom Line*: Research is limited, but the non-psychoactive substance of marijuana offers hope for those with schizophrenia.*

Case Study 104 – Rhodiola rosea and St. John's Wort (Depression)

Maggie, a 26-year-old graduate student, had been depressed for as long as she could remember. From age 15, she was prescribed a variety of psychotropics. The debilitating side effects she suffered included sexual dysfunction, intense anger, nausea, feeling "spacey", and rapid heartbeat, depending on which drug was involved.

On her own, she tried SAM-e, but that caused continual stomach and intestinal upset.

Then she tried a combination of 450 mg/day Rhodiola rosea and 600 mg of St. John's Wort (Perika) taken twice daily. Her depression went away without weight gain, sexual dysfunction, or other troublesome side effects.[15]

Case Study 105 – Kava kava (Anxiety)

At 37, Lucelena was diagnosed with generalized anxiety disorder, a simple phobia, and one specific social phobia. She was treated with Kava kava. Within four weeks, symptoms improved by 75%, and by six months her practitioners observed an almost total remission of symptoms. Kava kava was well tolerated.[1284]

WHAT ARE ADDITIONAL RESOURCES?

- Herb Quality by Brand. www.ConsumerLab.com.
- Natural Supplements that work. http://goo.gl/cZSswN.
- National Ayurvedic Medical Association. www.ayurvedanama.org.
- Herb/CAM overviews and interactions with drugs. www.drugs.com.
- US Pharmacopeia standards organization. www.usp.org.
- Alternative Medicine Foundation database. www.herbmed.org.
- Natural Products database. www.NaprAlert.org.
- Natural Medicine database (Subscription). www.NaturalDatabase.com.

SOURCES FOR HERBS

The following can be used to help you determine quality sources for herbs. However, listing a resource does not guarantee quality, so work with your practitioners for the most appropriate sources. The supplier table is extracted from *Codex Alternus,*[22] courtesy of Mental Health Researcher Dion Zessin.

Supplier	Comments
Pacific Botanicals	Carries organic herbs and spices, and fresh non-dried herbs. www.PacificBotanicals.com.
Mountain Rose Herbs	Carries organic dried herbs, spices, essential oils, extracts, herbal capsules, teas, etc. www.MountainRoseHerbs.com.
Dragon Herbs	Carries a variety of Chinese herbs. www.DragonHerbs.com.
Mother Herbs	Provides Indian medicinal herbal products. www.MotherHerbs.com.
Blue Dragon Herbs	Grows and manufactures organic Chinese herbal formulas free of heavy metals. www.BlueDragonHerbs.com.
Himalaya Drug Company	Carries Geriforte, Mentat, Brahmi, Rauwolfia serpentine, and other Ayurvedic herbs. www.HimalayaWellness.com.
Orthomolecular Products	Offers a wide variety of Orthomolecular products, including Lithium Orotate. www.OrthomolecularProducts.com.
CannaVest	Hemp and cannabidiol products. www.cannavest.com.

Figure 31 – Sources of Herbs

Sensory Therapy

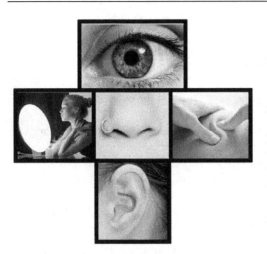

WHAT IS THE ESSENCE?

Sensory therapies seek to influence the brain and body by stimulating one or more of the senses, often creating calm and relaxation.

Of the five senses, four have therapies associated with them: *sight* (light/darkness therapy), *hearing* (sound therapy), *smell* (aromatherapy), and *touch* (hydrotherapy, massage). We have also included *anion therapy* in this group.

Chronotherapy studies daily (circadian), monthly, tidal, and seasonal rhythms. Manipulating biological rhythms and sleep can improve mood disorders quickly. Overall, the scientific evidence for *Sensory Therapy* is less rigorous than with other therapy groups, though each study should be evaluated on its own merits.

WHAT EVIDENCE SHOWS THIS IS EFFECTIVE?

Bright light therapy. Bright light therapy is based on the idea that sunlight can strongly influence mood. The therapy consists of sitting in front of a device called a light therapy box, which emits bright light that mimics natural outdoor light. It is typically only effective when used in the morning.

- For *depression*. A 2015 study found that bright light therapy was more effective than antidepressants for major depression.[1285]
- For *Seasonal Affective Disorder* (SAD). SAD is mood cycling that often results in fall or winter depression. Light therapy is the treatment of choice.[1286] A meta-analysis suggests that bright light treatment and dawn simulation for SAD and bright lights alone for non-seasonal depression are effective.[1287]
- For *schizoaffective disorder*. Light therapy improves depressive symptoms.[1288] Patients with panic disorder showed medium to high levels of aversion to bright light, however.[1289]
- For *insomnia*. Anecdotal evidence indicates daytime exposure to light with an intensity of 10,000 lux is sometimes helpful when insomnia is unrelated to circadian phase disturbance.[16]

Dark Therapy. *Dark Therapy*, in which complete darkness is used as a mood stabilizer for bipolar, is roughly the opposite of light therapy for depression. Data is limited, but one small study shows that being in complete darkness from 6:00 p.m. to 8:00 a.m. over three days can reduce rapid cycling manic symptoms.[1290] Instead of complete darkness, wearing amber colored glasses (which block blue light often emitted by computer screens and TVs) seems similarly effective and can preserve normal nocturnal melatonin levels.[1291] See Case Study 107, p. 242.

Chronotherapy. Chronotherapy seeks to align the circadian, or other rhythmic cycles, which are often considered our "internal clock".

- For *bipolar*. Circadian rhythms and sleep disturbances are core concerns. Adding morning light to antidepressants is an effective therapy. Short-term use of chronotherapy can induce long-term remission. After sleep deprivation, patients went to bed at 5:00 p.m., and then an hour later each night for the next six nights (which is called sleep phase advance). The combination of sleep deprivation and sleep phase advance resulted in long-term maintenance of health sleep patterns.[1292]

Audio Visual Stimulation (AVS). AVS uses flashing lights and pulsing sounds at different frequencies for symptom relief. The brain responds to this stimulation and synchronizes to it in a process called *entrainment*. In some cases, AVS is a combination of *Biofeedback* (p. 142) and *Bright Light Therapy* (p. 239).[1293]

- For *depression*. Thirty minutes of white light with AVS increases serotonin levels by 23% and norepinephrine levels by 18%, resulting in reduced depressive symptoms.[1294]
- For *Seasonal Affective Disorder*. One study[1295] found that depression was reduced in more than 80% of the patients using AVS; 84% of women and 100% of men had no clinical anxiety remaining by the end of treatment. In addition, AVS appears to have potential for avoiding the weight gain often associated with SAD.

Sound Therapy. Sound therapy includes white noise or binaural sound (using headphones to listen to slightly different frequencies of tones in each ear); this can cause shifts in brain waves, resulting in relaxation. The external sound involved in *Sound Therapy* also appears to interrupt inner auditory hallucinations for some people. (See

- For *insomnia*. Nighttime exposure to white noise may improve sleep, since it appears to increase the threshold of perceived sounds during sleep.[1296]
- For *dementia*. A white noise generator appears to decrease psychological symptoms in dementia patients with schizophrenia.[1297]

Tinnitus Therapy. Tinnitus is the perception of sound, like "ringing in the ears," or buzzing, when no external noise is present. It is not a mental health diagnosis. Success has been found in treating tinnitus with external noise to counteract the perception of sound.

- For *schizophrenia.* Limited case studies have found that using a sound generator designed to treat tinnitus can eliminate audio hallucinations.[1309] (See Case Study 106, p. 242.)

Music Relaxation. Music relaxation improves overall psychopathology, including *depression.*

- For *anxiety.* A significant correlation was found between reducing the level of situational anxiety and improving sleep efficiency through music.
- *More broadly.* The findings suggest that music relaxation is effective as a treatment for insomnia and emotional distress in people living with schizophrenia.[1298]

Aromatherapy. Aromatherapy uses essential oils and fragrant plant essences to sooth and relax. The oils can be heated in oil burners, rubbed onto pillows, or massaged onto the skin.

- For *stress.* Rose oil has been shown to significantly reduce the breathing rate, blood oxygen saturation, and blood pressure, resulting in greater calm.[1299] In a small study, lavender oil reduced agitation in 60% of dementia patients.[1300] A variety of small trials suggest aromatherapy benefits people suffering from dementia by improving sleep, agitated behaviors, and resistance to care.[1301] The plant varieties used for aromatherapy include lemon balm, lavender, chamomile, bergamot, neroli, valerian, and rose oil.

Hydrotherapy. Hydrotherapy employs hot or cold water, often as showers or baths, to calm, at least temporarily, people experiencing mania or psychosis. Used long before the advent of psychotropics, hydrotherapy is resurging in popularity.[1302] Warm showers are soothing. Bracing cold showers may interrupt unhelpful thought patterns by jolting and diverting thoughts, to focus on the sensation of cold rather than troubles. Spending fifteen or thirty minutes in a sauna at between 140 and 190 degrees Fahrenheit, with humidity between 10% and 50%, has been effective in treating *depression* and *neuropsychiatric disorders.*

Anionization. When air molecules naturally become charged particles, they are called air ions. These ions are odorless and tasteless, and we inhale them in abundance in certain environments, particularly in the mountains and near waterfalls and beaches. These air ions improve breathing by increasing cilia activity in the trachea, which helps minimize the introduction of foreign particles into the lungs, thereby reducing stress. Air ions can be artificially produced with an anion generator through a process called Ambient Air Anionization (AAA) or negative air ionization.

- For *bipolar.* One study showed AAA had significant anti-manic effects.[1303]
- For *depression.* High-density ions act as an antidepressant and can be considered a possible alternative to light therapy; it may result in reducing a person's reliance on antidepressant drugs.[1304]

- For *Seasonal Affective Disorder*. One study found that high-density ionization was as effective as light therapy.[1305] In another, depressive symptoms improved by at least 50% in half the patients using high-density ionization for thirty minutes daily.[1306]

   Massage. There are many different types of massage, including *Swedish* (full body for general relaxation), *deep tissue* (for muscle damage), *sports* (to prevent athletic injury), and *chair* (upper body only, while fully clothed).
- For *PTSD*. Studies indicate that massage can be therapeutically helpful for combat veterans.[1307]
- For *insomnia*. A variety of massage techniques have been extensively investigated and found beneficial in inducing sleep[1308] after inducing a relaxed state.

WHAT CONSIDERATIONS SHOULD I KEEP IN MIND?

   One of the outcomes of sensory therapy is a calm, relaxed state. Consider other techniques that achieve the same result, including *Progressive Muscle Relaxation* (p. 74), *Mindfulness* (p. 74), *Meditation* (p. 78), and *Autogenic Training* (p. 74).

   Sensory Therapy can be used in combination with psychotropics. No serious adverse side effects from these therapies have been reported.

REAL-WORLD EXPERIENCE

Case Study 106 – Sound Therapy (Schizoaffective Disorder)

   When Carmela first visited a psychiatrist, she complained about visual and auditory hallucinations that started after the birth of her first child. She was diagnosed with schizoaffective disorder. Her doctor prescribed antipsychotics and hospitalization. After eighteen months in the hospital, nothing seemed to help.

   As a last resort, her doctor suggested using sound therapy for as long as possible in a month. Carmela's hearing was normal, but a Tinnitus Control Instrument (TCI) sound generator was used at 10db of pink noise. Within a week, her auditory hallucinations decreased. In two weeks, the frequency of hallucinations dropped by 80%. After three weeks, the hallucinations rarely occurred, so she stopped using the TCI. The hallucinations completely disappeared by six weeks.[1309]

   Bottom Line*: Interrupting hallucinations with controllable sound may be a gateway to eliminating them.*

Case Study 107 – Dark Therapy (Rapid cycle bipolar)

   Carol, 70, was diagnosed with rapid cycle bipolar and was hospitalized on and off for 24 years. Endless psychotropics, ECT, estrogen therapy, lithium, and other treatments were largely ineffective.

She then decided to try a novel treatment of daily 10-14-hour periods of complete darkness and rest, plus a self-selected 1-hour midday nap. Rapid cycling immediately stopped. Depression gradually improved when midday light therapy was added. Soon she became very near normal after light therapy was shifted to the morning.[1310]

___**Bottom Line**___*: Carol decided on a path of therapy experimentation. For 24 years this experimentation used conventional psychiatric approaches. Only when she chose alternative treatments did she find recovery.*

WHAT ARE ADDITIONAL RESOURCES?

- Chronotherapy. http://goo.gl/uArGyU.
- Light Therapy. NAMI SAD factsheet, http://goo.gl/9YiHBl.

Electroconvulsive Therapy

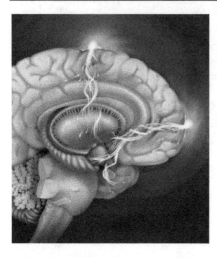

WHAT IS THE ESSENCE?

Electroconvulsive Therapy (ECT) is the most controversial treatment in psychiatry.[1311] It creates electrically induced seizures in anesthetized patients, to reduce serious mental health symptoms. Scientists don't know why it works.[1312]

Usually ECT starts unilaterally (on one side of the brain), but when patients don't respond to this treatment, ECT may be done bilaterally (on both sides). Most people will have between four and six treatments prescribed, though some have many more before their symptoms show significant improvement. Typically, ECT is administered twice a week until the symptoms are significantly improved or until no further improvement is noted in two successive sessions.

> "ECT is the most controversial therapy in psychiatry...
> "Although it may quickly and temporarily reduce depressive symptoms for some people, memory loss is common."

By experimentation, the practitioner determines the size of the electric charge needed to induce seizure–individuals can vary 50-fold. Once the seizure threshold is determined, the brain is charged between 2.5 and 6 times the threshold.[1313]

For subsequent ECT treatments, the seizure threshold often needs to increase to gain results. Practitioners typically attempt to induce a physical seizure for between twenty and sixty seconds.

Most commonly, charges are delivered in short bursts ("brief-pulse") of constant current, up to a massive 500 volts,[1314] (over four times the voltage in house wall sockets) although more recently, ultra-brief-pulse ECT has been available.

A therapy of last resort for patients with no improvements from drug therapy, ECT is used most commonly in the treatment of severe depression and depression with psychosis, but also with bipolar and schizophrenia. Immediately after ECT, people are often less depressed, but this has been interpreted differently by ECT's proponents and opponents. Proponents claim that ECT clearly relieves depression. Opponents claim that the improvement is a post-concussion, post-sedation euphoria that is short-lived.

WHAT EVIDENCE SHOWS THIS IS EFFECTIVE?

Remission Rates. Different trials found very different remission rates. (See *Glossary*, p. 337.) A large study of 347 ECT patients in New York community hospitals found remission rates of between 30% and 47%. However, of those who saw substantial improvement, 64% relapsed during the trial, on average after two months.[1315] The researchers made their position clear: "It was evident that only a small percentage of patients who received ECT achieved a sustained remission. Many did not see significant benefit from ECT, and even those who did found the benefits unsustainable."

In all mental health trials, the best evidence is based on gold-standard meta-analyses of trials that are randomized and placebo-controlled. For ECT, the best placebo control is to have people go through the normal pre- and post-ECT protocol (including sedation, muscle relaxants, and practitioner care) without receiving the shock; the process is called sham ECT.

A 2006 meta-analysis of sham ECT found, "No study demonstrated a significant difference between real and placebo ECT at one month post-treatment. Many studies failed to find a difference... even during the period of treatment. Claims in textbooks and review articles that ECT is effective are not consistent with the published data."[1316] A 2010 ECT literature review agreed, noting, "Given the strong evidence of persistent, and for some, permanent brain dysfunction... the cost-benefit analysis of ECT is so poor that its use cannot be scientifically justified."[1317] A 2017 meta-analysis of recent studies reaffirmed, "there is still no evidence that ECT is more effective than placebo for depression reduction or suicide prevention. Given the well-documented high risk of persistent memory dysfunction, the cost-benefit analysis for ECT remains so poor that its use cannot be scientifically, or ethically, justified."[1318]

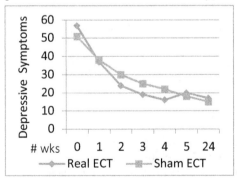

Figure 32 - Real vs. Sham ECT

A commonsense look at the details of one sham study[1319] is enlightening. Figure 32 highlights the similar depressive symptom decline in both real and sham ECT recipients over 24 weeks. In weeks two through four, real ECT shows slightly better results; a fact that is *statistically significant* but lacking in *practical significant.*

Would someone notice such a small difference in symptoms? Studies rarely consider such practicalities, but individuals considering ECT should *always* do so.

ECT Side Effects. The primary reason ECT is so controversial is its side effects. A large-scale study examining patients six months after receiving ECT found that "adverse cognitive effects...can persist for an extended period."[1323] A meta-analysis shows that persistent memory loss is experienced by between 29%-79% of people receiving ECT, averaging about one-third.[1320]

Memory loss and cognitive impairment from ECT varies. A 2003 meta-analysis of 73 trials found greater cognitive impairment from more frequent ECT administration.[1321] Additionally, the larger the ECT charge placed on the brain, the more effective the treatment, but also the more severe the cognitive impairment.[1322] Some researchers maintain that virtually all patients experience persistent memory loss.[1323]

The professional psychiatric organization of the United Kingdom indicates:

> *Patient-led surveys [indicate that about] half of those having ECT [experience long-term memory problems]... Some memory problems are probably present in everyone receiving ECT... Most people feel better after the course of ECT has finished and a few weeks have passed. However, some people do complain that their memory has been permanently affected, that their memories never come back... Some people have complained of more distressing experiences, such as feeling that their personalities have changed, that they have lost skills, or that they are no longer the person they were before ECT. They say that they have never gotten over the experience and feel permanently harmed.[1324]*

Furthermore, bilateral ECT produces greater amnesia than the other electrode placements, at a level proportional to the number of bilateral treatments during acute ECT. Consequently, little evidence justifies the continued first-line use of bilateral ECT in the treatment of major depression.[1323]

Brief-pulse vs. Ultra-brief-pulse. A 2015 meta-analysis confirmed that brief-pulse ECT is much more effective than ultra-brief-pulse in treating depression but showed significantly more cognitive side effects (less global cognition, difficulty in learning new concepts, difficulty in recall and memory).[1325]

ECT for schizophrenia. One extensive review found insufficient evidence to support the use of ECT for core schizophrenia symptoms.[1326] The Cochrane collaboration, the most respected source of medical research summarization, indicates, "The initial beneficial effect [of ECT for people with schizophrenia] may not last beyond the short term."[1327]

Never tested by the FDA. Surprisingly, ECT machines have never undergone safety testing for FDA approval. Rather, they were given grandfathered FDA approval as high-risk devices in 1976.[1328] Since then, new ECT devices have been approved automatically if they were similar to old ones. In evaluating ECT safety in 2010, the majority view of an FDA panel recommended retaining the high-risk classification.[1329] The panel's chair, representing the Mayo Clinic, recommended standard testing for the devices.[1330] Overwhelming public response agreed, citing memory loss issues.[1331]

WHAT CONSIDERATIONS SHOULD I KEEP IN MIND?

Opinions are polarized on ECT, even when researchers and psychiatrists look at the same evidence. Those who strongly support ECT claim that the benefits far outweigh the risks. Those who strongly oppose it claim the opposite. Some view it as "far and away the most effective treatment that currently exists for depression,"[1332] while others believe ECT offers no benefit beyond a few days—and those are not worth the risk involved.[1317]

The National Institute for Health Care and Excellence in the U.K. weighed the evidence and recommends caution and a very limited applicability: "ECT (should be) used only to achieve rapid and short-term improvement of severe symptoms after an adequate trial of other treatment options has proven ineffective… in people with catatonia or prolonged/severe mania."[1333]

In the end, your calculus is the one that counts. Evaluating the evidence, here is the author's view:

Avoid ECT to avoid persistent memory loss. Engage Integrative Mental Health practitioners to explore all reasonable alternatives including nutrient therapy and very-low-charge electromagnetic techniques. Meta-analyses have found that ECT has a poor cost-benefit calculus.

ECT subjects the brain to intense electrical shock that induces a grand mal seizure. It is ineffective in the mid- to long-term, although it can reduce depressive symptoms during treatment. In gold-standard trials, real ECT is only slightly better than sham ECT, and this advantage fades very quickly. Preliminary studies find that sedation therapy[1334]* using an ECT sedation drug appears to offer rapid depressive symptom relief similar to ECT.*

ECT relapse is common. Symptoms often return to pretreatment levels. ECT has troubling cognitive side effects: some memory loss occurs in all cases; larger and persistent memory loss in about one-third of the cases; and very severe cognitive dysfunction more rarely. The cognitive impact of ECT is cumulative: future shocks must be larger than previous ones, and the more powerful and frequent the shocks, the greater the side effects.

REAL-WORLD EXPERIENCE

Case Study 108 – Electroconvulsive Therapy (Depression)

Sue Cunliffe, a doctor, received 21 sessions of electric shock. After ECT her hands shook, she had very poor balance and slurred speech, she couldn't read or retrieve words well, and could no longer use money. 14 years later she still cannot drive. She can no longer practice medicine and she has lost most of her independence.

She refuses to call ECT therapy since it damaged her brain as confirmed by a neurologist. Today she is an outspoken critic of ECT.[1335]

> ***Bottom Line****: Memory loss from ECT is very common and its cognitive impact is sometimes devastating and life-long.*

Case Study 109 – Electroconvulsive Therapy (Major Depression)

After a significant trauma, Ruth became severely depressed and psychotic; her mind was constantly overworking. She was unable to work. She received psychotropics and counseling and had slight improvement, but toward the end of the two years, she was almost catatonic.

Ruth and her family decided to try bilateral ECT. The headaches she experienced at the beginning of ECT subsided. After 16 treatments, her anxiety was reduced, but she still felt depressed and had no motivation and no empathy for people. Ruth felt a change through sessions 17 to 23. She became more engaged and felt she was becoming herself again.

Ruth does not remember many things (vacations, films she saw, people she met) during an entire year, but, she adds, she is happy. She returned to work six months after the therapy ended. She says ECT was lifesaving for her, and she recommends that people consider ECT for severe depression.[1336]

Bottom Line*: Ruth was offered limited options. ECT provided benefit, but with significant memory loss. Don't limit your options. Consider the many therapies in this book to help you avoid the ECT side effects.*

Case Study 110 – Electroconvulsive Therapy (Major Depression)

Mary says, "I got my first bolt of electricity just three days after childbirth. This continued twelve more times while I was being drugged into oblivion. My treatment was without informed consent. I was transformed from a twenty-eight-year-old, happy, optimistic woman to a person who could not think or feel. My capacity to be myself was severely diminished.

"Electroshock damaged my brain and made it very difficult to be a mother to my newborn daughter. I was separated from her for over four months. My heart was broken. When we were finally united, I was filled with fear and suffering from the adverse effects of the psychotropic drugs I had been prescribed."

Mary is a founding member of MindFreedom Ireland and is an outspoken advocate for "mental health victims."[1337]

Bottom Line*: No other medical procedure creates such a strong and vocal opposition as ECT. Consider this significant social evidence.*

WHAT ARE ADDITIONAL RESOURCES?

- Mental Health America on ECT. http://goo.gl/hoNpZI.
- Royal College of Psychiatrists on ECT. http://goo.gl/ZS5oWK.

Transcranial Magnetic Stimulation

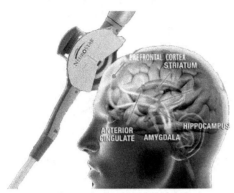

WHAT IS THE ESSENCE?

Repetitive Transcranial Magnetic Stimulation Therapy (rTMS) uses a magnetic field generator, or coil, placed near the head to produce small electrical currents, typically to the frontal cortex. This impulse is a much smaller electric current than *Electroconvulsive Therapy* (ECT, p. 244), and does not result in seizure or loss of consciousness. Each procedure lasts approximately forty minutes and is given daily over four to six weeks. The FDA has cleared rTMS for treatment-resistant depression.

WHAT EVIDENCE SHOWS THIS IS EFFECTIVE?

Overall, the evidence supporting rTMS is not compelling though some individual studies show benefit.

- For *depression*. The 2002 Cochrane meta-analysis of 16 *Repetitive Transcranial Magnetic Stimulation Therapy* (rTMS) trials for people with depression found no strong evidence of benefit from using rTMS—"although the small sample sizes do not exclude the possibility of benefit."[1338] The results from this therapy weren't different from those taking sham rTMS.

- For *treatment resistant depression*. One small trial found that rTMS produced a strong improvement in depression scores, as compared to the control group.[1339] However, a study of 164 veterans with treatment resistant depression, found that rTMS provided no value over placebo – both groups experienced a 39% reduction in symptoms.[1340]

- For *schizophrenia*. A 2015 Cochrane meta-analysis of 41 trials using rTMS for schizophrenia found insufficient evidence to support or refute the therapeutic use, noting that overall quality of evidence was very low, due to risk of bias; in addition, a relatively small number of patients participated in the studies.[1341] One meta-analysis found that although rTMS was shown to be very effective for negative symptoms in one trial,[1342] overall, the evidence of benefits for negative and positive symptoms is modest.[1343] However, in one study, repeated sessions of 1 Hz rTMS delivered to the left temporoparietal area of the brain suppressed auditory hallucinations, in some cases for weeks after treatment ended.[1344] Some evidence suggests that rTMS may be useful for negative symptoms of schizophrenia.[1345] A small study found that 34% of voice hearers receiving rTMS targeted at the speech area of the brain had over a 30% reduction in audio hallucinations.[1346]

- For *bipolar*. A very small study found that rTMS given daily for fourteen days improved manic symptoms dramatically, without side effects.[1347] The most effective placement appears to be over the right dorsolateral prefrontal cortex; mania worsened with left prefrontal rTMS.[1348]

- For *substance abuse*. Patients reduced cigarette smoking without change in the level of craving[1349] when receiving rTMS over the left dorsolateral prefrontal cortex (DLPFC). Cocaine-dependent patients receiving rTMS over the right DLPFC felt cravings diminish within four hours.[1350]

- For *other diagnoses*. TMS has beneficial effects in the treatment of post-traumatic stress disorder and obsessive-compulsive disorder.[1351]

- *Safety*. The most common rTMS side effect is scalp pain at the site of stimulation. Most patients find this mild to moderate, and it usually fades after the first week. However, in rare cases it can cause seizure and death.[1352]

- In the *long-term*, one study found that rTMS gains were maintained for a year in 26% to 37% of the patients; however, additional treatment beyond the standard protocol timeframe was given when deemed necessary.[1353]

- In terms of *limitations*. Some studies suggest that rTMS may not have a substantial benefit over a placebo.[1354] The most common deficiency in rTMS studies is the relatively small sample sizes of these studies (from six to seventy, with most less than twenty).[1351] *Repetitive Transcranial Magnetic Stimulation Therapy (rTMS) is not indicated for individuals who have bipolar, depression with psychosis, or a high risk of suicide.*

WHAT CONSIDERATIONS SHOULD I KEEP IN MIND?

There is little evidence that supports that rTMS works better than placebo, with no evidence supporting the use of it as an ongoing "maintenance treatment". The Cochran Collaboration, one of the most respected research groups, found no strong evidence that it works for depression or schizophrenia.

Although rTMS is called "noninvasive", we do not fully understand its impact on the brain. It is also an expensive treatment.

Unlike *Electroconvulsive Therapy* (p. 244), rTMS does not require sedation, and its low rate (~ 5 percent) of discontinuation seems to be influenced by its rather minor adverse effects (most commonly, headache).

Consider *Other Electromagnetic Therapy* options (p. 253) as alternatives to rTMS.

People who have metal (aneurism clips, pacemaker, a VNS device, etc.) near the device may not use the treatment.

Vagus Nerve Stimulation Therapy

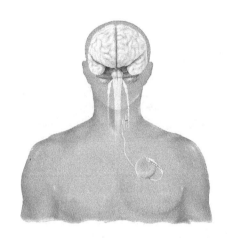

WHAT IS THE ESSENCE?

Two vital cranial nerves called *vagus nerves* exit the brain stem and branch to the heart, lungs, digestive tract, liver, kidneys, adrenal gland, and more; 80% of the vagus nerve fibers carry information from the body up to the brain, sending signals to our emotional centers (limbic system) and our thinking centers (including the frontal cortex).[15]

As a result, the vagus nerves are a direct and immediate pathway for bodily sensations and stresses that influence our thoughts and emotions. These nerves serve as a pathway of influence to our mood and mental health.

Vagus Nerve Stimulation (VNS) uses a device similar to a cardiac pacemaker. Implanted under the skin of the collarbone, the small device sends pulses to one of the vagus nerves in the neck, which then sends a message to the brain. Its implantation requires neurosurgery. In addition, transcutaneous VNS (tVNS) – stimulating the vagus nerve on the outer canal of the ear – is a non-invasive and more recently developed therapy. Little is understood about exactly how vagal nerve stimulation modulates mood, however.

The FDA approved use of VNS for adults with depression in specific situations: 1) for treatment of long-term chronic depression (lasting two or more years), in conjunction with standard treatments; 2) recurrent or severe depression; 3) depression that hasn't improved after the use of at least four other treatments, such as four different antidepressants.[1355]

WHAT EVIDENCE SHOWS THIS IS EFFECTIVE?

VNS Studies. Studies have shown that VNS therapy significantly helps about 30% of the patients who have chronic depression or Type II bipolar.[1356] One small study found response rates during the acute phase of the study were very low: only one patient responded after three months. By the end of a year, 55% had responded to treatment, suggesting that long-term follow-up is required to realize VNS potential.[1357] Similar findings came from a second small study: depression improved, but it took several months. The researchers saw very large changes in brain metabolism occurring before any improvement in mood—"as if there's an adaptive process that occurs. First, the brain begins to function differently. Then, the patient's mood begins to improve."[1358] If patients feel an improvement after twelve months, research shows that they have almost a 70% chance of keeping that positive response after two years.[1359]

tVNS. In one small study, patients with major depression receiving five treatments of tVNS per day for two weeks showed a significant improvement in depressive symptoms.[1360]

VNS controversy. Many studies agree that VNS is effective in treating depression. However, these findings do not consider improvements over time in patients without the device. In the only randomized controlled trial, VNS failed to perform any better when the device was turned on than when the devices were not turned on.[1361] Not all scientific studies have shown that vagus nerve stimulation is an effective treatment for depression. Some studies have suggested it's no more effective than a placebo.[1362]

The vagus nerve and the gut/brain connection. Ninety percent of the fibers in the vagus nerve carry information from the gut to the brain. Given the tie between the nerve and our emotional state, emotions may well be influenced by nerves in the gut,[1363] emphasizing the importance of digestion for mental health. (See *Diet & Digestion*, p. 62.) Research shows that people with high vagus nerve activation in a resting state are more prone to feel compassion, gratitude, love, and happiness. Children with high baseline vagus nerve activity are more cooperative and likely to share.[1364]

WHAT CONSIDERATIONS SHOULD I KEEP IN MIND?

VNS is known to affect blood flow to the brain, but scientists don't know how it works to alleviate the symptoms of depression. To become a candidate for VNS, patients must have tried at least four different medication therapies for depression from two different classes (which means the medications must have at least two different mechanisms of action in the body's chemistry).

VNS has side effects, but patients often find them minor, and they decrease with time. The frequencies and currents of VNS electrical impulses can be adjusted to help minimize side effects.

Since tVNS appears to offer symptom relief without the risk of neurosurgery, it should be evaluated prior to choosing an implanted VNS device.

WHAT ARE ADDITIONAL RESOURCES?

- VNS Overview. www.psych.med.umich.edu/vns/.

Other Electromagnetic Therapy

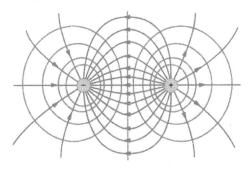

WHAT IS THE ESSENCE?

This section on *Other Electromagnetic Therapy* includes a cluster of approaches that employ magnetism, low levels of electricity, radio waves, or electrical grounding to influence changes in the brain.

Some appear to be able to change brain wave patterns, while one might cause endorphin release. The therapies include:

- Echo-planar Magnetic Resonance Spectroscopic Imaging (EP-MRSI)
- Impulse Magnetic Field Therapy (IMFT)
- Transcranial Direct Current Stimulation (tDCS)
- Transcranial Alternating Current Stimulation (tACS)
- Low-Energy Emission Therapy (LEET).
- Paraspinal Electrical Stimulation (PES)
- Earthing

WHAT EVIDENCE SHOWS THIS IS EFFECTIVE?

Echo-planar Magnetic Resonance Spectroscopic Imaging. EP-MRSI uses oscillating magnetic fields similar to those used in functional magnetic resonance imaging (fMRI), except they differ in field direction, waveform frequency, and strength.

- For *bipolar*. Preliminary data suggest that the EP-MRSI scans are associated with mood improvement, as reported by 23 out of 30 people who received EP-MRSI (77%). Of the 30, all those who were not taking medication showed greater response (100%), compared to those on medication (63%). These results were not seen in bipolar patients receiving sham EP-MRSI and healthy individuals receiving EP-MRSI.[1365] The findings are similar to those for rTMS depression treatments.[1366]

Impulse Magnetic Field Therapy. Magnetic fields may improve *insomnia*. In one study, 70% of the patients reported significant improvements or full remission from nightly IMFT treatment for four weeks, in contrast to 2% in the control group.[1367]

Transcranial Direct Current Stimulation (tDCS). A small cell-phone sized device that costs a few hundred dollars gives a low-intensity electrical current to stimulate the brain via two electrodes placed on the head. Although tDCS is not currently FDA-approved, Johns Hopkins indicates that this therapy, tDCS, is non-invasive, painless, safe, easy to administer, and may have several advantages over other brain stimulation techniques.[1368] tDCS can be given in both anodal and cathodal forms.

- For *major depression.* A meta-analysis concludes that tDCS has consistent positive impact on major depression.[1369] However, as with other antidepressive techniques, tDCS can induce mania/hypomania in some patients.[1370]

- For *bipolar.* A small study found anodal stimulation decreased depressive symptoms after five sessions, with sustained benefit one month later.[1371]

- For *schizophrenia.* Small studies have shown that tDCS offers patients a reduction in hallucinations[1372] and negative symptoms[1373] as well as improvements in working memory and executive function.[1374] Most studies report an overall improvement in the patient's general state, functioning, social interaction, and insight.[1379] (See Case Study 111, p. 255, and Case Study 112, p. 256.)

- For *substance abuse.* Bilateral cathodal stimulation of the frontal-parietal-temporal area resulted in a significant decrease in cigarette consumption.[1375] Stimulation of the left dorsolateral prefrontal cortex (DLPFC) can reduce cravings in heavy drinkers.[1376] tDCS reduces acute substance craving in drug addicts.[1377] Right anodal/left cathodal tDCS of DLPFC significantly diminishes cravings for marijuana.[1378]

- *Safety.* tDCS appears very safe for people with schizophrenia, including one case of twice-daily use for three years without side effects.[1379]

Transcranial Alternating Current Stimulation (tACS). tACS is the external application of low level oscillating (alternating) current to the brain. tACS appears to influence cortical excitability and activity, but a Cochrane analysis found no high-quality studies supporting its use.[1380] tACS has variants including Cranial Electrotherapy Stimulation.[1381]

- For *obsessive-compulsive disorder (OCD).* A small set of patients with treatment-resistant OCD were given tACS and each improved substantially.[1382] (See Case Study 113, p. 256.)

Low Energy Emission Therapy. LEET delivers low-frequency radio waves through a mouthpiece; its goal is to induce relaxation. Little sensation is experienced during treatment, which may increase the release of melatonin. It is currently not available in the U.S. and requires special training to administer.

- For *insomnia*, a study of more than 100 patients found that twenty-minute LEET treatments given three times a week for four weeks significantly increased total sleep time and reduced the time needed to fall asleep for chronic insomnia. It was well tolerated. The sleep pattern following LEET resembles normal sleep.[1383]

Paraspinal Electrical Stimulation. For *PTSD.* A single case report[1384] suggests that pulsing microcurrents along the paraspinal muscles from the base of the skull to the sacrum will alleviate symptoms in refractory PTSD. A complete loss of all symptoms occurred after the third fifteen-minute session. (See Case Study 114, p. 256.) Adverse effects included transient tingling and loss of sensation in areas of the feet, but did not impede walking. Researchers attributed success to a massive release of endorphins.[16]

Earthing. *Earthing* is electrically grounding the body to the Earth and its continuously available supply of electrons. Grounding – whether being outside barefoot or indoors connected to grounded conductive systems – appears to affect a variety of bodily processes that influence mental health. Earthing can be used to address sensitivity to *Electromagnetic fields* (p. 213) associated with mental health issues.

Evidence for *Earthing* is small but growing. Pilot studies show that it can increase free thyroxine and thyroid-stimulating hormone,[1385] improve mood,[1386] and influence inflammation and the immune response.[1387] It also appears to reduce and resynchronize cortisol (a stress hormone) levels to more align with the natural 24-hour circadian rhythm,[1388] improve sleep and reduce stress.[1389]

A variety of earthing products are available including grounded sheets, pillowcases, and wrist straps, as well as grounded mats for use under electronic equipment.

WHAT CONSIDERATIONS SHOULD I KEEP IN MIND?

The Electromagnetic therapies in this group should be considered before *Electroconvulsive Therapy* (p. 244), since side effects are much less severe. Transcutaneous Electrical Stimulation (TENS) applies electrical current through electrodes attached to the skin, but it has not yet been extensively tested.

Although preliminary studies are positive for these therapies, there is concern since the results have been difficult to consistently reproduce.[1390] Therefore, consider the results suggestive, but yet-to-be-proven. The low cost and apparent lack of side effects of these therapies, however, weighs in favor of their consideration.

REAL-WORLD EXPERIENCE

Case Study 111 – tDCS (Schizophrenia)

Jon, 24, was diagnosed with schizophrenia. In time, he became reluctant to take previously effective antipsychotic medication. His practitioner decided to try tDCS, and reported,

"After five days of twice-daily tDCS treatment, Jon had complete cessation of hallucinations, improved concentration ability, and significant improvement in his interpersonal interactions. Additionally, the patient's insight into his illness improved markedly, to the point that he agreed to take medications for residual symptoms."[1391]

Case Study 112 – tDCS (Schizophrenia)

Jaime, now an adult, was diagnosed with schizophrenia as a teenager. She had been hearing near-constant background noise ever since her illness surfaced at age 15. Drugs never managed to eliminate it.

She tried tDCS with a steady two milliamps of direct current for twenty minutes. Following her first treatment, she said she felt better than she could remember ever feeling in her entire adult life.[1392]

Case Study 113 – tACS (OCD)

Peter, 17, had severe treatment-resistant OCD for three years. Cognitive Behavioral Therapy worked for a few days, but he soon relapsed. His symptoms were so severe he was hospitalized for 18 months.

He agreed to tACS treatment and found immediate results. After two tACS stimulations he quickly transitioned to out-patient care. He continued to improve. Peter has since gone back to high school and is currently symptom free.[1382]

Case Study 114 – Paraspinal Electrical Stimulation (PTSD)

Raul, a 34-year-old victim of war who had survived torture, suffered from panic attacks, chronic abdominal pain, nightmares, insomnia, and intrusive thoughts. He was diagnosed with post-traumatic stress disorder. He tried psychotropics and talking therapy, with no success. His condition worsened over five years and he became depressed to the point of considering suicide.

And then his therapist suggested PES. Raul experienced almost complete pain relief after a single fifteen-minute PES treatment. PTSD symptoms completely disappeared after the third treatment. His mood lifted markedly, and his work, marriage, and social life improved significantly.

Raul received another seven treatments. At last report, he had remained symptom-free for ten months.[16]

WHAT ARE ADDITIONAL RESOURCES?

- Supplier of tDCS devices. www.soterixmedical.com.
- Omron maker of TENS device. www.OmronHealthCare.com.
- TENS devices. www.TENSPros.com.

7 – Over-care Avoidance

Over-Care Avoidance (Figure 33) is the fourth and last category in the *Wellness Continuum* (Figure 9, p. 47).

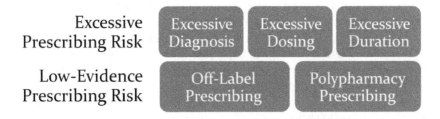

Figure 33 - Over-care Avoidance

Unlike the three previous stages, you won't find suggestions here of possible therapies to try. Instead, you will find **a dose of caution: avoid too much intervention.** *Over-Care* can lead to unnecessary treatment, the stigma of being labeled mentally ill, and a waste of resources—financial and personal.

But more importantly, overuse of psychotropics can lead to escalating side effects and premature death. In fact, in the U.S., **far more people die from high doses of psychiatric drugs than from heroin overdoses.**[1393] The American Psychiatric Association (APA) was concerned enough about over-care risk to launch a continuing program to curb psychiatric over-care practices.[1454]

Dr. Steven Sharfstein, past president of the APA, emphasizes:

> *There is widespread concern about the over-medicalization of mental disorders and the overuse of medications. Financial incentives and managed care have contributed to the notion of a 'quick fix' by taking a pill and reducing psychotherapy and psychosocial treatments.... despite the strong evidence base that many psychotherapies are effective.*[1394]

Dr. James Scully, past APA Medical Director and CEO, indicates:

> *Physicians and patients together should be thinking carefully, 'Are the medications really needed and are there downsides and negative consequences for overuse?'... Patients really need to be a part of the decision... of their own treatments.*[1403]

Over-care is also a problem outside of the U.S. The British Medical Association (BMA), noticing an alarming growth in psychotropic-dependency and withdrawal issues, launched a project to understand and address the practice. In their report,[1395] they highlight a troubling reality.

> *In undertaking this project, it was clear... that this subject was contentious and emotive. It is characterised by a mistrust of the medical profession... by those affected, who describe meeting a denial of the problem and too little help from their doctors.*

The leaders of the APA and BMA are both saying loudly and publicly: *we have an over-care problem in psychiatry that we must fix.*
This chapter urges you to claim the self-determination that Dr. Scully suggests. It also urges you to recognize the contentious nature of this problem as highlighted by the BMA. Ultimately, you must make the decisions for your own recovery, guided by trusted practitioners. As you make those decisions, be aware that you may encounter the very prescribing patterns that the APA and BMA are working vigorously to change.

The best way to frame *Over-Care Avoidance* is in the context of risk. When we engage in *Over-Care*, we accept elevated risk in two broad categories:

- **Excessive Prescribing Risk**, prescribing too many psychotropics too often, in dosages that are too high, for time periods that are too long.
- **Off-Label & Polypharmacy Risk**, where there is little or no evidence that individual drugs work for the purpose for which they are prescribed, or that multiple drugs work in combination.

Excessive Prescribing Risk

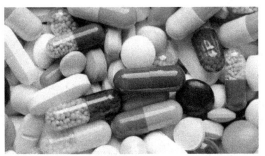

WHAT IS THE ESSENCE?

There are three types of **Excess Prescribing**: *Excessive Diagnosing, Excessive Dosing,* and *Excessive Duration.* These risks often result in an over-use of psychotropics with their associated long- and short-term side effects.

Excessive Diagnosing involves prematurely classifying someone as having a mental disorder. Sometimes our difficulties are transitory and will go away on their own. At other times, mental difficulties such as grief and anxiety are a natural part of life. Many situations *could* create a diagnosis, but not every situation *should* create a diagnosis—which is too often a starting point for guessing which pill to prescribe instead of a starting point for an integrated plan for healthy living.

Excessive Dosing means taking drugs in amounts higher than is needed – above the trade-off point where symptom relief is balanced optimally with side effects. *Excessive Dosing* should be evaluated *for* an individual *with* the individual actively participating in a process of prudent experimentation.

Excessive Duration means taking a medication for longer than is needed.

WHAT IS THE EVIDENCE?

Prescribing to vulnerable populations. Excessive prescribing is most common with our most vulnerable: foster children, young people in juvenile detention, the elderly, and those with intellectual and developmental disabilities.

According to one study, 13.5% of children in child welfare were taking psychotropic medications, a rate between two and three times that of other children in the same community.[1396] Texas reports a rate of 20%.[1397] Overall, the percentage of foster children on psychotropic medication fluctuates dramatically between 0% and 40%,[1398] not so much based on needs of the children, but based on where they live.[1399] The antipsychotic prescription rate for foster children is 4.5 times greater than that of other children on Medicaid.[1400]

There is also concern over the increased mortality risk of elderly patients treated for dementia-related psychosis.[1401] The U.S. Department of Health and Human Services launched a national effort to "safeguard nursing home residents from unnecessary antipsychotic drug use." They set a goal: reduce the number of people in nursing homes using antipsychotics by 15%.[1402]James Scully,

American Psychiatric Association Medical Director and CEO, states, "The [dosages of] antipsychotics in nursing homes… need to be really reduced."[1403]

Additionally, people with intellectual and developmental disabilities are at risk. One study found that 29% of those who were prescribed antipsychotics had no psychiatric diagnosis.[1404]

Excessive prescribing to cope with inadequate services. Over 80% of the general practitioners in the United Kingdom admit to over-prescribing antidepressants to patients with depression, anxiety, and stress, indicating they do this because psychological therapies or social care are not available.[1405]

Excessive prescribing before considering all options. Patients often receive psychotropic medications without being evaluated by a mental health professional.[1406] Most psychotropic drugs are prescribed by general practitioners (GP) [1417] who lack the in-depth mental health training of psychiatrists. As a result, many Americans receive antidepressants from their GP without being aware of other evidence-based treatments that can offer as good or better outcomes without the risk of psychotropic side effects.

Excess prescribing for non-severe situations. There is little justification to prescribe antidepressants for mild depression since a meta-analysis shows that they are no better than placebo for this level of symptoms.[1407]

Excessive diagnosing based on patient requests. Direct-to-consumer advertising is a powerful and effective approach to increase drug sales. Patients who request advertised drugs from their doctors are over sixteen times more likely to receive them than patients who do not request any drugs.[1408] In this situation, the patient is effectively self-diagnosing and self-prescribing.

Excessive diagnosing for normal life situations. Psychiatrist Patrick Landman notes, "[*The Diagnostic and Statistical Manual of Mental Disorders*] has led to a growing medicalization of emotions, whereby the distinctions between normality, its variations, and its pathologies have all but disappeared."[1409] Dr. Peter Gøtzsche gives a startling example, noting the dramatic escalation of the medicalizing of bereavement. [1410] In 1980, one full year of bereavement was considered within the normal realm of coping with grief. In 1994, anything longer than two months was considered a depressive disorder. In 2013, this was shortened to two weeks. The DSM also has a caffeine intoxication disorder from drinking two or three cups of coffee.[1411] The Director of the National Institute of Mental Health felt the DSM was so flawed that he directed the NIMH to "re-orient its research away from DSM categories."[1412]

Excessive diagnosing for catch-all disorders. According to Landman, the DSM "has also caused an inflation in psychiatric diagnoses that are both clinically and scientifically questionable and that include 'catch-all' categories… that are the source of artificial epidemics." For example, some psychiatrists think that *Generalized Anxiety Disorder* (GAD) is over-diagnosed. One reason for this is that screening for GAD produces many false positives. One study found that 7% of all patients met GAD criteria, but only one-third of those truly had a diagnosis that could be confirmed.[1413]

Excessive dosing for first episode psychosis. Prescribing guidelines for first episode psychosis emphasize using the lowest effective doses possible,[1414] since these individuals have increased sensitivity to the adverse effects of drugs. However, the National Institute of Mental Health indicates that many patients with first episode psychosis are prescribed contrary to these guidelines.[1415]

Excessive dosing with neuroleptics. Evidence suggests that patients often receive neuroleptic (tranquilizer) doses that exceed the maximally effective range.[1416] Excessive dosing is widely prevalent in Canada, East Asia, and the U.S.[1417] One study found that 20% of the patients receiving antipsychotics in an inpatient setting were given dosages that exceeded guidelines.[1418]

Excessive duration of psychotropic prescribing. There is a knowledge gap[1224] between the practice of long-term drug prescribing and the fact that most psychotropics lack sufficient proof of long-term effectiveness. We simply don't have evidence that they are required long term. In fact, a large survey of long-term psychotropic users found that over half of those who attempted to withdraw from drugs were successful in doing so, and 82% of those who ended their drug use were satisfied or very satisfied with their decision to discontinue.[1419]

WHAT CONSIDERATIONS SHOULD I KEEP IN MIND?

The presence of these many systemic flaws in our mental health system calls loudly for strong self-advocacy to avoid the risks of over-prescribing.

It might seem natural to routinely follow your practitioners' recommendations and allow them to manage the over-care risks. But in an environment where over-prescribing is recognized as a potentially life-threatening problem, patients must exercise caution. Patients should collaborate with practitioners who respect the patients' choices of risk. Whenever psychotropics are prescribed, patients and their supporters should discuss why the drugs and dosages are being recommended. (See *Questions for Your Practitioners*, p. 328.) In these discussions, ask them for the exit plan for the drugs and what withdrawal effects may appear when the plan is executed.

Also evaluate any other prescription drugs you may be taking. There are over 200 drugs that have depression as a potential side effect. In the U.S., over 37% of the population are taking these drugs.[1420]

Additionally, everyone in the recovery process should experiment prudently with proven non-drug approaches. Often these will reduce symptoms with few or no side effects, and they may also reduce the psychotropic dosages needed. Reduced symptom levels can avoid *Over-Care* scenarios.

Throughout history, humans have had to deal with loss, grief, disappointment, changing life circumstances, and bad days without drugs. We should, too. Review with your practitioners all reasonable options of care and choose the ones you think best fit your risk profile.

REAL-WORLD EXPERIENCE

Case Study 115 – Over-prescribing

Mary, 72, was put on antipsychotics while she was living at home because she had outbursts of screaming. The medication reduced her screaming, but her daughter noticed that Mary also lost her emotions. "She would be sleeping all the time. She just wasn't there," she told Mary's doctor. But Mary continued on antipsychotics for two more years.

She was then moved to a long-term care home where she spent many days in a deep sleep, and when she was awake, she didn't talk. Mary's daughter consulted with the doctors, and they agreed to reduce and eventually stop Mary's antipsychotics.

Mary perked up immediately. "It was like she was back," her daughter said. Stopping the medication made Mary more alert. Although she had difficulty communicating at times, at others times she was smiling and laughing.

One day, Mary was able to go to her daughter's house for a family lunch. Mary looked at her daughter and said, "I love you." Her daughter beamed with excitement. It was the first time in years that her mother had spoken.[1421]

Bottom- Line*: The elderly are a vulnerable population and are often over-medicated. Once doctors prescribe medication, often inertia keeps the elderly on the medication. Simple advocacy, working with doctors, can sometimes bring a quick and positive end to over- prescribing.*

Practitioner's Story 6 – Overmedication

Dr. Allen J. Frances is a psychiatrist known for chairing the task force that produced the fourth revision of the psychiatric "bible", the Diagnostic and Statistical Manual of Mental Disorders.

"My own experience [has been] with hundreds of over-medicated patients — 'deprescribing' has often resulted in marked improvement," he tells audiences. *"But this doesn't generalize to everyone. No one size fits all. I heartily support [the] crusade against over-medication when it is inappropriate, but… it can be harmful when extended to those who really do need medication to stabilize symptoms."*[1422]

Bottom Line*: Dr. Frances sees the harm of overmedication and seeks change. But, he cautions, don't throw the baby out with the bath water.*

WHAT ARE ADDITIONAL RESOURCES?

- Psychotropic Withdrawal Resources. http://goo.gl/GH3pzI
- Drug Tapering. http://goo.gl/B0TJWJ.
- Difficulties in psychotropic withdrawal. http://goo.gl/VuBX2B.

Off-Label & Polypharmacy Risk

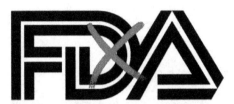

WHAT IS THE ESSENCE?

Off-Label & Polypharmacy Risk stems from two common prescribing practices that are poorly supported by evidence. Unlike most mental health prescribing, these two practices have not been proven safe and effective; they represent a risk borne by those with mental health issues.

Off-label Prescribing is when a practitioner prescribes drugs that have not been approved by the FDA for the specific disorder for which they are prescribed. Currently, this is a legal and common practice, with more than 20% of American outpatient prescriptions being given off-label. This stems from the fact that the FDA regulates drug approval, but not drug prescribing. Doctors are free to prescribe a drug for any reason they think is medically appropriate.

Polypharmacy Prescribing is most commonly defined as the simultaneous use of multiple drugs to treat a single condition.

WHAT EVIDENCE SHOWS THESE PRACTICES ARE RISKY?

Issues and evidence of off-label prescribing.

The American Psychiatric Association has a reasonable policy on off-label prescribing, supporting it "when such use is based on sound scientific evidence in conjunction with sound medical judgment.[1423] **Unfortunately, 94% of psychiatric off-label prescribing has little or no sound scientific evidence supporting it.**[1424]

People who are given off-label prescriptions assume a substantial risk: a 57% higher chance of adverse side effects.[1425] Despite the lack of evidence to support the practice, it is common. One study found that the off-label prescription rate was 28.5% for mood stabilizers[1426] and 40% for antipsychotics.[1427] Perhaps more concerning, 72% of all antidepressants are prescribed without any psychiatric diagnosis, driven primarily by a surge in the prescribing by nonpsychiatrist providers.[1428]

The United States military is often the target of off-label prescribing in significant proportions: although only antidepressants are FDA-approved for PTSD,[1429] in 2009, more than 81,000 veterans diagnosed with PTSD received second-generation antipsychotics. A subsequent trial found them ineffective for military-related PTSD.[1430] In addition, the practice of off-label prescribing for elderly veterans is evident in long-term nursing facilities.[1431]

The elderly is another population at risk. In Germany, antipsychotic prescribing for older patients is almost exclusively off-label.[1432] Part of the reason for excessive off-label prescribing is due to the practitioners' lack of continuing education. One study of 1,200 primary-care physicians and psychiatrists asked them to assess whether certain prescriptions were off-label or not; 45% of the time they were wrong.[1433]

Issues and evidence of polypharmacy prescribing.

Psychiatric polypharmacy poses a risk because it is based more on educated guess than scientific evidence,[1434] a vital consideration for those seeking scientifically-validated care. Very few studies examine polypharmacy, but those that focus on antipsychotic polypharmacy suggest avoiding it.[1435] Even though some forms of polypharmacy are less dangerous than others, nearly all forms "venture beyond the evidentiary base."[1437]

Reports of polypharmacy's adverse effects are common. Polypharmacy can increase psychotropic side effects, drug interactions, patient treatment noncompliance, and medication errors.[1436] It is also associated with longer hospital stays[1437] and polypharmacy numbers among the major causes of drug-related deaths.[1438]

This is not surprising given that one drug can affect another drug's absorption, distribution within the body, as well as its metabolism or excretion, thereby changing the blood levels of other drugs.[1439] For example, combining the psychotropics valproate and carbamazepine may lead to neurotoxicity.

One detailed analysis found, "Polypharmacy often becomes a cycle of treating one condition, experiencing side effects, and treating the side effects, until the patient and the clinician cannot remember where the cycle began."[1440]

Researchers have called this the *prescribing cascade*,[1441] and it has become an area of growing concern, especially considering that Americans now spend six times more on prescription drugs than they did in 1990.

To underscore the point, Figure 34 (p. 265) highlights an extreme example of potential *prescribing cascade*.[1442] Each drug prescribed in this cycle can be justified based upon its ability to address specific symptoms. However, the larger picture highlights how individuals can spin around this wheel, being prescribed an ever-increasing cocktail of drugs with ever compounding side effects.

The American Society of Consultant Pharmacists goes as far as to advise, "[A]ny new symptom in an older adult should be considered a drug side effect until proven otherwise. Unfortunately, medicines are often overlooked by clinicians as a likely cause of new symptoms in older adults."[1443]

The frequency of polypharmacy makes the situation even more precarious. Studies repeatedly show a high frequency of polypharmacy for seriously ill psychiatric patients.[1436] The simultaneous use of four or five medications is not uncommon, especially in the treatment of bipolar.[1444]

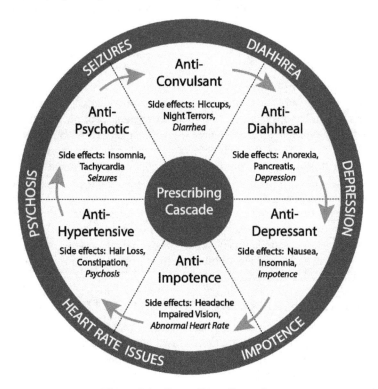

Figure 34 – Prescribing Cascade

Antipsychotic polypharmacy (APP) deserves special attention. APP is not evidence-based.[1445] In fact, there has been only one combination of antipsychotics that has been thoroughly evaluated—clozapine and risperidone—and the findings failed to support their use together.[1326]

The evidence on APP is grim. The greater the number of antipsychotics given concurrently, the shorter the patient will live.[1446, 1447, 1448] Taking multiple antipsychotics is associated with higher rates of metabolic disorders,[1449] diabetes, and Parkinson's-like movement disorders.[1450] It also lowers HDL ("good cholesterol") levels. This is becoming all the more alarmingly since APP is becoming increasingly common.[1326]

Moreover, a study examining 42 different combinations of an antipsychotic with a second psychoactive drug found that none had consistent evidence to support their use together.[1451]

Rational Polypharmacy – the prescribing of multiple drugs based on selected clinical experience instead of RCTs – is sometimes considered a reasonable middle ground. However, it is more of an "art of prescribing"[1452] than science. Although there is room for art in medicine, rational polypharmacy lacks strong evidence. Given the significant proven downsides of polypharmacy, those who value a strong evidence base should view *Rational Polypharmacy* with a healthy dose of skepticism.

Polypharmacy occurs much too frequently, caused by fear (for instance, the clinician is afraid to allow a patient to withdraw from a drug), laziness, sloppy diagnosis, unknowns in switching drugs, and more.[1436]

There has been a recent significant increase in polypharmacy involving antidepressants and antipsychotics.[1453] The median number of medications prescribed in each psychiatric visit increased from one in 1996-1997 to two in 2005-2006. Over one-third of psychiatric visits result in three or more meds being prescribed. While some combinations are supported by clinical trials, many are unproven and put patients at increased risk with uncertain gains in clinical outcomes.

The polypharmacy problem is well recognized in psychiatry. As part of its Choosing Wisely® campaign, the American Psychiatric Association identifies limiting antipsychotic polypharmacy as one of the five major goals of the program.[1454] Drug audits and electronic prescribing systems are also being implemented to curb the practice.

WHAT CONSIDERATIONS SHOULD I KEEP IN MIND?

Doctors are working hard to satisfy the needs of their patients, and off-label and polypharmacy prescriptions are tools available to them. However, both practices often undermine evidence-based care and can increase patient risk.

For this reason, a growing number of doctors are deprescribing – helping patients taper, stop, discontinue, or withdraw from drugs, with the goal of managing polypharmacy and improving outcomes.[1455] A variety of organizations and resources are available to encourage and assist in psychiatric deprescribing (see p. 341).

The need for deprescribing can often arise from insufficient communication as people switch doctors. The latest practitioner often has little information about why specific drugs were prescribed, when and by whom, and with what result.[1456] As a result, many doctors are reluctant to alter an individual's current prescription set. They often choose to add new drugs to address the patient's current situation. As they do, polypharmacy, and its risks, accelerate.

If your doctors recommend polypharmacy or off-label prescriptions, or if you are unsure why you are taking a specific prescription, be cautious. This is especially true for the elderly, since 60% of them are taking at least one potentially inappropriate drug.[1457]

Ask your doctors about each drug's risk/reward profile and evidence that supports their prescribing recommendations. Especially inquire about the evidence that supports using your prescribed set of drugs in combination. This conversation can naturally lead to a discussion of potential deprescribing. For a more extensive list of potential questions to ask your practitioners, see *Questions for Dialogue with your Mental Health Practitioners* (p. 328).

If in doubt, seek a second opinion, especially from an integrative mental health practitioner. Such assertive action is not only appropriate, but recommended by researchers to limit the risks of polypharmacy and off-label practices.[1458]

Integrative mental health professionals can help reduce polypharmacy. They typically start by adding appropriate non-drug approaches to decrease overall symptoms and increase core wellness. Then, working with the prescribing physician, they can help the individual reduce to *minimum effective dosages* for all necessary drugs over time, while potentially eliminating others.

There are many examples of how using customized combinations of non-drug approaches can dramatically improve outcomes (See Practitioner's Story 7, p. 268).

REAL-WORLD EXPERIENCE

Case Study 116 – Polypharmacy (Schizophrenia)

Mark, 46, was diagnosed with schizophrenia. His situation was chronic. He had been hospitalized many times and was taking standing doses of four antipsychotics, an antidepressant, a mood stabilizer, an anti-seizure medication, and a medication to reduce Parkinson's-like side effects.

His physician noted in his admission note, "Mark is on too many meds."

Mark frequently engaged in verbal altercations with his peers and with medical staff members. Following these encounters, he would be given additional doses of antipsychotics. He began showing signs of overmedication. He had an unsteady gait. He fell several times, resulting in head injuries. The family expressed concern, but no significant changes were made. When Mark was found dead in his bed, an autopsy concluded that the cause of death was "polypharmacy overdose."[1459]

__Bottom Line__: Although this is an extreme example, polypharmacy can run out of control, even with well-intending practitioners. Few suitable guidelines exist for polypharmacy. We must all be assertive about minimizing polypharmacy. The downsides can be significant.

Case Study 117 – Polypharmacy (Schizophrenia)

Paulette stopped me in the hallway at a conference to say, "You mentioned animal therapy in your workshop as one potential therapy. I wanted to tell you that if it wasn't for my cat, I would have committed suicide. You may think it odd to decide to live for something as small and insignificant as a cat, but that's why I'm alive today."

> *Paulette continued her story and told me that she had been on a cocktail of as many as six psychotropics for many years, to treat schizophrenia.*
> *Her life became unmanageable. Finally, she decided she had no choice but to find a new psychiatrist to significantly scale back her psychotropics.*
> *She found a psychiatrist who listened to her concerns and acted. Paulette is now stable, working, and managing well on a single psychotropic. She still loves her cat dearly.*
> *__Bottom Line__: Paulette found purpose (a Wellness Basic) in her cat. That purpose kept her alive and gave her a sense of self-determination (another Wellness Basic) to find a new practitioner who could help her experiment to end her serious polypharmacy risk (a part of Over-Care Avoidance).*

Practitioner's Story 7 – Tailored Treatment (Bipolar)

Seven case studies were selected from the practice of an Integrative Psychiatrist. All were patients with bipolar, aged 17 to 28, who had a poor response to, or significant side effects from, psychotropics.

Treatment was tailored to the patient. Each used multiple approaches, including herbs, nutrients, amino acids, acupuncture, diet, homeopathy, stimulation reduction, sleep/wake cycle changes, psychosocial therapies, guided imagery, and self-regulation with meditation and mindfulness.

All seven were gradually and safely withdrawn from medication and stable for at least ten months with virtually no symptoms. A very slow psychotropic tapering process was vital, averaging forty-three weeks.[1460]

__Bottom Line__: Customizing treatment with a variety of non-drug treatments can speed recovery and eliminate the need for long-term psychotropic use. Find practitioners who consider all the recovery tools available.

WHAT ARE ADDITIONAL RESOURCES?

- Polypharmacy in psychiatry. p. 341, http://goo.gl/t6pu8E.
- What can you do about polypharmacy? http://goo.gl/W3y3aA.
- Polypharmacy: The Good, the Bad, and the Ugly. http://goo.gl/vL4NzC.

8 – Most Promising Therapies

This chapter contains the most promising non-drug therapies for seven major mental health diagnoses:

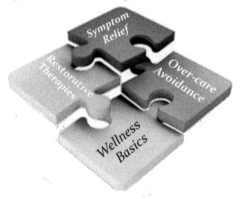

- Depression
- Schizophrenia
- Bipolar
- Anxiety
- Dementia
- Substance Abuse
- Insomnia

These therapies span the full *Wellness Continuum* (Figure 9, p. 47) and have been distilled from the 27 broad approaches and 294 individual techniques found in chapters 3-7.

Figure 35 – Simplified Wellness Continuum

In this chapter we winnow the mountain of *possible* approaches down to a list of the *most promising* things to try. In this context, *most promising* means those therapies that have the strongest evidence of efficacy and safety. It doesn't mean they are the best for you, but they are the ones that research suggests you should try first.

The list of what is *most promising* for each diagnosis is condensed, giving a bird's-eye view of therapy options. Page references will send you to earlier chapters, where you will find the detailed description and evidence for the therapy.

With your practitioners, use *Most Promising Therapies* as an evidence-based menu, selecting approaches that best fit your diagnosis, lab test results, personal history, and preferences. Your selections will become part of your individual recovery plan, which will naturally evolve over time as you find what works for you.

To prepare for the work ahead, attitudes are critically important:

- *Be sensible* – consider the probable benefits/risks, costs, and availability of approaches prior to experimentation.
- *Be realistic* – know that some approaches won't work for you. We each respond differently to various approaches.
- *Be hopeful and optimistic* – know that some approaches will work for you—and you will find them through experimentation.
- *Be patient* – give your therapies a chance to work. Find success in even the small steps of recovery.
- *Be persistent* – develop an attitude of "leaving no stone unturned".
- *Be kind* – Plans never seem to work out as expected. False starts and setbacks are part of the process. Understand and forgive both yourself and those around you for the inevitable hiccups.

Building your Recovery Plan

Before you consider the *Most Promising Therapies* in this chapter, it is important to get grounded in key concepts related to your recovery plan.

- **Always consult with practitioners**. Trained, certified, empathetic practitioners are vital to every recovery process. (See *People of Recovery*, p. 35.) When you choose professionals skilled in mental health recovery and the specific approaches you select, trust them to do their job. *Do not self-diagnose or self-treat—that can be dangerous.* This point cannot be over-emphasized. Your practitioners are your partners and advisors in recovery.
- **Own your plan and lead it, to the greatest extent possible**. The U.S. Substance Abuse and Mental Health Services Administration (SAMHSA) emphasizes, "Individuals optimize their autonomy and independence...by leading, controlling, and exercising choice over the services and supports that assist their recovery."[1461] In short, SAMHSA is advocating *Self-determination* (p. 87); this is crucial to recovery. Practitioners typically don't integrate the parts of your recovery plan for you—you must do that.[1462]
- **Use effective assessments to target experimentation.** Your practitioners should use the best assessment tools to look for possible causes of your mental health issues. They should investigate your personal/medical history, symptoms, past traumas and stresses, blood/urine chemistry, and much more. These assessments include *Biomedical Test Panels* (p. 323) and an evaluation with a psychotherapist. You and your practitioners should choose therapies that best address the issues discovered in these assessments.

- **Understand your chosen approaches.** Learn about your chosen approaches before using them. Follow the many links in this book to find details and gain insight from practitioners and people who have used the approaches.
- **Choose approaches that match your symptoms and diagnosis.** You may want to consider multiple diagnosis categories (for example, bipolar and insomnia) if your symptoms don't fit neatly into a single category.
- **Choose approaches that match your stage of recovery.** (See p. 32.) For instance, *Housing & Security* (p. 57) are necessary in the first recovery stage. Many approaches can be used in multiple stages.
- **Choose both general and targeted approaches.** Your recovery plan should start with general approaches that are helpful to nearly everyone with mental health issues. (See *Template of Recovery*, p. 273.) Then add targeted approaches that have been found particularly beneficial for your specific diagnosis. (See the section devoted to each diagnosis.)
- **Experiment in tier order.** Approaches targeted to specific diagnoses are tiered based on the strength of supporting evidence. In general, Tier 1 approaches have good meta-analyses showing they are effective, Tier 2 approaches have multiple well-designed studies, and Tier 3 approaches have more suggestive evidence. Consider Tier 1 approaches first, with your practitioners' advice. The foundational work of Psychiatrist Dr. James Lake, MD[16, 18] and Researcher Dr. Jerome Sarris, PhD.,[1463] as well as the works of the professional psychological associations of the United States, United Kingdom, Australia, and Canada strongly influenced this tiering. Both Lake and Sarris have used similar tiering strategies to distill research and make it more accessible and actionable for both practitioners and lay people.
- **Experiment across the *full* Wellness Continuum.** We often need simultaneous efforts in all four categories of the *Wellness Continuum*. Improve your *Wellness Basics* (p. 55) while you and your practitioners evaluate *Restorative* approaches (p. 115 and p. 165). In addition, you may need *Symptom Relief* (p. 221) to help you manage the process, while ensuring *Over-care Avoidance* (p. 257).
- **Focus *early* in the Wellness Continuum.** Often, the more you focus early in the *Wellness Continuum* (improving out-of-balance *Wellness Basics* and using *Restorative* approaches), the more complete your recovery. This isn't easy, since it means changing ingrained habits and working with therapies that require more effort than popping a pill. But, the payoff can be substantial. Generally, the more diligently you use *Wellness Basics* and *Restorative* approaches, the less you need *Symptom Relief.*
- **Plan each experiment.** Experimenting with a therapy means trying it for a reasonable period to assess its impact. Typically, experimenting within a therapy group (for instance, herbs) is best done one at a time; trying three things at once might yield improvements, but you won't know what caused the improvement. Consider a crossover technique;[1464] if your symptoms

improve after you start one approach, then worsen when you stop, you have a good sign that the approach works for you.

- **See each experiment through**. Therapies show results at different times, so try them long enough to see if they work for you. Follow the plan agreed upon with your practitioner, provided you don't experience troublesome side effects or have other issues. For instance, *Nutrient Therapy* (p. 167) targeting a pyrrole disorder can often show improvement in as little as a week, but addressing copper overload with nutrients can take up to a year.
- **Track your results**. Track your symptoms and side effects and try to make connections between the changes you feel and the specific approaches you use. This helps you determine what works and what doesn't.
- **Stick with what works**. Unfortunately, most often there is no single silver bullet. Stick with approaches that work for you and experiment with new approaches. The things that help you get well are likely the things that can help you stay well.
- **Use common sense**. Watch for therapy interactions, especially *Biomedical* and *Herbal* approaches with psychotropics. Discuss with your practitioners what you are doing and experiencing.
- **Use psychotropics cautiously, only as needed**. If psychotropics are a part of your recovery plan, seek your minimum effective dosage where symptom relief and side effects balance. This can be done by either a "start low and go slow" approach, or if you are already taking meds, a *very slow* taper down from your current dosage. (See
- Practitioner's Story 7, p. 268, that highlights a ten-month taper.) In either case, only change dosages under your practitioner's guidance. Understand psychotropic benefits and limitations, as well as their long- and short-term side effects and withdrawal difficulties. (See *Changes in Treatment*, p. 24.) Psychotropics that are particularly effective at relieving symptoms often come with heightened side effects.[1465]
- **Consider self-help tools**. Those who prefer self-led approaches should consider the many *Recovery Models & Tools* (p. 327).

This spirit of experimentation is best exemplified by the great inventor Thomas Edison. Before inventing the lightbulb, Edison stated, "I know 10,000 ways that don't work." He found inspiration and hope in his failures, since he realized that his failures narrowed the field of options down to the ones with the best chance for success. We should do the same. To get started, consider the *Template of Recovery*.

Template of Recovery

With the dizzying array of non-drug options available, how do we best sort through them all?

A good place to start is the *Template of Recovery* – a set of general approaches helpful to everyone with mental health issues, regardless of diagnosis. *The Template of Recovery* is laid out simply below. There are tables for each category of the *Wellness Continuum* (Figure 9, p. 47). Within each table, non-drug approaches are clustered into the *Recovery Stage* (p. 32) in which they are most helpful.

For instance, if you or your loved-one is in the *Distress* stage, think about engaging practitioners (a *Wellness Basic*) who can run a full-protocol biomedical exam (a *Biomedical Restorative* task) and perform a full evaluation for trauma, stress, and emotional issues (a *Psychosocial Restorative* task).

The *Template of Recovery* is the starting point for your individual recovery plan and is a foundation for the *Most Promising Therapies* for each major mental health diagnosis found later in this chapter.

Stage	*Wellness Basics for All Diagnoses*	
	Approach	**Comments**
Distress	Crisis intervention	Call 911 if in danger; consider *Peer Respites* (p. 132), *Hospitalization* (p. 327), and psychotropics to stabilize.
	Befriending	Supporters should talk with the individual but avoid excess questioning or confrontation; listen; show *companionship* (p. 99), *recovery attitudes* (p. 37), and *unconditional love* (p. 100). Use the language of the individual's experience.
	Engage practitioners	Engage qualified practitioners (p. 35) who expect recovery and have a history of aiding *personal recovery* (p. 31).
	Baseline care	Ensure continuous *Housing & Security* (p. 57), *Emotional Sanctuary* (p. 101), access to nutritious food (p. 61), and ability to sleep.
	Reduce stressors	Reduce obligations, stimulation, stress, toxic relationships, and *Expressed Emotions* (p. 79). Relax expectations (p. 39).
	Substance avoidance	Work substance-abuse issues (p. 305) and mental health issues together. Consider *Addiction Co-Therapy* (p. 332).
Awareness	Hope & Knowledge	Gain recovery *Knowledge* (p. 40); develop hope and recovery *expectation* (p. 106); foster *self-compassion* (p. 86).
	Foster self-management	Start doing things that are positive and self-affirming; foster 3 *Awareness Stage* perspectives (p. 33).
	Initial self-care	Start *Calm Awareness* technique (p. 73) of 5 min/day. Get outside often and walk. Address diet (p. 61)—especially avoid junk food. Get sufficient sleep. Avoid social isolation.

Stage	Wellness Basics for All Diagnoses	
	Approach	**Comments**
Preparation	Identify 1st approaches	Review *Recovery Tools/apps* (p. 327) and *Most Promising Therapies* for your diagnosis (this chapter); identify ones you think are best for you.
Preparation	Commit to plan with practitioners	Review recovery ideas with practitioners; accept their counsel; agree on initial recovery plan; find new practitioners for chosen approaches as needed; lead the effort to the greatest extent possible.
Preparation	Improve self-care	Expand *Calm Awareness* (p. 73) practice to 15+ min/day; further improve diet; curb use of addictive substances; get 6+ hours of sleep/day; develop daily routines; notice thoughts and emotions that get in your way (p. 84).
Preparation	Exercise (p. 62)	Choose some form of exercise with goal of 3+ times/week of moderate exertion for 30-45 min/session; consistency at lower exertion (e.g., brisk walking) is more important than high exertion.
Rebuilding	Healthy diet (p. 62)	Eat Mediterranean-like diet: about 40% carbs (whole grains, green vegetables, berries), 40% protein, 20% fat; ensure high Omega-3 intake and B vitamins; consider fatty fish (see Figure 13, p. 65) and nuts; restrict alcohol, refined sugar, saturated fat, and processed foods; avoid junk food; take ample probiotics for digestive health.
Rebuilding	Execute & evolve plan	Stick with and evolve your plan as best you can; forgive yourself for stumbles. Continue symptom tracking. Know this takes time.
Rebuilding	Social interaction	Become more oriented to externals, engaging with supportive friends and peers (p. 99); consider support groups (p. 131).
Rebuilding	Mind-Body hygiene	Continue some form of *Calm Awareness* (p. 73) and *Exercise* (p. 62). Consider *a Mind-Body Discipline* (p. 111) that combines both; they are best done 2-4 times/week, 30-90 minutes each. Learn from qualified teacher.
Maintenance	Relapse avoidance	Maintain *Emotional Sanctuary* (p. 101) and approaches that work; be careful with stressors; ensure health services access.
Maintenance	Self-management	Refocus occasionally on *Attitudes* (p. 37) that promote wellness; monitor unhelpful thoughts/emotions (p. 84).
Maintenance	Purpose, Meaning & Engagement	Extend yourself *slowly*; clarify your *Purpose* (p. 94); engage in *creative activities* you enjoy (p. 137); look beyond solely self-interest (see *Self-transcendence*, p. 105).

Stage	Biomedical Restorative Approaches for All Diagnoses	
	Approach	**Comments**
Distress	Full-protocol biomedical lab testing	**Consider this mandatory** to create a good differential diagnosis (p. 21) and target treatment. Work with an *Integrative Biomedical Practitioner* (p. 320) who uses robust *Biomedical Test Panels* (p. 323). Start individualized therapies based on test results; retest periodically to assess progress.
All	Nutrient Plan	Customize nutrient plan based on biomedical testing. Consider *Food Allergy Tests* (p. 210), especially for gluten & dairy – even mild intolerance may affect symptoms.

Stage	Psychosocial Restorative Approaches for All Diagnoses	
	Approach	**Comments**
Distress	Psychosocial evaluation	**Consider this mandatory**. A therapist assesses for trauma, stress, and other emotional factors. Find one you respect, who seeks your self-determination and with whom you have rapport; a strong relationship is often more important than a specific therapy. Consider psychosocial therapies - *they are often as effective as or more effective than psychotropics.*
Awareness	Psycho-education	Builds awareness, hope, and self-empowerment, either self-directed or face-to-face for individuals and families (p. 126).
	Motivational Interviewing	Consider help in clarifying goals and increasing motivation, to jump-start commitment to recovery (p.126).
	Self-management	Learn to identify and alter unhelpful thought/emotional responses for better *Effective Self-Management* (p. 83). *CBT* (p. 117) can be very helpful (online, app or face-to-face).

Stage	Symptom Relief for All Diagnoses	
	Approach	**Comments**
All		Currently, no approaches appear to be generally effective in relieving symptoms for all diagnoses. Rather, see the targeted *Symptom Relief* approaches for each diagnosis later in this chapter.

Stage	Over-care Avoidance for All Diagnoses	
	Approach	**Comments**
All	Over-care Avoidance	If psychotropics are used, target minimum effective dosages either with a "start low and go slow" mentality or, if already on them, consider a *very slow* reduction under practitioner care. Find the benefit/side effects balance point. Work with practitioners to avoid or minimize *polypharmacy* and *off-label prescribing* (p. 263). If you are concerned about your psychotropic prescriptions, consider getting a 2nd opinion.

Depression Therapies

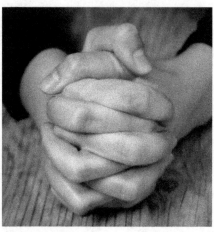

The most promising evidence-based therapies for depression should be considered in the context of *Building Your Recovery Plan* (p. 270). Depression symptoms include depressed mood, diminished interest in activities, weight loss, insomnia or excessive sleep, agitation, fatigue, feelings of worthlessness, and diminished ability to concentrate. Depression covers a variety of mental health diagnoses:

- Dysthymia (chronic depression)
- Bipolar depression (addressed in bipolar section)
- Seasonal Affective Disorder (SAD)
- Postpartum Depression (PPD)
- Atypical Depression (chronic overeating, oversleeping, and sensitivity)
- Major Depressive Disorder

Start your recovery plan with approaches selected from the *Template of Recovery* (p. 273), then add specific approaches for depression from the tables below. Work closely with your practitioners to create, execute, and evolve this plan.

Template for Recovery approaches especially important for depression are:

- **Biomedical Testing**. Robust biomedical testing (p. 323) should be considered mandatory. Work with an *Integrative Biomedical Practitioner* (*See People of Recovery,* p. 35) who can select the tests and assess potential underlying physical causes of depression. In cases of suicidal depression, test for elevated translocator protein levels, a marker for brain inflammation.[1466] For treatment-resistant depression, consider cerebral spinal fluid metabolic testing (p. 325) looking for deficiencies since a small study shows imbalances are relatively common. From 300,000 blood samples of people with depression, the Walsh Institute (see Figure 28, p. 168) has identified **five primary depression biotypes: undermethylation, folate deficiency, copper overload, pyrrole disorder, and toxic overload.** Knowing your biotype helps identify an appropriate nutrient response. An open-label trial indicates that 70% of people with depression who use customized *Nutrient Therapy* for six months based on the Walsh diagnostic and treatment techniques return to normal without psychotropics.[19] In nearly all the remaining 30%, symptoms can go into remission with lower psychotropic dosages. The biomedical options in the tables below will require greater experimentation if you don't use testing.

- **Psychosocial Evaluation.** Depression can be caused or influenced by past trauma, stress, unhelpful thinking, or other difficulties that can be effectively addressed with psychosocial therapy. Work with a psychotherapist you trust who can identify issues and recommend therapies.
- **Calm Awareness.** Find a *Calm Awareness* (p. 73) technique that works for you. Mindfulness is especially helpful for relieving depressive symptoms. An eight-week meditation class (p. 78) can be as effective as antidepressants.
- **Exercise.** *Exercise* (p. 62) is extremely important. If done consistently, it can significantly improve depression. Aerobic exercise can be as effective as antidepressants, with benefits in three and six weeks without antidepressant side effects and with add-on cardiovascular benefits. Try to establish a discipline immediately.
- **Mind-Body approaches.** Research has shown that yoga reduces depressive symptoms by combining exercise and mindfulness.
- **Diet.** Avoid diets high in carbohydrates, especially refined sugar, since carbohydrates are associated with greater depression. Especially avoid junk food. Omega-3 sources are helpful.

In addition to the above, see the targeted approaches for depression found in the tables below. With your practitioners, consider them in tier order.

Biomedical Restorative Therapies for Depression		
Approach	**T**	**Comments**
DHEA / 7-keto DHEA (p. 200)	1	Typical dose of 50-450 mg/day with benefit in 2-4 weeks. Can be used with antidepressants. *Men with prostate issues and women with estrogen receptor breast cancer should avoid.*
SAM-e (p.188)	1	Typical dose 300-1600 mg/day before meals in 2-3 dosages with benefit in 1-4 weeks. May be used with antidepressants. Often helpful for undermethylation biotypes. Best taken with B12 and folate (1 mg ea). Rarely causes agitation and mania.
Folate/ Methylfolate (p. 171)	1	Typical dose 7-15 mg/day L-methylfolate for moderate-to-severe depression. Can be used with antidepressants. Especially helpful for low-folate depression biotypes, but not for undermethylation biotypes. Ensure B12 levels are in bounds before use.
Vitamin D3 (p. 174)	1	Typical dose 400-800 IU/day up to 10,000 IU/day with benefit in 1-2 weeks. Often as good as antidepressants. One-time doses of 100,000 IU can be useful for SAD. Can be used with antidepressants. Usually well tolerated.
Omega-3 Fatty Acids (p. 187)	2	EPA may be as effective as antidepressants. Use as supplement or increase EPA in diet. Possible gastrointestinal issues. May affect glucose metabolism in diabetics.

Biomedical Restorative Therapies for Depression

Approach	T	Comments
Probiotics (p. 63)	2	Dose varies. Lactobacillus/bifidobacterium combo aids digestion. Can be used with antidepressants. Rare chance of infection.
5-HTP / L-tryptophan (p. 183)	2	Typical dose 300-600 mg/day 5-HTP in 2-3 doses, or 1-2 gm/day L-tryptophan with benefit in 3 wks similar to antidepressants. Generally safe. May sedate, take at bedtime. Can be used with antidepressants. Avoid with low-folate biotypes and MAOIs.
Acetyl-L-Carnitine (p. 181)	2	Typical dose 500mg-2gm/day in 3 doses, with benefit in 4 weeks for moderate depression. Generally safe and may be as effective as antidepressants; can be used with antidepressants. Especially helpful for the elderly with cognitive impairment.
Magnesium (p. 178)	2	Typical oral dose 125-300mg 4 times daily; also available intravenous or skin cream, with benefit in 2-4 weeks. Use with vitamin D3 increases cellular uptake. Can be used with antidepressants. Usually well tolerated.
Zinc (p. 179)	2	Dosages vary. Can be used with antidepressants. Mild side effects, but usually well tolerated.
Thyroid evaluation (p. 198)	2	Hypothyroidism is strongly associated with depression. Consider thyroid evaluation mandatory; even subclinical (not severe enough to cause symptoms) cases may contribute to depression.
Inositol (p. 171)	3	Typical dose 12-20 gr/day, including for treatment-resistant depression, with benefit in 2-4 weeks. Gastrointestinal issues may occur. Generally well tolerated but may produce mania.
Selenium (p. 179)	3	If blood tests show deficiency, 100 μg daily dose can significantly improve depression and anxiety.
DL-phenylalanine (p. 181)	3	If amino acid test shows deficiency, 75–200 mg dose per day (possibly up to 3-4 gr/day) may be as effective as antidepressants for depression.
Multivitamin (p. 175)	3	May improve antidepressant effectiveness. Multivitamins including B1, B2, B6, C, and E at 10 times the RDI may improve mood. Use B12 for low-folate biotype. Usually well tolerated.
Chromium (p. 176)	3	Typical dose 600μg/day chromium picolinate. Can be used with antidepressants. May influence cholesterol for those on beta blockers; typically well tolerated. *Avoid use with bipolar. Diabetic caution since it may lower insulin.*
Phosphatidyl-serine (p. 184)	3	Typical dose 200 mg/day may reduce depressive symptoms in 3-6 weeks.
Therapeutic Fasting (p. 64)	3	Fasting may reduce symptoms, perhaps by aiding bodily detoxification. Use only under the guidance of practitioners.
Folinic Acid (p. 186)	3	For treatment-resistant depression, if tests show low cerebral spinal fluid folate, folinic acid supplementation may help.

Psychosocial Restorative Therapies for Depression

Approach	T	Comments / Evaluation
CBT (p. 117)	1	Cognitive Behavioral Therapy (CBT) is as effective as antidepressants in a number of trials.

Psychosocial Restorative Therapies for Depression

Approach	T	Comments / Evaluation
Interpersonal Psy. (p. 132)	1	Interpersonal psychotherapy is effective as CBT and antidepressants, with significant improvement post-treatment.
Psychodynamic therapy (p. 127)	1	Shows significant benefit for depression. Somewhat less effective than Interpersonal Psychotherapy and CBT.
Psychoeducation (p. 126)	2	Provides information on depression, typical therapies, prognoses, and how to manage symptoms.
DBT (p. 120)	2	Dialectic Behavioral Therapy (DBT) can increase motivation and control thoughts that can influence depression.
EEG biofeedback (p. 142)	2	Dosage varies; safe with other therapies when used under guidance of trained therapist. An alternative to other *Calm Awareness* (p. 73) relaxation techniques.
Peer Support (p. 131)	2	Offers hope, belief in the possibility of recovery, incentive to move from social isolation and fosters self-determination - all vital in the *Awareness* stage of recovery (p. 33).
Acupuncture (p. 159)	2	Daily/weekly treatments lasting 20-60 minutes for moderate depression. Generally safe. Always use sterile needles. May be used with antidepressants.
MBCT (p. 121)	3	Mindfulness-Based Cognitive Therapy (MBCT) is used primarily to avoid depressive relapse. Helpful in preventing depressive episodes and reducing anxiety.

Symptom Relief Therapies for Depression

Approach	T	Comments / Evaluation
St. John's Wort (p. 229)	1	Typical dose 900-1800mg/day in 3 doses, with benefit within 6 weeks. Mild side effects. Potential toxic drug interactions. *Can lessen birth control pill effectiveness. Avoid use with MAOIs), protease inhibitors, immunosuppressive agents, and if pregnant.*
Saffron (p. 233)	1	Typical dose 30mg/day for mild-to-moderate depression, with benefit in 4-6 weeks. Can be used with antidepressants.
Bright Light Therapy (p. 239)	2	Typical dose 60-120 min in morning with white (10,000 lux) or dim blue/red (250 lux) light. Benefit in 2-3 weeks, especially for SAD. May be better than antidepressants for major depression. May cause hypomania (if bipolar) or insomnia (if used after morning); can be used with other therapies. Use with exercise, increases effectiveness. Avoid eye damage by avoiding light sources with UV; do not stare into light.
Sleep Deprivation (p. 70)	2	For moderate depression, one night without sleep, then sleep phase advance can quickly decrease depression. Can be used with antidepressants—under supervision only.
Borage (p. 224)	2	Typical dose 375 mg/day of E. amoenum aqueous extract for mild-to-moderate major depression, with benefit in 4 weeks. Side effects similar to placebo.
tDCS (p. 253)	2	Typical dose 30-45 min/day, with benefit in 3 weeks. Start daily, taper to twice weekly, as needed. Self-administered. Can use with antidepressants. May cause slight dizziness.

Symptom Relief Therapies for Depression

Approach	T	Comments / Evaluation
Anion Therapy (p. 241)	2	Typical dose 30 min/day for depression, with benefit in 2-3 weeks using negative ion generator for unipolar depression and SAD. Can be used with other therapies. No side effects.
Rhodiola Rosea (p. 228)	2	Typical dose 150-900 mg/day, with benefit in 2-4 weeks for mild-to-moderate depression. Can be used with antidepressants. Typically well tolerated, although may cause mild anxiety and insomnia. *Avoid for those with bipolar.*
Massage (p. 242)	3	To reduce stress, 20-min session 1-3 times/week. Increases immune function, with benefit in 4-6 weeks.
Chamomile (p. 225)	3	Typical dose 220 mg 2-4 times/day, with benefit in 2-4 weeks. Start with one capsule/day and increase as needed. Can interact with drugs. Mild side effects, though rare allergic reaction. Avoid use with substances that cause drowsiness.
Ayurvedic herbs (p. 234)	3	A variety of compounded herbs are available: Brahmi, Mentat, Geriforte, Withania somnifera, Mucuna pruriens, Acorus calamus, Convolvulus pluricaulis, and Celastrus panniculatus. Consult trained Ayurvedic practitioner.

WHAT CONSIDERATIONS SHOULD I KEEP IN MIND?

Safety is the #1 priority. If someone becomes a danger to themselves or others, call 911. Hospital emergency rooms can help the person stabilize, sometimes using the drug ketamine because of its rapid anti-depressive effects[1334] and suicidal ideation reduction[1484], though its long-term impact is unclear.[1467]

From a psychosocial perspective, *Cognitive Behavioral Therapy* (CBT, p. 117) is considered the most effective therapy for depression, on par with antidepressants without their many side effects. CBT teaches methods for controlling thoughts, influencing emotions, and improving depressive symptoms. *Interpersonal Therapy* (p. 132) and *Psychodynamic Psychotherapy* (p. 127) are similarly effective.

For symptom-relief with drugs, antidepressants have significant risks and limitations (Figure 3, p. 26) with up to 86%[1468] of people experiencing side effects. Within 6-months of starting antidepressant use, 53% discontinue use, 23% because of the side effects.[1469] Analyses of independent trials suggest that antidepressants include a surprisingly large placebo effect: 46% symptom relief with antidepressants and 38% symptom relief with placebos.[1470] At milder symptom levels, antidepressants have *no* advantage over placebo.[1407]

For symptom-relief with non-drug approaches, St. John's Wort has been well tested with favorable results. Consider also *Transcranial Direct Current Stimulation* (p. 253) or other minimally invasive Electromagnetic techniques, since they can often provide symptom relief and typically have few or no side effects. Avoid *Electroconvulsive Therapy* (p. 244)—many researchers have identified significant risks in the procedure.

Sub-types of depression have special considerations.

- *For Seasonal Affective Disorder (SAD).* SAD is a seasonal pattern that may occur with depression or bipolar. Spring/summer bipolar mania is often present with fall/winter depression, in a yearly cycle. [1471] Treating the mania can help minimize the depression. SAD treatments include *Bright Light Therapy* (p. 239), *Audio Visual Stimulation* (p. 240), *Vitamin D3* (p. 174), *Melatonin* (p. 202), *5-HTP/L-tryptophan* (p. 183), and exercise (p. 62). Light therapy in combination with exercise is especially helpful.
- *For postpartum depression.* Consider vitamins B2, B7, B9, B12, and D (both during and after pregnancy), iron (if found to be deficient), a healthy diet (p. 62) and Bright Light Therapy (p. 239). Estrogen (p. 204) has proven effective but is associated with higher risk of breast cancer.

See "Depression, Case Studies" in the index for individual stories.

REAL-WORLD EXPERIENCE

Case Study 118 – Undermethylation (Depression)
A successful executive, Charles had been depressed for fifteen years and had suffered with thoughts of suicide. When a doctor tested for physical symptoms, he showed signs of undermethylation, including hay fever, high libido, headaches, and anxiety. He had tried Zoloft, Paxil, and Prozac; each helped somewhat, but had side effects that caused him to stop taking them.
His blood work revealed an extremely high histamine level (142 ng/ml), mildly elevated pyrroles, and low-normal homocysteine. He was given SAM-e, methionine, zinc, serine, calcium, magnesium, and vitamins A, B6, C, D, and E.
He started improving in the third month of treatment. At twelve months, the depression had been insignificant for several months.[19]

WHAT ARE ADDITIONAL RESOURCES?

- University of Michigan Depression Toolkit. http://goo.gl/yMSJ6m.
- BlackDog Toolkit. http://goo.gl/nHe65a.

Schizophrenia Therapies

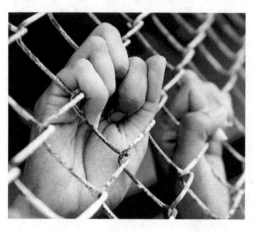

The most promising evidence-based therapies for schizophrenia should be considered in the context of *Building Your Recovery Plan* (p. 270).

Schizophrenia includes the following major mental health diagnoses:

- Catatonic schizophrenia (withdrawn and mute)
- Disorganized schizophrenia (incoherent speech and thought)
- Paranoid schizophrenia (feeling suspicious, grandiose, or persecuted)
- Schizoaffective (schizophrenia with a depression and/or mania)

Schizophrenia symptoms fall into three areas:

- *Positive symptoms* include hallucinations (see, hear, smell, or feel something that others can't, especially voices) and delusions (false beliefs held with evidence to the contrary).
- *Negative symptoms* include flat affect (no facial movement with speech, or dullness), lack of pleasure in life, and lack of ability to plan and execute.
- *Cognitive symptoms* include difficulty in understanding, focusing attention, and remembering.

Start your recovery plan with approaches selected from the *Template of Recovery* (p. 273) then add specific approaches for schizophrenia from the tables below. Work closely with your practitioners, leveraging their expertise and guidance. Approaches especially important for schizophrenia include:

- **Biomedical Testing.** Robust biomedical testing (p. 323) should be considered mandatory. Work with an *Integrative Biomedical Practitioner* who can select tests and assess for potential underlying physical causes. (See *People of Recovery,* p. 35.) From 3,600 blood samples of people with schizophrenia, the Walsh Institute[19] (see Figure 28, p. 168) has identified **five primary schizophrenia biotypes: overmethylation, undermethylation, pyrrole disorder, gluten intolerance, and a category that includes thyroid deficiency.** All biotypes involve severe *Oxidative Stress* (p. 52), and many involve *Methylation* (p. 54) issues. Over 85% of the people with paranoid schizophrenia have overmethylation; 95% of those with schizoaffective disorder have undermethylation; and abnormal blood levels of methyl and folate are found in 70% of those with schizophrenia. Knowing your biotype helps identify an appropriate nutrient response. When people with schizophrenia use customized *Nutrient Therapy* (p. 167) based on the Walsh Institute's protocols, 75%-80% report significant symptom improvement and the ability to reduce medication, while about 5% can eliminate medication altogether.[19] Further, a meta-analysis found that especially megadoses of B vitamins were consistently effective in reducing symptoms.[1472] The biomedical options in the tables below can be used without testing, but will mean more guesswork. Also consider evaluating for obstructive sleep apnoea since it is three times more common in people with schizophrenia[262] and can cause schizophrenia symptoms.

- **Psychosocial and Trauma Evaluation.** Childhood abuse and neglect appear to be causative factors in psychosis. [1473-1474] Those who had three types of abuse (e.g. sexual, physical, bullying) are 18 times more likely to have psychosis; those who experienced five types are 193 times more likely.[1475] In addition, 70% of people who hear voices had the voices begin after a very stressful triggering event.[658] A trusted psychotherapist can help evaluate for trauma and recommend trauma-informed therapies.

- **Diet.** *Diligently reduce saturated fat* and especially sugar *in the diet*; both are associated with worsening schizophrenia. Consider reducing red meat and eating more low-mercury fish (Figure 13, p. 65). Equally important, assess for gluten, dairy, and other food allergies (p. 209). People with schizophrenia have ten times the likelihood of having markers for gluten sensitivity and fifty times the likelihood of celiac disease than the normal population. They often see marked improvement on gluten/casein free diets.

- **Befriending.** It is vital to respect the individual with schizophrenia. (See *Honoring their Experience*, p. 38.) You needn't agree with what they're saying, but calmly accept it as their experience. This may be difficult, since the delusions and hallucinations of schizophrenia can seem strange and even frightening. Use the individual's words to talk about their experiences, recognizing the *Importance of Language* (p. 105). Offer *Companionship* (p. 99) and *Unconditional Love* (p. 100). Speak calmly, slowly, and simply and focus on only one topic at a time to effectively communicate with someone experiencing cognitive issues. Relax your expectations.

- **Calm Awareness.** Practicing *Loving Kindness Meditation*[302] for twenty minutes each day can be helpful. *Mindfulness-Based Cognitive Therapy* (p. 121) and *Controlled Breathing* (p. 75) are also helpful and generally quite safe, although multi-hour intense meditation in rare situations may cause a psychotic break. Mindfulness practices often improve self-awareness and the ability to manage psychotic symptoms; it also reduces social withdrawal.

- **Exercise.** Regular aerobic exercise at least three times a week can improve psychosis symptoms.

In addition to the above, see the targeted approaches for schizophrenia found in the tables below. With your practitioners, consider them in tier order.

Biomedical Restorative Therapies for Schizophrenia

Approach	T	Comments / Evaluation
Glycine (p. 181)	2	Typical dose 30-60 mg/day, with benefits for both negative and positive psychotic symptoms, cognitive function, and depression, in 4-6 weeks. Use with or without antipsychotics. Generally well tolerated; may rarely worsen psychosis taken in large dosages.
Melatonin (p. 202)	2	Typical dose 10 mg/day at bedtime for improving cognitive functioning and sleep. Can be used with antipsychotics. Generally safe. May cause drowsiness or headache; may reduce sexual side effects of antipsychotics.
Sarcosine (p. 184)	2	Typical dose 2 g/day may improve both positive and negative symptoms. Use with or without psychotropics. Generally well tolerated.
Omega-3 Fatty Acids (p. 187)	2	Typical dose 2-4g/day of EPA or EPA+DHA, to slow the progression of psychotic symptoms and decrease positive psychosis symptoms. Use with or without antipsychotics; may allow reduction in antipsychotic dosages. Possible side effects: gastrointestinal issues.
Estrogen (p. 204)	2	Typical dose 2mg/day oral Estradiol or 200 μg transdermal 1-2 times/week. Side effects include sexual dysfunction, feminizing (men), and headaches. *Avoid if pregnant or diagnosed with hormone-dependent cancer, a recent stroke, heart attack, or blood clot.*
Vitamin E (p. 174)	2	Typical dose 1200-1600 IU/day alpha tocopherol for extrapyramidal side effects of antipsychotics. Generally safe, but may cause headache and gastrointestinal issues. Avoid if taking blood-thinning drugs. High doses may increase risk of cancer and increased mortality.
Vitamin D (p. 174)	2	Typical dose 2,000 IUs daily, to improve mood and potentially reduce antipsychotic dosages. Virtually everyone with schizophrenia has sub-optimal Vitamin D levels.
Broad Amino Acid Therapy	3	Run comprehensive lab test for amino acids; certain amino acids can be helpful for schizophrenia, including D-Serine (p. 180), L-Lysine (p. 182), N-acetyl cysteine (p. 184), and L-Theanine (p. 182). D-serine may be helpful for people with treatment-refractory schizophrenia.
Vitamins B1, B3, B9	3	Typical doses are 3-8 gm/day of B3 (as niacinamide); 15 mg/day of B9 (as methylfolate); and 500 mg/day B1. Generally well tolerated, but B3 may cause flushing.
Vitamin C (p. 173)	3	Typical dose of 500mg-3gr/day, with benefit (decreasing severity of symptoms) within 4 weeks. May be used with antipsychotics. Generally safe. May cause mild gastrointestinal distress.
Vit. B12 (p. 172)	3	Typical dose 400 mcg/day may reduce negative symptoms. Serum B12 should be checked as standard care.
DHEA (p. 200)	3	Start with low dose to test tolerability; raise to 50-200 mg/day for benefit (reducing symptoms and extrapyramidal side effects, improved cognitive functioning) in 2-6 weeks. Take in morning. Generally safe with antipsychotics. May cause anxiety and insomnia, and men with prostate issues may have side effects.
Pregneno-lone (p. 200)	3	Typical dose 400-500mg with antipsychotics may significantly improve positive and negative symptoms.

Biomedical Restorative Therapies for Schizophrenia

Approach	T	Comments / Evaluation
Vitamins/ Nutrients	3	EMPowerplus (p. 185) and multi-vitamins (p. 175) have shown anecdotal ability to improve symptoms.
Selenium (p. 179)	3	Low selenium is associated with schizophrenia. Dosing is not clear; the U.S. RDA for people over 13 is 55mcg with a tolerable upper limit of 400 mcg/day. Generally safe, but it can worsen hypothyroidism, especially in people with iodine deficiency.
Therapeutic Fasting (p. 64)	3	Fasting may reduce psychosis, perhaps by aiding bodily detoxification and avoiding food allergies. Soviet clinics found 25-30 day water fasts (consuming ample water but very little food) with significant exercise and massage frequently effective. Use only under the guidance of full practitioner team.
Zinc (p. 179)	3	Test first for excess copper, which can cause psychotic symptoms—if found, zinc is effective in reducing copper.
Vitamin B6 (p. 170)	3	Typical dose 50mg 3 times/day (with psychotropics and B3) may significantly improve symptoms in 8-12 weeks.
Aspirin (p. 52)	3	Typical dose up to 1,000 mg/d for positive symptom relief as additive to antipsychotics; especially consider if elevated CRP levels or other markers for inflammation are present. May require additional medication to address stomach upset from aspirin.

Psychosocial Restorative Therapies for Schizophrenia

Approach	T	Comments / Evaluation
CBT for Psychosis (p. 118)	1	Cognitive Behavioral Therapy (CBT) is the most effective treatment for reducing depression in people with psychosis and can make voices less malevolent. *Recovery-Oriented Cognitive Therapy* (p. 120) can reduce negative symptoms.
Family Ther. (p. 132)	1	Can improve family interactions, which might reduce relapse rates and improve social functioning and insight.
Voice coping (p. 148)	2	Strategies include subvocalization, selectively listening to voices, ear buds with music, sound generators, modulating the degree of social interaction, and defining limits for voices.
Dialogue Therapy (p. 147)	2	*Voice Dialoguing* (p. 147), *Avatar Therapy* (p. 149), and *Open Dialogue* (p. 147) have shown some effectiveness in improving relationships with voices, and in some cases reducing or eliminating them.
Support Groups (p. 131)	2	*Hearing Voices Network* (p. 150) groups show anecdotal benefit with voice hearers. Conventional *Support Groups* can also help. Both can improve coping and social networking.
Peer Support (p. 131)	2	Peer support can offer hope and belief in the possibility of recovery, incentive to end social isolation, and foster self-determination - all vital in the *Awareness* stage of recovery (p. 33). Peer Support Specialists provide recovery models.
EEG Biofeedback (p. 142)	2	Small studies show that nearly all those with schizophrenia who use EEG improve in cognitive or behavioral areas. It appears to have long-term benefit. Generally safe with other therapies.

Psychosocial Restorative Therapies for Schizophrenia

Approach	T	Comments / Evaluation
Acupuncture (p. 159)	3	Studies show potential for significant symptom improvement. Treatments vary with benefit in days or weeks. Practitioners trained in TCM (see *Glossary*) should only use sterile needles. Laser acupuncture may be most beneficial for psychosis.
CET (p. 135)	3	*Cognitive Enhancement Therapy* can improve cognitive abilities of vigilance, attention, mental processing speed, memory, and planning—thereby improving social and vocational functioning.
Guided Self-determination (p. 150)	3	GSD can help those with delusions to trust others and feel empowered to understand their delusions. It tangentially helps install new perspectives/beliefs.
SFBT (p. 127)	3	*Solution-focused Brief Therapy* (SFBT) has helped some people change their beliefs about their delusions.
Creative Engagement (p. 137)	3	Anecdotal evidence suggests that art, dance, music therapy, involvement in sporting activities, and animal-assisted therapy may improve symptoms and create a more outward focus.

Symptom Relief Approaches for Schizophrenia

Approach	T	Comments / Evaluation
Bright Light Therapy (p. 239)	2	Typical dose 60-120 min in morning with white or dim blue/red light will benefit in 2-3 weeks. More effective if used with exercise. May cause hypomania or insomnia if used after morning.
tDCS (p. 253)	2	tDCS has shown consistent improvement with hallucinations; lesser benefits include cognitive functioning, social interaction, and insight. It appears to offer benefits similar to rTMS.
Ginkgo biloba (p. 231)	2	Typical dose of EGb 761 formulation 240-360 mg/day in 2-3 dosages with benefit (primarily in positive psychotic symptoms and cognitive functioning) in 2-4 weeks. May reduce antipsychotic dosages. Generally safe, though it may cause headache, dizziness, or stomach upset. *Avoid if using anti-clotting agents (e.g. aspirin).*
Ginseng (p. 226)	2	Typical dose 100mg American Ginseng twice daily with benefit (negative symptoms, memory, and lessening extrapyramidal effects of antipsychotics) in 2-4 weeks when used with antipsychotics. 500mg dried ginseng = 100mg non-dry. May cause agitation, diarrhea, insomnia, and (rarely) psychosis or allergic reactions. *Avoid if pregnant or nursing or taking blood thinners.*
Brahmyadi-yoga (p. 234)	3	Typical dose 8-16 mg/day of BR-16, with benefit in 2-3 months. Generally safe and well tolerated with antipsychotics. Use only with trained Ayurvedic practitioner.
Mentat (p. 235)	3	Dosage of 2 tablets 3 times/day, increasing to 3 tablets 3 times/day after one week, with benefit (typically negative symptoms) in 2-3 months. Generally safe and well tolerated with antipsychotics. Use with trained Ayurvedic practitioner.
Yokukan-san (p. 233)	3	Typical dosage in the range of 2.5-7.5 g daily. Use with or without psychotropics.
Cannabidiol (p. 225)	3	A clinical trial suggests CBD can reduce psychotic symptoms significantly, similar to antipsychotics. Dosages vary.

WHAT CONSIDERATIONS SHOULD I KEEP IN MIND?

Safety is the #1 priority. If the individual is unable to perceive reality, is experiencing severe psychosis, or is a danger to themselves or others, call 911. Hospital emergency rooms can help the person stabilize.

From a psychosocial perspective, *Cognitive Behavioral Therapy for Psychosis* (p. 118) and *Recovery-Oriented Cognitive Therapy* (p. 120) are among the most effective aids, helping psychotic depression, potentially decreasing hallucinations, and improving negative symptoms. In addition, *Family-Focused Therapy* (p. 132) has been shown to reduce the chance of relapse[1476] by improving family dynamics, often a source of stress. Various *Voice-coping strategies* (p. 148) may be very helpful, including using a sound source to interrupt voices. Many *Dialogue Therapies* (p. 147) directly engage with voices, accepting, confronting and working with them instead of ignoring them. Both voice coping and dialogue approaches can partially, and in some cases completely, stop the voices.

From a symptom-relief perspective, consider *Transcranial Direct Current Stimulation* (p. 253), since it may provide symptom relief with few or no side effects. Seek to avoid *Electroconvulsive Therapy* (p. 244), because many researchers highlight the procedure's significant risks.

Antipsychotic drugs are commonly prescribed for schizophrenia but should be used with caution because of their significant risks and limitations (Figure 4, p. 27). Although they can reduce symptoms in the short term for many people, long-term use appears to *reduce* cognitive performance[1477] and shrink the brain.[56] The past Director of the National Institute of Mental Health[52] notes that they appear to worsen the chance of long-term recovery[53] and may impede wellness.[54] A twenty-year study found that unmedicated schizophrenia patients had significantly *less* psychosis than those taking antipsychotics.[55]

People with first-episode schizophrenia should be especially careful since they have increased sensitivity to psychiatric drug side effects.[1415] Therefore, if antipsychotics are used for first-episode psychosis, people should be started at low dosages and increased only as required. Be especially cautious of using two or more antipsychotics together (see *Antipsychotic Polypharmacy*, p. 265).

One strategy is to slowly wean off antipsychotics after a prolonged stabilization. Paradoxically, this can lead to an increased risk of relapse in the first 6-10 months of being drug-free, but if relapse is avoided during this time, relapse rates appear to be considerably lower after that.[54]

There is good reason to remain hopeful since about half of those with schizophrenia become symptoms free. A five-year study found that 47% of people with psychosis improved considerably or recovered.[1478] One ten-year follow-up study found that almost half of people were symptoms free for the previous two years.[1479] Another found that 60% of people were in remission at 10-year follow-up.[1480] Other studies show extensive evidence of medication-free schizophrenia patients with favorable outcomes.[54]

See "Schizophrenia, Case Studies" in the index for many individual stories.

REAL-WORLD EXPERIENCE

Case Study 119 - Overmethylation (Schizophrenia)

Robert, age 25, was diagnosed with schizophrenia after experiencing auditory hallucinations and anxiety. After many unsuccessful attempts at finding help from therapy and psychotropics, he considered nutrient therapy.

An exam suggested overmethylation, since his symptoms included hallucinations, difficulty sleeping, and low libido. Biomedical testing revealed a low histamine level and confirmed overmethylation. He was placed on folic acid, vitamins B3, B6, B12, C, and E, with supplements of zinc, manganese, and chromium.

At his annual follow-up, Robert reported that the voices had disappeared, and he felt in good health. He faithfully returns for biochemical testing each year.[24]

Case Study 120 - Undermethylation (Schizophrenia)

David was a brilliant PhD candidate at Berkeley when, at age 22, he started believing that Russian agents were trying to kill him. He sat for hours with a blank expression on his face. Needless to say, he lost his job and had to drop out of school.

When admitted to the hospital, David was prescribed psychotropics, but he was still unable to return to work. A biochemical test pointed to undermethylation. Doctors suggested targeted nutrient therapy, including SAM-e, calcium, magnesium, zinc, and vitamins A, B6, C, D, and E.

David slowly improved over six weeks. At the end of a year of nutrient therapy, David reported almost a complete recovery. He was then weaned from three psychotropics to a single low dose of Zyprexa.

He is now employed and has no side effects from low dose Zyprexa.[24]

WHAT ARE ADDITIONAL RESOURCES?

- *Psychosis, Schizophrenia and Voices* resources (p. 342).

Bipolar Therapies

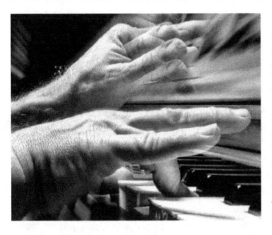

The most promising evidence-based therapies for bipolar should be considered in the context of *Building Your Recovery Plan* (p. 270).

Bipolar symptoms include episodes of mania (excessive energy, racing thoughts, euphoria, irritability, unrealistic belief in one's powers, uncharacteristic poor judgment, unusual sexual drive, and intrusive/aggressive behavior) and depression (see p. 276). Authors, poets, visual artists, and other groups of creative people experience higher rates of bipolar symptoms.[1481]

Bipolar encompasses four major mental health diagnoses:

- Bipolar 1 - severe mood episodes of mania with possible depression
- Bipolar 2 - milder mood elevation than bipolar 1, with severe depression
- Cyclothymia - milder bipolar with hypomania and milder depression
- Rapid cycling – four or more mood episodes in twelve months

Start your recovery plan with approaches selected from the *Template of Recovery* (p. 273), then add specific approaches for bipolar from the tables below. Work closely with your practitioners, leveraging their expertise and guidance to define, execute, and evolve this plan.

Template for Recovery approaches especially important for bipolar involve:

- **Biomedical Testing.** Robust biomedical testing (p. 323) should be considered mandatory. Work with an *Integrative Biomedical Practitioner* who will prescribe appropriate tests and assess underlying physical causes of bipolar. (See *People of Recovery*, p. 35.) From a database of more than 1,500 blood samples of people with bipolar, the Walsh Institute (see Figure 28, p. 168) has identified **five primary biotypes: overmethylation, undermethylation, copper imbalance, zinc imbalance, and severe oxidative stress.** [767] About 70% of bipolar patients exhibit a severe *Methylation* (p. 54) disorder. Knowing your biotype helps identify an appropriate nutrient response. One trial[767] indicated that 74% of the bipolar patients who follow customized *Nutrient Therapy* using the Walsh Institute's diagnostic and treatment techniques, report that they can reduce or eliminate (less common) psychotropics. The biomedical options in the tables below can be used without testing but will mean more guesswork.

- **Psychosocial Evaluation.** Bipolar can be influenced by past trauma, stress, or other difficulties that can be addressed with psychosocial therapy. People with bipolar are over twice as likely to have suffered emotional, physical or sexual abuse as children than the general population.[1482] Work with a trusted psychotherapist who can identify potential issues and recommend therapies.
- **Diet.** Poor diet is correlated with depression. Avoid diets high in carbohydrates, refined sugar, and especially junk food. A Mediterranean diet high in Omega-3 may be helpful. Also consider avoiding processed meat products since one study found that people hospitalized with mania consumed 3.5 times the levels of healthy controls.[1483]
- **Exercise.** People with bipolar often have poor exercise habits. Consistent exercise is important to help alleviate depressive symptoms of bipolar. Exercise can significantly improve mood. However, excess sweating can reduce the effectiveness of lithium.
- **Mind-Body Disciplines.** Many people with bipolar use yoga to help reduce agitation and regulate their mood swings. Working with a qualified teacher and keeping a regular discipline will offer the greatest benefits.

In addition to the above, see the targeted approaches for bipolar found in the tables below. With your practitioners, consider them in tier order.

Biomedical Restorative Therapies for Bipolar		
Approach	**T**	**Comments / Evaluation**
Branch-chain amino acids (p. 185)	2	Typical dose 60 gm/day of amino acid drink that excludes tyrosine, with benefit within hours for mania. Generally safe, including with mood stabilizers. May cause sleepiness. Monitor liver functioning while using.
Omega-3 Fatty Acids (p. 187)	2	Typical dose of 1-3 gm/day with benefit over several months for depression. Likely best to use more EPA than DHA (6:1 Omega-6 to Omega-3 ratio). Generally safe, including with psychotropics. May influence LDL cholesterol and blood sugar. May promote bleeding. Do not use with aspirin.
NAC (p. 184)	2	Typical dose: 1 gm twice/day. With antidepressant, will benefit over several months. Generally safe, including with psychotropics. Side effects include possible heartburn, headache, and intestinal issues.
Magnesium (p. 178)	2	Dosages vary with benefit in hours for rapid cycling. 125-300mg 4 times daily was found to improve mood. Use with vitamin D3 increases cellular uptake. Usually well tolerated. Possible lithiuim alternative. High doses may slow heart rate. Usually safe with mood stabilizers and antidepressants.
Coenzyme Q10 (p. 186)	2	Typical dose 200-1200 mg/day reduces bipolar depression with large impact in 8 weeks as adjunct to mood stabilizers.

Biomedical Restorative Therapies for Bipolar

Approach	T	Comments / Evaluation
Thyroid evaluation (p. 198)	2	Thyroid evaluation is vital for bipolar; 2/3 of bipolar patients in depressive states have subclinical hypothyroidism. Lithium can cause low thyroid hormone levels.
Choline (p. 175)	3	Typical dose 2-7gm/day of free choline and 15-30 gm/day phosphatidyl choline, in 2 doses with benefit for mania and depression in days to weeks. May cause mild diarrhea.
Lithium Orotate (p. 177)	3	Dosage of 150-200 µg/day (in 3 doses, at meals) may decrease manic and depressive symptoms. If prescription lithium carbonate causes renal failure, lithium orotate may provide benefit without toxicity. Maintain consistent salt intake if used.
L-tryptophan/ 5-HTP (p. 183)	3	Typical dose: 1-2 gm/day at bedtime. May reduce frequency of depressive mood swings, severity of mania, and insomnia. Generally safe. Mildly sedating, so take at bedtime.
Vitamin B8 (p. 171)	3	Vitamin B8 (Inositol) possibly helpful in reducing depression in those with bipolar.
Vitamin B12 (p. 172)	3	B12 injections may reduce the risk of manic episodes in bipolar patients with B12 deficiencies. Generally safe.
Vitamin B9 (p. 171)	3	B9 supplements can improve response to lithium. Generally safe, including with mood stabilizers.
Vitamin C (p. 173)	3	Vitamin C helps remove vanadium, which may be high in people with bipolar. Typical dose 3gm one time may improve manic and depressive symptoms if person has high vanadium.
EMPowerplus (p. 185)	3	Dosages vary, with benefit in weeks to months. Has shown reduction of manic and depressive symptoms; some patients can reduce or eliminate psychotropics. Generally safe, though possible toxicity with mood stabilizers.

Psychosocial Restorative Therapies for Bipolar

Approach	T	Comments / Evaluation
CBT (p. 117)	2	Cognitive Behavioral Therapy (CBT) can be a helpful add-on therapy to psychotropics.
MBCT (p. 121)	2	Mindfulness-Based Cognitive Therapy (MBCT) adds mindfulness to CBT and is an effective alternative.
IPSRT (p. 132)	2	Helps establish daily rhythms (routines and sleep cycles) and appropriate activity/social stimulation levels to help moderate mood and relieve symptoms. Helps avoid relapse.
Family Therapy (p. 132)	2	Family therapy with meds yields faster recovery and longer intervals of wellness for those with bipolar.
Psychoeduc. (p. 126)	2	Provides information on bipolar, typical therapies, prognosis, and ways to manage symptoms.
Peer Support (p. 131)	3	Offers hope and living example of recovery; fosters self-determination; provides incentive to move from social isolation, vital in the *Awareness* stage of recovery (p. 33).

Psychosocial Restorative Therapies for Bipolar

Approach	T	Comments / Evaluation
Creative Engagement (p. 137)	3	Those with bipolar are very visible in the fields of art, literature, and music. Creative therapies can help improve mood and promote stability.

Symptom Relief Therapies for Bipolar

Approach	T	Comments / Evaluation
Rhodiola Rosea (p. 228)	2	May reduce stress and improve cognition in mild-to-moderate depression of bipolar. Typically well tolerated. *Use caution and only use with mood stabilizers--they may cause cycling.*
tDCS (p. 253)	3	Mild electric stimulation. *Be cautious to avoid mania onset.*
Rauwolfia serpentina (p. 235)	3	Consider for treatment-resistant or acute bipolar mania potentially with psychosis. Generally safe, including with mood stabilizers/lithium. May result in reduction of doses of lithium needed. Use with trained Ayurvedic practitioner.
FEWP (p. 231)	3	Typical dose not established. This Chinese herb mixture provides depressive symptom benefit (not mania) in one month. Generally safe, including with mood stabilizers
rTMS (p.249)	3	rTMS (right dorsolateral prefrontal cortex) may significantly improve manic symptoms in 14 days, with no side effects.
Anion therapy (p. 241)	3	Can promote relaxation and relieve manic symptoms. Generally safe, including with psychotropics.
EP-MRSI (p. 253)	3	In a small study, those given an EP-MRSI experienced an improvement in mood, especially those not on psychotropics.

WHAT CONSIDERATIONS SHOULD I KEEP IN MIND?

Safety is the #1 priority. If the individual is a danger to themselves or others, call 911. Hospital emergency rooms can help them stabilize, sometimes with the anesthetic drug ketamine, that may offer rapid relief from depression[1334] and suicidal ideation[1484], though its long-term impact is unclear.[1467]

From a biomedical perspective, have your practitioner run a robust *Biomedical Test Panel* (p. 323) to look for specific issues. Deficiencies in vitamins B9 and B12 are common in those with bipolar, so supplementation may result in significant improvement.

From a psychosocial perspective, those with bipolar receiving intensive psychotherapy are 58% more likely to be well and have higher recovery rates.[1485] *Mindfulness-Based Cognitive Therapy* (p. 121) can strongly improve cognition and anxiety, helping to avoid mania. It is most effective in the *Maintenance stage* (p. 34) of recovery. *Interpersonal and Social Rhythm Therapy* (p. 132) helps re-sync the body's internal clock, often an issue with bipolar. Assessment for childhood emotional, physical, and sexual abuse should be performed since these traumas are associated with worsening bipolar symptoms.[1486] If past trauma is found, trauma-informed *Exposure Therapies* (p. 151) may prove helpful.

Bipolar Drugs
Benefits, Risks, and Limitations
Summary of gold-standard evidence of *attributable* benefit and harm[1]

BIG Picture *Trade-offs*

CRISIS USE

Bipolar drugs can sedate during suicidality and dangerous behavior.

PARTIAL RELIEF

Bipolar drugs offer *partial* but *inconsistent* symptom relief that varies by person.

LOW RECOVERY

On drugs alone, people rarely recover[6] and have symptoms half the year.[7]

STABILIZATION

Drugs can reduce the frequency of severe mania and depressive episodes.

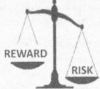

REWARD

RISK

NON-CURATIVE

Bipolar drugs can reduce *symptoms* but don't cure or address *causes.*

DRUG LOAD

2-5 drug combos are prescribed for bipolar.[2] High drug load is linked to higher suicide rates and worse outcomes.[3]

UNCERTAINTY

Bipolar drug combo testing is "practically nonexistent".[4] Prescribing is largely trial and error.[5]

SIDE EFFECTS

Sexual dysfunction, organ damage, diabetes, cognitive impairment, tremors, and addiction may occur.

Conventional
Bipolar Care

VS

Integrative
Mental Health

Bipolar drugs reduce symptoms, frequency of relapse, and may be vital in crisis. Some find them essential for stability but...

75-85% of the time people don't see substantial benefit due to drugs they take.[37]
2 of 5 drugs are controversial to use.[38]
3 of 5 drugs increase risks of suicide.[39]
5 of 5 carry FDA black box warnings.[40]
Drugs are poorly tested in combination.
Drug risks are usually dose-proportional, so long-term use is of greatest concern.

A paradigm shift is available today, embraced by many practitioners...

It uses the best of drug therapy and evidence-based nondrug options.
It reduces symptoms so drug dosages and their side effects can be reduced.
It often targets causative factors.[41]
It often supports sustainable wellness.
Not a panacea, but nondrug options have few side effects[42] and are crucial to long-term recovery.[43]

Figure 36 - Bipolar Drug Benefits, Risks, and Limitations
(see supporting studies[1487])

From a symptom relief perspective, standard care is often a combination of drugs (called polypharmacy) that may include antipsychotics, prescription lithium, anticonvulsants, antidepressants, and benzodiazepines - all of which have significant risks and limitations. See Figure 36 above and figures on pp. 26-28. For detail on the sizable and unique problems with each bipolar drug, review the infographic at www.OnwardMentalHealth.com/bipolar. Polypharmacy carries additional risk (p. 263).

Lithium appears to be a neuro-protectant involved in the expression of over 50 genes. It can reduce mania symptoms and may reduce the risk of suicide.[1488] However, prescription lithium is intolerable to some people and can cause kidney damage with long-term use. Non-prescription lithium (lithium orotate, p. 177) is showing promise at low dosages and appears to avoid kidney damage.

Consider *Transcranial Direct Current Stimulation* (tDCS, p. 253) or other minimally invasive Electromagnetic techniques that can provide symptom relief with few or no side effects. Seek to avoid *Electroconvulsive Therapy* (p. 244).

Tracking your moods with a mood diary can help you notice trends and detect hypomania before it becomes full mania.

If you have bipolar, consider <u>avoiding</u> **supplements for** *calcium*[1489], *chromium picolinate*[1490], *glutamine*[1491], *SAM-e* [1492], *vanadium* (**it is suspected as being one cause of bipolar**), *St. John's Wort*,[1493] **and** *ginseng.*[1494] When therapies are used to reduce the depressive symptoms of bipolar, caution should be exercised to avoid the onset of mania.[24]

See "Bipolar, Case Studies" in the index for a variety of individual stories.

REAL-WORLD EXPERIENCE

Case Study 121 – Lithium and Psychotherapy (Bipolar)

Kay is a clinical psychologist who has struggled with her own bipolar disorder. "I cannot imagine leading a normal life without taking lithium together with the benefit of psychotherapy," she said. "Lithium prevents my seductive but disastrous highs, diminishes my depressions... keeps me from ruining my career and relationships, keeps me out of hospital, alive, and makes psychotherapy possible.

"But, ineffably, psychotherapy heals. It makes some sense of the confusion, reins in the terrifying thoughts and feelings, returns some control and hope and possibility of learning from it all ... [I]t is where ... I might someday be able to contend with all of this."[1495]

Bottom Line: Kay knows the vital difference between clinical recovery (the elimination or reduction of symptoms) and personal growth (finding meaning in it all). Personal Recovery requires both. See Figure 38 (p. 315).

WHAT ARE ADDITIONAL RESOURCES?

- Mood Tracker tools (https://goo.gl/kuR1wp) and apps (p. 328).
- Beating bipolar interactive course. http://www.beatingbipolar.org.
- Bipolar UK. www.BipolarUK.org.
- Depression & Bipolar Support Alliance. www.dbsalliance.org.

Anxiety Therapies

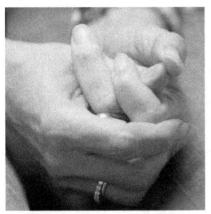 The most promising evidence-based therapies for anxiety should be considered in the context of *Building Your Recovery Plan* (p. 270).

Anxiety symptoms include heart palpitations, sweating, trembling, shortness of breath, chest pain, dizziness, nausea, numbing, chills/hot flushes, feelings of unreality, and fears.

Anxiety covers the following major mental health diagnoses:

- Generalized anxiety disorder (GAD)
- Panic disorder
- Acute stress disorder
- Social/specific phobias
- Obsessive-compulsive disorder (OCD)
- Post-traumatic stress disorder (PTSD)

Start your recovery plan with approaches selected from the *Template of Recovery* (p. 273), then add specific approaches for anxiety from the tables below. Work closely with your practitioners to create, execute, and evolve this plan.

Template for Recovery approaches especially important for anxiety include:

- **Biomedical Testing**. Consider full protocol biomedical lab testing as mandatory. Many people report that customized *Nutrient Therapy* using the Walsh Institute protocols (See Figure 28, p. 168) significantly improve anxiety symptoms. The biomedical options below can be used without such testing but will mean more guesswork and will likely take you more time to discover what works for you.
- **Psychosocial Assessment**. An evaluation by a trained psychotherapist should be mandatory for cases of anxiety, especially post-traumatic stress disorder and obsessive-compulsive disorder. Trauma and stress can be a directly influence anxiety—and these may be unknown to family members and supporters.
- **Calm Awareness**. *Calm Awareness* techniques (p. 73) can be very effective for anxiety, likely as effective as psychotropics, and in some cases, more effective. Consider especially *Mindfulness-Based Stress Reduction* (p. 77),

Controlled Breathing (p. 75), *Meditation* (p. 78), and *Guided Imagery* (p. 79) as Tier 1 treatments. *Meditation* may be especially helpful for veterans with PTSD who find the re-experiencing of trauma in exposure therapies too difficult. *Mindful Awareness in Body-oriented Therapy* (p. 77) has proven especially effective for female veterans with PTSD. Also consider *Mind-Body Disciplines* (see below) that include mindfulness components.

- **Exercise or Mind-Body Discipline**. Some form of consistent movement between 30 and 45 minutes per day in the form of either exercise or a *Mind-Body Discipline* is important. Yoga can significantly reduce generalized anxiety and panic attacks and may be somewhat more effective than *Qigong* and *T'ai Chi Chuan*.
- **Diet**. Avoid excess refined sugar, junk food, and caffeine, to reduce the severity of generalized anxiety as well as the frequency of panic attacks.

In addition to the above, see the targeted approaches for anxiety found in the tables below. With your practitioners, consider them in tier order.

Biomedical Restorative Therapies for Anxiety

Approach	T	Comments / Evaluation
L-Theanine (p. 182)	1	Typical dose 50-200 mg 1-2 times/day (for moderate anxiety) or 100-200 mg 3-4 times/day (severe anxiety), with benefit in days. Generally safe, including with psychotropics. May allow decrease in psychotropic dosages. Does not cause drowsiness.
Omega-3 (p. 187)	1	Dosages $\geq$ 2000 mg/day (<60% EPA) are modestly effective in reducing anxiety with greater benefit the worse the anxiety.
L-tryptophan and 5-HTP (p. 183)	2	Typical dose of 1-3gm/day L-tryptophan or 50-100mg 3 times/day 5-HTP for generalized anxiety, with benefit in days. Additional bedtime dose can aid sleep. Generally safe, although it may interact with psychotropics, so start doses low and ramp up. Best taken at bedtime, due to mild sedentary effects.
Vitamin B8 (p. 171)	2	Typical dose of 12-20 gm/day (for panic, obsessions, agoraphobia, and compulsions), with benefit in 2-4 weeks. May be as effective as psychotropics for panic attacks. Generally safe, including with other therapies, although it may cause gastrointestinal issues, insomnia, and headaches. *May cause mania with bipolar.*
Pregnenolone (p. 200)	3	400mg pregnenolone reduces self-reported anxiety.
Amino Acid Supplement	3	Phosphatidylserine (p. 184), L-lysine (p. 182), and L-arginine have all been associated with the relief of anxiety symptoms.
Vitamins & Minerals	3	Vitamins B1, B3 (2-3 gm/day), B6, B12, C, E, or multi-vitamins and minerals (phosphorus, magnesium, selenium, p. 179) for generalized anxiety, with benefit in weeks to months. Vitamin B3 alone, 2.5 g gm/day, showed significant reduction in anxiety in a case study, with no serious side effects.

Biomedical Restorative Therapies for Anxiety

Approach	T	Comments / Evaluation
DHEA and 7-keto DHEA (p. 200)	3	Typical dose of 100 mg/day to reduce anxiety. Generally safe, including with psychotropics. Test for DHEA-sulfate levels especially in older patients; if low, DHEA supplementation may also improve depression. Consult with practitioners.
D-cycloserine (p. 180)	3	Typical dose of 50 mg/day for anxiety increases effectiveness of exposure therapy. Generally safe.

Psychosocial Restorative Therapies for Anxiety

Approach	T	Comments / Evaluation
Biofeedback (p. 142)	1	Use 1-3 times/week, self-administered or with practitioner, for benefit in days/weeks. Both EEG and EMG biofeedback can be as effective as medication for generalized anxiety; HRV is also effective. Generally safe, including with other treatments. Most effective if combined with *Calm Awareness* techniques (p. 73).
Exposure therapy (p. 151)	1	Many therapies (e.g., EMDR, VRET, etc.); EMDR often best for trauma. CBT (p. 117) is an alternative (see CBT for anxiety). In vivo (direct confrontation) or VRET (virtual computer-based) often best. In weeks or months, 1-3 sessions/week will benefit generalized anxiety, phobias, and PTSD. *Avoid if having psychosis, seizures, or substance-abuse issues.*
Energy Therapies	2	Use typically 1-3 times/week for moderate anxiety, with benefit in days/weeks. Consider *Emotional Freedom Technique* (p. 161), *acupuncture* (p. 159), *Reiki* (p. 160) and *Healing Touch* (p. 160). Work with trained practitioners. Generally safe, including with psychotropics. Especially helpful for PTSD.
Peer Support / Psycho-education	2	This includes local *mental health support groups* (p. 131) and *mental health training*. (See *Educate Yourself*, p. 50.) Consider techniques to connect with others who faced similar situations while you learn, work, and enact your recovery plan.
Creative Engagement (p. 137)	3	Nature, dance, music, art, literature, and animals—have shown effectiveness for anxiety. Choose an activity, or variety of activities, most appealing to you.

Symptom Relief Therapies for Anxiety

Approach	T	Comments / Evaluation
Kava (p. 227)	1	Can be as effective as psychotropics for anxiety. Typical dose 70-300 mg/day of 70% kava lactones in three doses with benefit in 2-4 weeks. Best for low/moderate anxiety. Generally safe, including with psychotropics. Side effects: possible skin rash and gastrointestinal issues, serious liver toxicity (rare). *Avoid alcohol, Tylenol, and sedatives when using.*

Symptom Relief Therapies for Anxiety

Approach	T	Comments / Evaluation
Passion-flower (p. 232)	2	Typical dose of 45 drops of concentrated P. incarnata extract 1-2 times/day for moderate generalized anxiety, with benefit in weeks to months. Generally safe but may cause depression. Interacts with anti-anxiety meds. *Consult doctor if using psychotropics. Avoid if pregnant or breastfeeding.*
Galphimia glauca (p. 226)	2	Although dose is individualized, 350-700 mg/day of dry standard prep, used for moderate anxiety, will benefit in days. Likely as effective as psychotropics for moderate anxiety. Generally safe, does not cause sedation or lead to dependence.
Massage (p. 242)	2	Use typically 1-3 times/week for 30 min., with benefit in 2-6 weeks for generalized anxiety. Use with other treatments. Avoid or modify if experiencing chronic pain or joint/muscle issues.
Music & binaural sound	2	Typical binaural sound dose 30 min., 2-3 times/week, with benefit in days/weeks for moderate generalized anxiety. Generally safe, including with other therapies. May cause fatigue or dizziness. Also consider relaxing music at a low-to-medium volume; enjoyable instrumental music is often most relaxing.
Chamomile (p. 225)	2	Multiple doses of 220-1100 mg/day of M. recutita in the form of tea or oil will benefit in 2-4 weeks for moderate generalized anxiety. Generally safe, including with other treatments, although possible mild gastrointestinal issues.
Ginkgo biloba (p. 231)	2	Typical dose of 240-480 mg/day for generalized anxiety, with benefit in 2-4 weeks. Generally safe, although may cause gastrointestinal issues, headache, or dizziness. *Risk of bleeding or other issues when used with psychotropics. Consult with doctor before use.*
Bacopa monniera (p. 234)	2	Although doses are highly individualized, the typical dose is 300mg daily for chronic generalized anxiety. Use with trained Ayurvedic practitioner.
Centella Asiatica (p. 230)	2	Dosages vary. Historic use in Chinese and Ayurvedic medicine is considered effective in reducing anxiety symptoms, including the startle response to loud noises.
Withania somnifera (p. 235)	2	Typical dose for chronic generalized anxiety is 150-300mg 2 times/day, with benefit in 2-6 weeks. Use with trained Ayurvedic practitioner. Generally safe, although it may have sedating effects.
Geriforte (p. 235)	2	Doses vary. May reduce symptoms of generalized anxiety. Use under care of an Ayurvedic practitioner.
tACS (p. 254)	3	Transcranial Alternating Current Stimulation (tACS). A small trial found each OCD patient improved substantially.
Lavender and Rosemary oil (p. 227)	3	Typical aromatherapy dose of 2-4 drops daily in aromatic diffuser or cup of boiling water for generalized anxiety. Generally safe, may cause drowsiness. May be rubbed into skin, but this should be limited if also using sedating psychotropics.

Symptom Relief Therapies for Anxiety

Approach	T	Comments / Evaluation
Echinacea (p. 226)	3	Typical dose of 40mg/day of extract concentrate Echinacea for moderate generalized anxiety, with benefit in 1-2 weeks. Generally safe, including with other treatments.
Lemon Balm (p. 227)	3	Typical dose of 300-500 mg/day (or 60 drop tincture) for moderate generalized anxiety. Generally safe, may interact with sedatives and thyroid meds. *Avoid if pregnant or breast feeding.*
Milk Thistle (p. 228)	3	For OCD, 600mg of Milk Thistle daily was found to be as effective as Prozac. Generally safe, with mild or no side effects.
American Skullcap (p. 224)	3	Typical dose of 3-9 gr/day for moderate generalized anxiety and restlessness. Generally safe but may cause liver toxicity. For tea, put 1-2 tsp of dried extract in a cup of boiling water and steep 10-15 min.
Drugs for inner ear issues	3	Some sources indicate a strong tie between panic/anxiety attacks and inner ear issues;*[1496]* Drugs for dizziness or motion sickness have helped some people significantly (for example, Dramamine, Meclizine).
Damiana (p. 226)	3	Clinical trials have not established doses, but historic doses are 2 gm. *Potentially toxic in high doses.*

WHAT CONSIDERATIONS SHOULD I KEEP IN MIND?

Safety is the #1 priority. If the individual is a danger to themselves or others, call 911. Hospital emergency rooms can help them stabilize, often with psychotropics.

Some form of psychosocial therapy is very often helpful, since anxiety is often rooted in unhelpful thinking. In fact, strong evidence shows that *Cognitive Behavioral Therapy* (CBT, p. 117) is especially useful for *all* types of anxiety, including PTSD, OCD, phobias, and panic. It is a first-line treatment. Online and app-based CBT are available, but be sure to have access to a trained therapist either by phone or email if you use these approaches. *Biofeedback* (p. 142) and *Exposure Therapies* (p. 151) help people learn to control their stress response to anxiety. Psycho-therapy and *Neuro-Linguistic Programming* (p. 128) have been shown effective. Find a therapist you like and trust. Learn the latest on MDMA- and ketamine-assisted psychotherapies, an area of study that is changing rapidly. These drugs appear to improve trust and compassion, and significantly improve the results of psychosocial therapies.

From a biomedical perspective, nutrients and/or herbs can help reduce symptoms while psychosocial approaches are being explored.

From a symptom relief perspective, both antidepressants and benzodiazepines can relieve anxiety symptoms, but both come with serious risks and limitations (Figure 3, p. 26 and Figure 5, p. 28). Especially use caution with benzodiazepines. Their addictive nature results in guidelines that typically limit their use to short time spans of a few days to a few weeks.

The various sub-types of anxiety have special considerations.

- For *PTSD*. A meta-analysis found psychosocial therapies more effective and more acceptable than drugs.[27] A variety of *Exposure Therapies* (p. 151) have been very effective and appear to deliver similar results. Select an approach that you find most acceptable and available in your area. Virtual reality versions of these therapies can provide realistic visual exposure to war experiences for veterans. In addition, *Meditation* (p. 78) has been shown to be broadly beneficial for mental health and can significantly reduce trauma symptoms. Research indicates that PTSD nightmares are among the most common symptoms: 60%- 80% of PTSD patients suffer from them. As such, addressing nightmares while they occur via lucid dreaming shows promise, but few studies have explored that possibility. Be cautious with meds since vets with PTSD who took either antidepressants or antipsychotics had a significantly greater risk of later developing dementia than those who did not take these drugs.[1555] Consider MDMA-assisted psychosocial therapy for PTSD; it has been granted "breakthrough" status by the FDA.

- For *obsessive-compulsive disorder and phobias. Exposure and Response Prevention Therapy* (p. 151) is one of the most effective therapies. It carefully exposes the individual to situations that trigger obsessive thoughts, helping individuals learn how to choose better responses. In addition, consider Inositol (p. 171). Transcranial Alternative Current Stimulation (p. 254) which has shown success in a small number of case studies.

Individual stories of recovery from anxiety can be found by looking in the index under the appropriate diagnosis (OCD, panic, anxiety, or PTSD).

WHAT ARE ADDITIONAL RESOURCES?

- Anxiety Disorders Toolkit. http://goo.gl/PFEB5t.
- Anxiety Tools. www.anxietyBC.com.
- Mood Tracker Apps (p. 328).
- PTSD Coach, an app designed to help those with PTSD.

Dementia Therapies

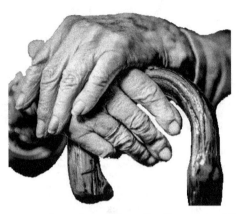

This section provides the most promising evidence-based therapies for dementia. Consider them in the context of *Building Your Recovery Plan* (p. 270).

Dementia and cognitive impairment symptoms include memory loss, problems with thinking and language, disorientation in time or space, poor judgment, changes in mood or behavior, and loss of initiative.

Start your recovery plan with approaches selected from the *Template of Recovery* (p. 273), then add approaches for dementia from the tables below. Work closely with your practitioners to create, execute, and evolve this plan.

Template for Recovery approaches that are especially important include:

- **Diet.** A healthy diet, including foods high in antioxidants, is the first line of prevention for dementia and Alzheimer's Disease (AD). A Mediterranean diet may reduce the chances of AD by as much as 40%.[1497] Blueberries are especially helpful in reducing the severity of dementia. Avoid sugar beverages, since they are associated with increased risk of AD. Moderate caffeine consumption is associated with improved cognition. Drinking one glass of wine or beer a day is associated with a reduced risk of dementia.

- **Exercise.** Consistent exercise, adjusted to any physical disabilities, helps to avoid the cognitive impairment of dementia. Simple activities, such as walking, can make a positive impact. Exercise encourages brain health because it causes nerve cells to multiply. A six-year study of more than 1,700 people found that exercise lowered the risk of developing dementia.[1498]

- **Social Engagement.** Keeping socially active is as important as keeping physically active. Social engagement and absorbing leisure activities may delay or prevent dementia.

In addition to the above, see the targeted approaches for dementia found in the tables below. With your practitioners, consider them in tier order.

Biomedical Restorative Therapies for Dementia

Approach	T	Comments / Evaluation
Idebenone (p. 186)	1	Typical dose of 120-360 mg/day, with benefit (reduced symptom severity of dementia and Alzheimer's) in 3-6 months, for mild-to-moderate symptoms. Generally safe.

Biomedical Restorative Therapies for Dementia

Approach	T	Comments / Evaluation
Acetyl-L-carnitine (p. 181)	2	Typical dose of 1,500-3,000 mg/day with benefit (slow the progress of dementia, improve memory) for mild-to-moderate dementia in months. Acts as neuroprotectant. Generally safe, including with drugs, although may cause gastrointestinal issues or headache. Use with or without psychotropics.
Combination Supplement	2	ALC 500mg, folate 400mg, SAM-e 400mg, NAC 600mg, vitamin B12 6mg and vitamin E 30 IU, with benefit (reduced rate of cognitive decline and improved depression).
Vitamin B1, B2, B3, B9, B12 (p. 169)	2	Typical dose of 50 mg/day methyl-folinic acid (B9) to decrease dementia in early stages and depression; 1 mg/week B12 to reduce cognitive decline; and 3-8 gm/day B1 to decrease mild-to-moderate symptoms, with benefit in weeks to months. Generally safe. B9 may cause nervousness or insomnia. Test nutrient levels before starting, especially folate.
DHEA (p. 200)	2	Taking 25-400 mg/day of DHEA for up to six months or a 200mg/day injection of DHEA-S for 4 weeks can yield significant cognitive improvement.
Lithium (p. 177)	2	Appears to reduce brain plaque. Standard dose is associated with reduced dementia. Low dose may benefit cognition.
CDP-Choline (p. 175)	3	Typical dose: 500mg-1000 mg/day, with benefit (neuroprotection and better brain metabolism, improving memory and cognition). Generally safe.
Resveratrol (p. 188)	3	Doses vary. Found in skins and seeds of red grapes and red wine. They are anti-inflammatory and antioxidant and provide neuroprotection and cognitive improvement. Generally safe, but studies have not been done on humans.
Melatonin (p. 202)	3	Take 3-24 mg of fast-release preparation 30 min before bed, with benefit (reduced agitation, slower rate of cognitive decline, and improved sleep) in weeks for dementia and mild cognitive impairment. Mildly sedating. Generally safe.
Vitamin C (p. 173) and E (p. 174)	3	Typical dose: 500mg+/day vitamin C and 400+ IU/day vitamin E with benefit (reduce odds of dementia) in months. High dose of Vitamin C may reduce plaque in the brain. Generally safe. May increase bleeding risk; avoid if on blood thinners.
Phospha-tidylserine (p. 184)	3	Typical dose: 100mg 3 times/day with benefit (cortisol-lowering that leads to improvement in memory, concentration, and mood) in 12 weeks. Generally safe.
Lipoic Acid (p. 187)	3	Typical dose: 600 mg/day with benefit (improve cognition) in weeks to months. Generally safe.
Periwinkle (p. 228)	3	Typical dose: 10-20mg 3 times/day vinpocetine with benefit (cognitive improvement) in 16 weeks. Generally safe.

Psychosocial Restorative Therapies for Dementia		
Approach	**T**	**Comments / Evaluation**
Creative Engagement (p. 137)	3	Therapies include dance, music, woodworking, painting, sculpting, nature, and animals have been shown effective for dementia. Choose a variety of activities that are most appealing.

Symptom Relief Therapies for Dementia		
Approach	**T**	**Comments / Evaluation**
Ginkgo biloba (p. 231)	1	Typical dosage of EGb 761 of 120-600 mg/day in 2-3 dosages, with benefit (improved memory and cognition) in weeks/mos. Can reduce depression and anxiety. With ginseng, can improve cognition. Typically well tolerated. May cause gastrointestinal issues or dizziness. An anticoagulant, so do not use with aspirin or other anticoagulants.
Yokukansan (p. 233) and Chotosan (p. 231)	2	Typical dose: 7.5 g/day each of dry herb with benefit (improved cognition, decreased agitation and confusion of dementia) in 4-6 weeks. Yokukansan may also reduce depression and anxiety associated with dementia. Generally safe, including with psychotropics; may allow reduction in psychotropic dosages used to treat behavioral issues.
Huperzine-A (p. 232)	2	Typical dose: 200-400 µg/day with benefit (neuroprotectant to delay progression of dementia and improve cognition and memory) in several weeks. Generally safe, though may cause dry mouth, gastrointestinal issues, or mild dizziness. *Avoid if pregnant or nursing.*
Galantamine (p. 226)	2	Can offer significant cognitive support to Alzheimer's Disease patients and can slow neurological degeneration.
TENS (p. 255)	3	Typical dose: 30-45 min/day, 5 days/week of 0.5-2 Hz at 10-100 micro-amps connected to mid-back (TENS) with benefit (improved memory, cognition, and sleep) in 3 weeks. Self-administered. Generally safe, including with other therapies.
Curcumin (p. 234)	3	Typical dose: 100mg-4gm/day with benefit (aid cognition and memory, reduce agitation and apathy) in months. Generally safe, including with drugs. May have additive benefit with Ginkgo biloba. Side effects may include headache or diarrhea.
Lavender, Lemon Balm (p. 227)	3	Rub 1ml oil of lavender or lemon balm (30%) concentrate into arms/face 2 times/day or use via aromatherapy with benefit (reduce agitation and stress, promoting calmness) in 2-4 weeks. Generally safe, including with psychotropics. *Avoid if pregnant.*
Bright light therapy (p. 239)	3	Brief exposure to 2500-10000 lux full spectrum light or all-day ceiling lights (1000 lux) for dementia with benefit (improved sleep and mood; decreased agitation) in weeks. Generally safe, including with psychotropics.
Massage (p. 242)	3	A 10-15 min gentle massage to head, shoulders, and hands with immediate benefit (increased calmness and reduced agitation) for dementia. Generally safe, including with psychotropics.
Music (p. 137)	3	From daily to weekly. Listening to music, playing instruments, or singing improves mood and cognition in weeks to months for dementia, especially in residential care setting.

Symptom Relief Therapies for Dementia		
Approach	**T**	**Comments / Evaluation**
Saffron (p. 233)	3	Typical dose: 30mg/day with benefit (antioxidant and neuroprotection that can slow cognitive decline) for moderate-to-severe Alzheimer's; may be as effective as prescription meds for cognitive issues. Also provides antidepressant benefits. Generally safe, including with psychotropics.

WHAT CONSIDERATIONS SHOULD I KEEP IN MIND?

Safety is the #1 priority. If the individual is a danger to themselves or others, call 911. Hospital emergency rooms can help them stabilize.

Typically age-related, dementia affects about 10% of Americans over 65 and between 25 and 50% of those over 85. Decline in memory and cognition are considered a normal progression of aging, but dementia is a deterioration of intellectual function and other cognitive skills. Alzheimer's Disease, which accounts for two-thirds of all cases of dementia, is characterized by a build-up of plaque in the brain. Researchers estimate that one in eight baby boomers will develop Alzheimer's in the United States.

A healthy diet and an active physical, mental, and social life are among the most pragmatic things that can help avoid or slow dementia. See "Dementia, Case Studies" in the index for a variety of individual stories.

There is an alarming amount of evidence of the over prescribing of antipsychotic medication for those with dementia. The British Psychological Association states that "the use of antipsychotic medication for people with dementia needs to be reduced to limit the risk of harm of medications in this frail and vulnerable group of people".[1499] The United States Department of Health and Human Services launched a national effort to "safeguard nursing home residents from unnecessary antipsychotic drug use".[1402] James Scully, American Psychiatric Association Medical Director and CEO, states, "The [dosages of] antipsychotics in nursing homes... need to be really reduced".[1403] It is therefore vital that you take individual responsibility to work with care providers to avoid inappropriate prescribing of antipsychotics for the elderly.

WHAT ARE ADDITIONAL RESOURCES?

- Alternatives to Antipsychotics for Dementia. https://goo.gl/HU5W7v.
- Alzheimer's Association. www.alz.org.
- National Institute on Aging. https://goo.gl/DOR3JC.
- Alzheimer's disease overview. www.Alzheimers.gov.

Substance Abuse Therapies

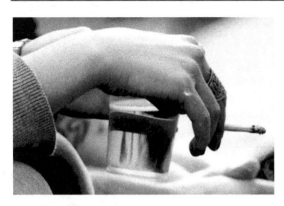

This section provides the most promising evidence-based therapies for substance abuse. Consider them in the context of *Building Your Recovery Plan* (p. 270).

Abused substances include alcohol, caffeine, nicotine, illegal drugs (including cocaine, heroin, methamphetamines, and others), prescription drugs (for example, sedative-hypnotics and narcotics), and chemicals. One of the challenges of discontinuing substance abuse is that it is often associated with withdrawal symptoms.

Start your recovery plan with approaches selected from the *Template of Recovery* (p. 273), then add specific approaches for substance abuse from the tables below. Work closely with your practitioners, relying upon their expertise and guidance to create, execute, and evolve this plan.

Template for Recovery approaches that are especially important include:

- **Housing & Safety**. Homelessness and crime often go hand-in-hand with substance abuse. It is vital that the individuals have safe and stable housing. This must be a top priority.

- **Diet**. Most people with substance abuse issues fail to have healthy diets; they do not consume enough amino acids, omega-3 fatty acids, and protein, and they are often cross-addicted to sugar, caffeine, and nicotine. To further complicate matters, alcohol and substance abuse interfere with fundamental nutritional processes. **Correction of the basic diet is a powerful tool for substance abuse recovery and should be one of the first steps taken.** In one study, 60% of dual-addicted (alcohol and drugs) patients who had a history of being unable to recover achieved abstinence for at least a year by focusing on a good nutritional diet.[1500] Switching to a diet of whole foods and avoiding junk food, coffee, and dairy products can dramatically improve the chances of remaining sober.[1501] Especially reduce the intake of refined sugar, trans-fats, and caffeine, while increasing omega-3 fatty acids and protein.

- **Biomedical Testing**. Start with full-protocol biomedical lab testing. The biomedical options below can be used without such testing but will mean more guesswork and will likely take longer to find what works. People with substance abuse often have nutrient deficiencies that can be corrected if they follow the nutrient plan.

- **Psychosocial Evaluation.** Past trauma, stress, and unhelpful thinking often accompany substance abuse. Psychosocial therapy can help with this. Work with a psychotherapist who can identify issues and recommend therapies. A strong and trusting relationship with your therapist is vital to recovery.
- **Calm Awareness.** Spending between 20 and 45 minutes each day will reduce withdrawal symptoms and cravings and help regulate thoughts and emotions. The benefits will become evident in two to four weeks. Training is sometimes available with twelve-step programs.
- **Exercise.** Consistent aerobic or moderate exercise of at least a half hour to 45 minutes a day at least three times a week provides many benefits, among them a sustained reduction in cravings for alcohol, nicotine, and narcotics. Exercise can also improve depression.
- **Mind-Body Disciplines.** Yoga and other disciplines can benefit those with substance abuse issues. Avoid external Qigong if agitated.

In addition to the above, see the targeted approaches for substance abuse found in the tables below. With your practitioners, consider them in tier order.

Biomedical Restorative Therapies for Substance Abuse

Approach	T	Comments / Evaluation
Vitamin B (p. 169)	2	Daily B1 may reduce alcohol cravings; 1gm B3 before drinking may protect the liver. Brewer's yeast, two tablespoons twice a day, is good source of B vitamins and trace minerals. Generally safe, though a mild flush possible with B3. Metadoxine helps alcoholics maintain abstinence a d decrease alcohol cravings.
Amino Acids (p. 180)	2	Amino acid therapy including L-tyrosine, L-glutamine, and L-tryptophan with multi-vitamins and minerals can reduce alcohol withdrawal symptoms and decrease stress; 1gm 3 times/day taurine may decrease the severity of alcohol withdrawal and reduce the risk of cocaine addiction. Safe with other therapies.
ALCAR (p. 181)	3	Typical dose of 2-3gm/day may improve alcohol withdrawal, craving, and memory in alcoholics, with benefit in weeks. Safe with other therapies.
Vitamin A (p. 169)	3	Typical dose: 700-900 µg/day. Those with alcohol abuse issues should be tested for Vitamin A deficiency because alcohol overuse often depletes this vitamin, possibly resulting in vision problems.
Omega-3 Fatty Acids (p. 187)	3	Typical dose of 6000 mg/day can reduce alcohol cravings, withdrawal symptoms, anxiety, and depression associated with substance abuse. Rely on a healthy diet, which can improve general brain function. Safe with other therapies.
Antho-cyanins (p. 224)	3	Daily ingestion of anthocyanins, found in blueberries, raspberries, and other sources have antioxidant properties and may reduce the toxic effect of alcohol. Safe with other therapies.
Melatonin (p. 202)	3	Typical dose: 2mg of controlled release formula at bedtime with benefit (helps withdrawal from prescription sedatives and nicotine, protects kidneys from alcohol abuse, and reduces agitation), with benefit in days to weeks. Generally safe even at very high doses (300mg/day). May reduce need for potentially addictive sedatives.

Biomedical Restorative Therapies for Substance Abuse

Approach	T	Comments / Evaluation
Magnesium (p. 178)	3	Typical ongoing dose of 500-1500 mg/day with benefit (reduce cravings, improve abstinence in drug abusers, and improve mental functioning), with benefit in days to weeks. Supplements can improve depressed mood in alcoholics. Safe with other therapies.
Zinc (p. 179)	3	Typical ongoing dose up to 40 mg/day with benefit (may help alcohol-related cognitive problems) in days to weeks. Generally safe. May cause gastrointestinal issues and increase risk of prostate cancer (men). Taking B6 supplement increases zinc effectiveness.
SAM-e (p. 188)	3	Typical dose of 400-800 mg/day with benefit (may reduce alcohol consumption, improve liver damage from alcohol abuse, and improve depression often found with substance abuse) in days to weeks. Generally safe, although possible gastrointestinal issues. *Avoid use for those with bipolar, since it may cause mania.*
NAC (p. 184)	3	Typical dose of 2400 mg/day may reduce cocaine craving.

Psychosocial Restorative Therapies for Substance Abuse

Approach	T	Comments / Evaluation
CBT (p. 117)	1	Cognitive Behavioral Therapy (CBT) and Dialectic Behavioral Therapy (p. 120) effective in controlling addictive behavior.
reSET app (p. 328)	2	Phone app. Use with outpatient therapy and a contingency management system to improve abstinence.
Acupuncture (P. 159)	2	Typically 20-40-min sessions. Benefit in 2-5 treatments. Electro-acupuncture may be most effective form for substance abuse. Use with or without other treatments. Generally safe, has sedating effect.
EEG Biofeedback (p. 142)	2	Typical dose: 30 min, 1-3 times/week, with benefit (decrease alcohol, cocaine, methamphetamine, and other substance consumption) in 10-15 treatments. Use with or without other treatments. Generally safe. Can also reduce anxiety and PTSD symptoms possibly associated with substance abuse. Can be self-administered or with practitioner.
Matrix Model (p. 328)	2	A 16-week intensive program of education, support groups, counseling, and drug testing appears to have a 70% success rate. Accepted as evidence-based by SAMHSA.
12-Step Programs (p. 133)	2	Weekly meetings in 12-step programs can increase abstinence from both alcohol and narcotics—however, less frequent meetings do not. Gaining a peer sponsor is vital to success. The 12-step programs or approaches with spiritual focus can aid recovery.
Exposure Therapy (p. 151)	3	Reduces cravings and aids in avoiding nicotine, alcohol, and cocaine by desensitizing to abuse-stimulating situations. Benefit in days or weeks. Often used with Cognitive Behavioral Therapy (p. 117). Use with or without other therapies.

Symptom Relief Therapies for Substance Abuse

Approach	T	Comments / Evaluation
tDCS (p. 253)	2	Typical dose: 30 min/day with benefit (improved sleep; reduced cravings, anxiety, depression and withdrawal symptoms) in 3-5 weeks. Shows benefit for tobacco abuse; may improve effectiveness of meds used for substance withdrawal. Typically well tolerated.

Symptom Relief Therapies for Substance Abuse		
Approach	**T**	**Comments / Evaluation**
Kudzu (p. 232)	2	Typical dose of 3g/day of Kudzu extract with 25% isoflavone content may help reduce alcohol craving. Interactions with drugs are not clear. Widely used in Chinese medicine.
Aralia elata (p. 230)	2	Dose varies, but benefits include reducing symptoms of acute alcohol intoxication. Little is known of interactions with other drugs/substances. Chinese herbal formula.
Mentat (p. 235)	2	Dose varies in helping to reduce alcoholics' risk of relapse once they stop drinking. Little is known of interactions with other drugs/substances. An Ayurvedic herb.
rTMS (p. 249)	3	Typical dose is daily; showed significant reduction in cigarette smoking and cocaine craving.

WHAT CONSIDERATIONS SHOULD I KEEP IN MIND?

Safety is the #1 priority. If the individual is a danger to themselves or others, call 911. Hospital emergency rooms can help them stabilize.

People with mental health issues are much more likely to have substance-abuse issues than the general population. The multipliers are significant: people with major depression are 4.1 times more likely to abuse substances; people with bipolar are 14.5 times more likely; those with OCD are 3.4 times more likely; those with panic disorder, 4.3 times; and schizophrenia, 10.1 times.[778] Substance abuse issues must be addressed simultaneously with mental health issues—they can rarely be overcome separately.

Overprescribing sedative-hypnotics and psychotropics has resulted in a growing population of people dependent on prescription drugs. (See *Excessive Prescribing Risk*, p. 259.)

People with severe substance abuse issues are among the most vulnerable people in our society. Do not impose abstinence as a condition for support in those areas. When individuals are stabilized, thorough biomedical and psychosocial assessments can help identify underlying issues.

From a psychosocial perspective, *Cognitive Behavioral Therapy* (p. 117) or *Mindfulness Based Sobriety* (p. 122), help adjust maladaptive behavioral patterns. *Biofeedback* (p. 142) and *Acupuncture* (p. 159) can also help.

Strongly consider avoiding SSRIs in cases of alcohol abuse. They appear to increase alcohol consumption, not decrease it.[1393]

See "Substance Abuse, Case Studies" in the index for individual stories.

WHAT ARE ADDITIONAL RESOURCES?

- See Addiction Co-Therapy (p. 332)

Insomnia Therapies

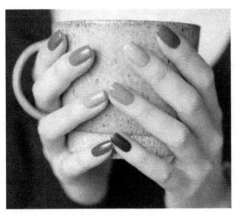

This section provides the most promising evidence-based therapies for insomnia. Consider them in the context of *Building Your Recovery Plan* (p. 270).

Insomnia symptoms include difficulty in falling asleep, recurring nightmares, continually awakening from sleep at night, awakening too early, and feeling unrefreshed from sleep.

Insomnia covers the following major mental health diagnoses:

- Sleep-onset insomnia (difficulty in falling asleep)
- Sleep-maintenance insomnia (difficulty in staying asleep)
- Sleep phase insomnia (inability to sleep until the early morning hours)

Start your recovery plan with approaches selected from the *Template of Recovery* (p. 273), then add specific approaches for insomnia from the tables below. Work closely with your practitioners, leveraging their expertise and guidance to create, execute, and evolve this plan.

Template for Recovery approaches especially important for insomnia include:

- **Biomedical Testing.** Full protocol biomedical lab testing is mandatory.
- **Calm Awareness.** Doing this 30 to 45 minutes each day can produce calm, which can decrease insomnia.
- **Exercise.** At least three times per week of moderate exertion for at least 30 minutes per session will help individuals fall asleep more quickly and stay asleep, in less than six weeks. May help depression and anxiety that accompany insomnia.
- **Diet.** Food impacts sleep. Low blood sugar at night is a common cause of insomnia, stimulating hunger pangs and signaling to the body an urge to eat. Foods high in carbohydrates should therefore be avoided before bed. Foods that contain tyramine (bacon, cheese, chocolate, eggplant, ham, potatoes, spinach, tomatoes, wine, and others) stimulate the brain and should be avoided.[1502] Food allergies can also cause sleep disorders.[1503] Foods with L-tryptophan (eggs, milk, grains) should be part of your diet. Avoid caffeine in all forms (coffee, tea, caffeinated sodas, etc.), since insomnia can be caused by caffeine withdrawal. Avoid or minimize alcohol, especially at bedtime.

- **Sleep Hygiene**. Various techniques help: restrict time spent in bed, go to bed only when you are sleepy, get out of bed if you are unable to sleep, reduce noise or light where you sleep, and get up at the same time every morning. Avoid using electronic screens (TVs, computers, tablets, or cell phones) within an hour before bed (p. 70).

In addition to the above, see the targeted approaches for insomnia found in the tables below. With your practitioners, consider them in tier order.

Biomedical Restorative Approaches for Insomnia		
Approach	**T**	**Comments / Evaluation**
Melatonin (p. 202)	2	Typical dose: 0.3-1 mg immediate release (for getting to sleep more quickly), 0.2-2 mg controlled-release (for longer sleep times), or 0.5-5 gm for jet lag (taken in destination time zone), with benefit in days. Take at bed time. Can resynch wake-sleep cycle. Consider in combination with Bright Light Therapy. Generally safe, though larger doses may cause drowsiness.
5-HTP and L-tryptophan (p. 183)	2	Typical dose: 300 mg/day 5-HTP split in 2-3 doses or 1-2 gm/day L-tryptophan, with benefit in days. Generally safe. May sedate, so take at bedtime. Can be used with antidepressants, but consult with doctor. *Avoid use with low-folate depression biotypes and MAOI antidepressants.*
Allergy diets (p. 209)	2	Run *Food Allergy Tests* (p. 324) to assess food sensitivities, especially dairy.
Vitamin B12 (p. 172)	3	Even if serum B12 levels are within normal bounds, B12 deficiencies can be present, causing insomnia. Typical therapeutic dose: 1.5-4.5 mg /day. Generally safe.
Magnesium (p. 178)	3	Typical dose 400-500 mg/day. Choose chelated form (such as citrate, ascorbate, orotate, glycinate, or a mix of them). Avoid oxide salts. Generally safe. Higher doses of citrate form make cause diarrhea.
Other nutrients	3	Adding B1 B9, C, E, zinc, and iron may help daytime drowsiness. B12 may help earlier sleep onset. Start with biomedical lab testing to assess deficiencies, realizing that certain individuals may have deficiencies even if lab results are within normal ranges.
Indole-3-acetic acid (p. 187)	3	Typical dose: 200-300 mg may improve symptoms of mild or situational insomnia. Generally safe.
DHEA (p. 200)	3	Typical dose: 500mg DHEA may increase REM sleep. Possibly effective when insomnia and depression occur together.

Psychosocial Restorative Approaches for Insomnia

Approach	T	Comments / Evaluation
Biofeedback (p. 142)	1	Daily 20-minute sessions will benefit in 1-2 weeks; longer, if weekly. Especially SMR (alpha-theta training) can increase sleep duration when insomnia is caused by sleep apnea or narcolepsy. May allow decrease in sleep meds. Generally safe, though may cause dizziness.
CBT for Insomnia (p. 119)	1	Delivered in a variety of forms, including mobile app, CBT-I can change sleep habits and improve sleep duration, quality, and latency in 1-3 months. Can be more effective than sleeping meds. Online/App versions more effective with therapist involvement via email/chat. Safe with other therapies.
Acupuncture (p. 159)	2	Widely used for insomnia in countries that value Traditional Chinese Medicine (TCM). Treatment frequencies vary, lasting 20-60 minutes, with benefit in 2-3 weeks that may last months. Has sedating effect. Generally safe. Always use sterile needles. Use a TCM-trained practitioner.
Massage (p. 242)	3	A 15-30 minute massage can induce relaxation and benefit sleep. Safe with other therapies.
Lucid Dreaming (p. 151)	3	If insomnia is tied to anxiety/trauma, confronting memories via lucid dreaming can reduce anxiety while awake and improve sleep. Very preliminary research. Lucid dreaming skill takes time to develop.

Symptom Relief Approaches for Insomnia

Approach	T	Comments / Evaluation
Bright Light Therapy (p. 239)	1	Typical usage: 30-40 min in morning with white (10,000 lux) light benefits in days. Generally safe and can be used with other therapies, particularly exercise. May cause hypomania (if bipolar) or insomnia (if used after morning). Avoid eye damage by avoiding light sources with UV. Do not stare into light.
Valerian (p. 229)	2	Typical dose: 600-900 mg prior to bed, with benefit in 2-6 weeks. Has sedating effect and can be as effective as sedatives, but without dependence risk. Generally safe. Combine with Kava for stress-induced insomnia. *Avoid use with alcohol or sleep meds, or if pregnant or breastfeeding. Large doses may impact liver.*
Sensory Therapies (p. 239)	3	Listening to soothing music 20-45 minutes before bed will benefit in 1-2 weeks. Safe with other therapies. Also, warm Hydro Therapy (p. 241) and *Sound Therapy* (p. 240).
Ginkgo Biloba (p. 231)	3	Typical dose of EGb 761 formulation: 240-360 mg/day in 2-3 doses, with benefit in 2-4 weeks. Generally safe, though may cause headache, dizziness, or stomach upset. *Avoid if using anti-clotting agents (e.g. aspirin).* 240 mg/day with antidepressants can reduce nighttime awakenings.

Symptom Relief Approaches for Insomnia

Approach	T	Comments / Evaluation
St. John's Wort (p. 229)	3	Typical dose: 900-1800mg/day in 3 doses, with benefit within weeks. Usually mild side effects, but potential toxic drug interactions. *Can lessen birth control pill effectiveness. Avoid use with protease inhibitors, immunosuppressive agents, MAOI antidepressants, and if pregnant.* It may improve sleep in depressed patients.
Ginseng (p. 226)	3	Typical dose: 200-600mg may help daytime wakefulness. May cause agitation, diarrhea, and (rarely) psychosis or allergic reactions. *Avoid if pregnant or nursing or taking blood thinners.*
Earthing (p. 255)	3	Grounded sheets/pillowcases may reduce the impact of electromagnetic fields and balance cortisol levels, aiding sleep.
Yokukan-san (p.233)	3	Typical dose 7.5 g/day for 3 days to be split between 3 daily doses will increase sleep time and quality while decreasing time to fall asleep. Generally safe.
Corydalis (p. 225)	3	Typical dose 100-200 mg/day of cdl-tetrahydropalmatine extract promotes relaxation and sleep. Generally safe.
Hops (p. 227)	3	Doses vary; dried strobile (hop cones) in doses of 1.5-2 g possibly in "hop pillows" to increase sleep times. Can facilitate vivid dreams. Generally safe, including with psychotropics.
Yohimbine (p. 236)	3	Typical dose 8mg/day may be effective for daytime drowsiness or narcolepsy. May cause diarrhea, insomnia, gastrointestinal issues, and flushing.
LEET (p. 254)	3	Typical dose: 20 min treatment 3 times/week for 4 weeks, with possible benefit of significantly increased sleep time and reduced time to fall asleep.

WHAT CONSIDERATIONS SHOULD I KEEP IN MIND?

Some people with insomnia have a confused sleep-wake cycle (circadian rhythm). Approaches that reset this cycle, like bright light therapy, are often effective. Light treatment affects the timing of melatonin released into the brain, which can reduce depression. In addition, insomnia is often associated with problems in thinking clearly, so therapy can improve cognitive function.

From a biomedical perspective, *Melatonin* (p. 202) is the most effective solution, but other nutrients are helpful. From a psychosocial perspective, both *Cognitive Behavioral Therapy for Insomnia* (p. 119) and *Biofeedback* (p. 142) offer more conscious control over our sleep patterns. See "Insomnia, Case Studies" in the index for a variety of individual stories.

9 – Looking Onward

In researching all the current knowledge in the field of mental health, the therapies available—and unavailable—for people suffering with mental health issues, it would have been easy for me to get disappointed in what we don't know and don't have; disappointed in a broken mental health system that delivers far less than what is needed; and disappointed with pills that sometimes cause the very problems they are designed to fix.

And there was certainly a dose of that disappointment.

But, in the end, I found that we know more, and we have more help than I first realized. I found that it isn't my job or your job to fix the broken system; our job is to navigate the system well enough to fix ourselves. I found that we don't need a myopic focus on pills; we can turn our attention to the broad palette of *Integrative Mental Health* treatments and recognize pills for what they are: one option for partial symptom relief. And most important of all, I found that thousands of people live in mental health recovery using the scientifically-grounded techniques of the emerging paradigm of *Integrative Mental Health*.

And that's not bad.

The book's preface started with an assertion: *people need options*. The remainder of the book provided many—294, to be precise.

But, I'll make another assertion: these options can only work for us if we work with them. All the options in the world aren't worth much unless we accept the responsibility to evaluate them and prudently experiment with them to map our own road to recovery.

And that's hard work. We must carefully weigh the evidence, so we experiment with the options that are most likely to help our individual situations. We must be patient and vigilant during those experiments, to assess for ourselves if the options work for us. Or not. We must persevere and keep turning over new stones when initial experiments don't bear fruit. We must work very hard at a time when we are already exhausted from simply managing the situations we face each day.

This personal effort is needed since there are many dynamics that can impede our efforts (Figure 37). But, since our focus is on individual recovery, our job is not to oppose these dynamics, but to understand and sidestep them, working both within and beyond the system.

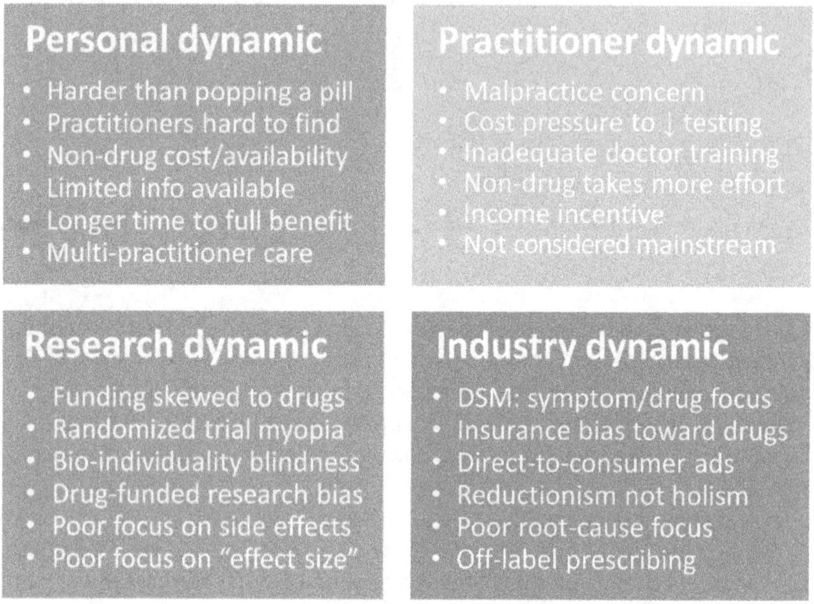

Personal dynamic
- Harder than popping a pill
- Practitioners hard to find
- Non-drug cost/availability
- Limited info available
- Longer time to full benefit
- Multi-practitioner care

Practitioner dynamic
- Malpractice concern
- Cost pressure to ↓ testing
- Inadequate doctor training
- Non-drug takes more effort
- Income incentive
- Not considered mainstream

Research dynamic
- Funding skewed to drugs
- Randomized trial myopia
- Bio-individuality blindness
- Drug-funded research bias
- Poor focus on side effects
- Poor focus on "effect size"

Industry dynamic
- DSM: symptom/drug focus
- Insurance bias toward drugs
- Direct-to-consumer ads
- Reductionism not holism
- Poor root-cause focus
- Off-label prescribing

© 2017 Craig Wagner – OnwardMentalHealth.com

Figure 37 - Impediments to Integrative Mental Health

Fortunately, emerging paradigm *Integrative Mental Health* practitioners make our job easier. Their discipline offers significant, even extraordinary, hope. Their root-cause-seeking diagnostic techniques and expanded treatment options give us many more avenues for personal recovery. They streamline our experimentation when they help us identify our individual body chemistry and ways to tailor therapies to our individual needs. They leverage the best of conventional psychiatry and psychology while adding an array of scientifically-validated alternatives. And with these alternatives, they help minimize our symptoms with little or no side effects.

That is very good news.

But recall what we discussed in Chapter 2: we want much more than the absence of symptoms. We want the presence of life's most positive things.[380] We want well-being, a state that encompasses quality of life, self-acceptance, purpose, autonomy, strong personal relationships, social contribution, personal meaning, and a sense of belonging. We want *personal recovery*. We want to be better than we've ever been before.

Figure 38 provides an expanded concept of recovery.[1504] It shows that

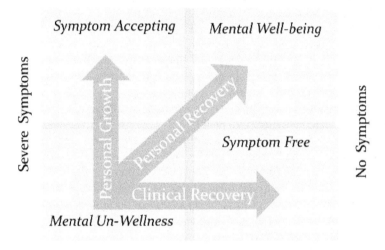

Figure 38 – Mental well-being model

clinical recovery is a one-dimensional activity that entails eliminating or significantly improving symptoms. However, *personal recovery* is two-dimensional; it adds a dimension of personal growth on top of *clinical recovery*.

The point is this: while we diligently work to reduce our symptoms, we should also focus on the important task of personal growth. Why? Personal growth enables clinical recovery—and vice-versa.

Healing our personhood gives us the necessary insight to more assuredly create our own mental wellness. And as Paramahansa Yogananda notes, when

> *"You gain strength only when you wrestle with a strong opponent. One who doesn't have difficulties is one who doesn't grow."*[1505]
>
> - Paramahansa Yogananda

we engage in the difficult work of personal growth, we become a stronger, more capable person. (See Case Study 121, p. 294.)

Practitioners of conventional psychiatry —those who stick almost exclusively to drug-based therapies (see Chapter 1)—tend to see personal growth as a fuzzy goal outside the scope of their discipline. *Integrative Mental Health* practitioners, however, are often grounded in the vital importance of integrating personal growth with mental well-being.

This framework helps explain why people can consider themselves recovered even while some of their mental health symptoms persist. These people have experienced enough personal growth to accept residual symptoms as their current reality and find joy and meaning despite them. In fact, personal growth can be a central theme for those pursuing mental health recovery. (See Case Study 11, p. 91.)

More broadly, placing personal growth into the context of mental health helps bring greater nuance to two realities.

First, *Wellness Basics* (p. 55) are likely more effective and more widely applicable than we think. Many *Wellness Basics* proven to aid clinical recovery also facilitate personal growth. These tools include mindfulness, managing our *Thought-Emotion-Action cycle* (Figure 16, p. 84), establishing meaningful relationships, meditation, and developing a sense of purpose, among others. The broad value of these tools suggests that mastering them may enhance our lives in stunning and unexpected ways.

Second, we must be careful not to confuse the disruption of personal growth with the symptoms of mental illness. New evidence suggests that a variety of experiences considered normal transformative growth in many cultures are now labeled and treated as mental illness. In some cases, we try to cure people when we should be trying to help them through a significant growth stage. Sometimes we seek to stop a disruption when the disruption may be a part of the growth process. *Transpersonal and Positive Psychology* (p. 104) offer approaches to recognize and facilitate these growth opportunities.

Frontiers of Mental Health

New frontiers in mental health research and practice hold great promise:

- **Genetics**. Considerable research is underway to identify how our DNA can predispose us mental health issues.
- **Imaging**. Scientists and engineers are extending our ability to create high-quality MRIs and other images that can shed light on both the static and dynamic states of the brain.
- **Expansion of Integrative Psychiatry**. The paradigm shift toward Integrative Psychiatry is accelerating, with an expanded menu of non-drug options.

- **Microbiome**. Significant work is underway to understand how the human microbiome – the living bacteria, fungi, and other organisms found naturally in a healthy human body – affects mental health. This includes the potential development of psychobiotics – brain-influencing bacteria that can be planted in the gut to provide mental health benefits.
- **Epigenetics.** Researchers are finding that the expression of genes, not just DNA sequencing, can have a profound effect on mental health. Methods to influence gene expression, lilke nutrient therapy, are able to target specific causes of mental health symptoms.
- **Person-centered care**. The field of mental health sees a strong movement toward more engaged, compassionate, and individualized care for those with mental health issues.
- **Transpersonal and Positive Psychology**. Efforts are underway to integrate these psychologies into the broader realm of personal recovery.

What can these new directions mean to us all?

Tom Insel, past Director of the National Institute of Mental Health, indicates, "Despite high expectations, neither genomics nor imaging has yet impacted the diagnosis or treatment of the 45 million Americans with serious or moderate mental illness each year." [1506] Indeed, examining 547 studies of fMRI imaging found that anatomical views of brain looked fairly similar across a wide variety of psychiatric disorders.[1507] For this reason, we find hope knowing research is underway on genetics and imaging—but we can't look to them to aid recovery immediately.

However, we can leverage the other elements of the frontier now. We can choose to engage practitioners who embrace the new paradigm of *Integrative Mental Health* and use therapies customized to our unique bio-individuality. We can keep a healthy microbiome by changing our diets to whole foods and sufficient probiotics to help ensure digestive health. We can use epigenetic-informed nutrient therapy to optimize gene expression. We can choose to work with practitioners who offer more personalized care than a fifteen-minute medication review. And we can choose to explore the growth opportunities in *Transpersonal and Positive Psychology*.

Let us begin

Although mental health is a universal goal, everyone seeking mental health recovery follows a unique path to a unique destination. Recovery is a deeply human effort deserving all the deeply human attributes we can bring to it.

Two attributes stand above the rest.

First, **we must be tremendously respectful – and indeed, loving – to ourselves and everyone involved in recovery.** To support someone with mental health issues, we must infuse these attributes into every interaction. We must be prepared to explore the uncomfortable center of many issues – physical, mental, and emotional. And when we reach this point of proximity, we must not only accept what we find, but embrace it with all the insight and tenderness we can muster.

From our position of closeness and respect, we can listen intently and compassionately as a loved-one in pain reveals a unique and often terrifying individual experience. As we listen, we must identify individual needs and strengths (in ourselves as well as our loved-one). And then we must become an ally on what could well be the loneliest journey in the world if a person travels it all alone. Along the way, we should take the time to marvel at the courageous humanity of the person we are supporting. As we do this, we can be more helpful as someone we love trudges, trips, and travels along the path of mental health recovery.

Second, **if we are the people in crisis, we must act. We must move. We must accept responsibility. We need to understand that no one can recover for us. We must experiment. And we must work. Hard.** We don't need to create a mountain of energy that will propel us to the end of our journey, but we must find a nugget of energy that can start us on our journey. We need to center ourselves enough to be able to take our next confident stride forward. (See *Recommitment*, p. 344.)

Unfortunately, there is no free lunch in mental health. The path to recovery is often a crooked one, with an occasional dead-end. But with the help of the information contained in this book, I hope you find the path better lit, easier to traverse, and in the end, a more assured way home.

The very best of luck to you.

> *"Whatever you can do or dream you can, begin it. Boldness has genius and magic and power in it. Begin it now."*
>
> - Johann von Goethe

__Bottom Line__: *Recovery is not found in a book, but in your passion-infused self-determined efforts.*

Appendices

Integrative Biomedical Practitioner Finder

See the latest version of this appendix at www.OnwardMentalHealth.com (Resources).

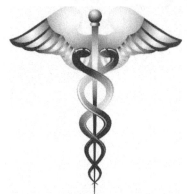

Integrative Mental Health embraces both conventional and alternative practices and includes several practitioner roles. (See *People of Recovery*, p. 35.)

One role has a biomedical focus. These practitioners use *Biomedical Test Panels* (p. 323) to assess for possible underlying physical causes for mental health symptoms, among them, nutrient imbalances, hormonal issues, amino acid irregularities, food allergies, pathogens, inflammation, and toxicities. Customized therapies can then be prescribed targeted at the specific issues identified in the lab results. These practitioners go by many names:

- *Integrative Psychiatrists* - psychiatrists who offer both drug and non-drug options
- *Orthomolecular Practitioners* – professionals who provide nutrient-oriented therapies based in orthomolecular principles
- *Integrative Medicine Doctors* - MDs who offer drug and non-drug options for overall health, including mental health
- *Functional Medicine Doctors* – MDs who focus on cause-based approaches to health.
- *Naturopathic Physicians* – holistic practitioners with a naturopathic degree
- *Specialists* – MDs such as endocrinologists or allergists who focus on a subset of biomedical causes. Specialists are brought in if initial testing indicates their expertise is required or when very detailed testing is desired.

It is vital to include practitioners on your team who are focused on the biomedical aspects of mental health, since more than one-quarter of mental health issues have underlying biomedical causes or influencers. Although primary care physicians often prescribe psychotropics, they typically do not fulfill this more specialized biomedical role focused on mental health.

Perhaps the most comprehensive and proven biomedical protocol for mental health was developed by the Walsh Institute (Figure 28, p. 168). Open-label trials indicates that over 70% of people with mental health diagnosis who use customized Nutrient Therapy for six months based on the Walsh protocol experience a significant decrease in symptoms and can often reduce medication dosages. A directory of Walsh-trained clinicians is found below.

Be aware that it is hard to find these new-paradigm biomedical practitioners. If you can afford to travel, you have more options.

Before calling for an appointment, do your homework: check out the practitioners' specialties and approaches on their websites, and read evaluations of people who recommended the practitioner. When you call, if you are told that the doctor is not accepting new patients, switch gears. Tell the scheduler why this doctor is very important to you: that he or she comes highly recommended by someone you trust; their area of specialization is something you have a good reason to explore; the approach mentioned on the website is something that resonates with you; et cetera. Such respectful assertiveness is an act of advocacy and may help you get an appointment. If it doesn't work, be sure to ask for a reference for another practitioner with similar standards who is accepting patients. Then when you call that practitioner's office, you have a referral to mention.

For a list of questions you may want to consider asking potential practitioners, see *Questions for Dialogue with your Mental Health Practitioners* (p. 328).

Consider the following directories, clinics, and practitioners as you look for a biomedical practitioner. Start by getting a referral from a medical professional or friend you already know and trust. You can also seek referrals at nearby clinics and hospitals. Americans living near Canada may consider leveraging the larger base of orthomolecular practitioners there.

Directories of Integrative Psychiatrists.
- APA Caucus on Complementary, Alternative, and Integrative Medicine www.IntPsychiatry.com.
- Integrative Medicine for Mental Health Registry. www.integrativemedicineformentalhealth.com/registry.php.
- American College for Advancement in Medicine. www.acam.org.

Directories of Naturopaths.
- Find a Naturopath. www.findanaturopath.com.
- American Association of Naturopathic Physicians. www.naturopathic.org.
- Canadian Association of Naturopathic Doctors. www.cand.ca.

Directories of Alternative/Integrative Medicine practitioners.
- Walsh Institute Clinicians. www.walshinstitute.org/clinical-resources.html.
- International College of Integrative Medicine. www.icimed.com.
- AlternativeMentalHealth.com Practitioner Directory, http://goo.gl/13q2LK.
- American Board of Integrative Holistic Medicine. http://www.abihm.org/search-doctors.
- Academy of Integrative Health Medicine. www.aihm.org.
- International Network of Integrative Mental Health. https://inimh.org.
- American Holistic Health Association Practitioner Directory. www.ahha.org/holistic-practitioners.

- Mad in America Provider Directory for withdrawing from psychiatric drugs. https://goo.gl/kvstV0.

Functional Medicine Practitioners. www.FunctionalMedicine.org.

Hospitals with Integrative Psychiatry focus.
- CA http://goo.gl/UpSEl4.
- PA http://goo.gl/FsnMx4.
- OH http://goo.gl/LmXtcc.
- MN http://goo.gl/QV3Nm9.
- NY http://goo.gl/idUun5.

Integrative Psychiatry clinics/practices.
- AZ www.mypassion4health.com.
- IL www.mensahmedical.com, www.chicagointegrative.com.
- MA http://goo.gl/lyWQ6f.
- MD www.wholepsychiatry.com, www.holisticpsychiatrist.com.
- MI https://goo.gl/cWYkh2 (www.OnwardMentalHealth.com → Resources).
- NY http://goo.gl/0V4xrV.
- CO http://goo.gl/fKhfzD.
- CA http://goo.gl/bfO3eG.
- KY http://goo.gl/ti9sW.
- UT www.paulthielkingmd.com.

Anthroposophical health centers www.steinerhealth.org.

Orthomolecular practitioners.

- Worldwide Practitioner Directory. www.orthomolecular.org/resources/pract.shtml.
- Canadian Practitioner Directory. https://ionhealth.ca/public/find-a-practitioner.
- Canadian clinic (Toronto). www.nmrc.ca.

In addition, search the internet for practitioners in your area, typing the following into your web browser (replacing "CITY" with the name of your city).

> *"integrative psychiatry" OR "Integrative psychiatrist" OR*
> *"integrative medicine" OR naturopath OR alternative OR*
> *complementary OR holistic CITY*

Biomedical Test Panels

See the latest version of this appendix at www.OnwardMentalHealth.com (Resources).

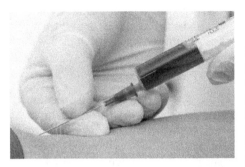

WHAT IS THE ESSENCE?
Mental health lab tests look for markers that may identify physical causes of mental health symptoms. A robust set of blood and urine tests should be run, with hair and cerebral spinal fluid potentially evaluated. Regrettably, baseline testing of numerous important physical ailments is not as common as it should be for people diagnosed with serious mental illness.[1508]

With your practitioner, select a reasonable set of tests based on your symptoms and medical history. See a list of possible tests below. Lab tests should be run by labs with CLIA certification (see *Glossary*, p. 337). Often a baseline test panel is the first choice, and additional tests are run as needed.

Individual lab tests synthesized from *Test Protocols* (p. 325).

- **Biochemical imbalance tests.** It is important to discover if any of the six most common mental health biochemical imbalances are present (copper overload, Vitamin B6 deficiency, zinc deficiency, methyl/folate imbalances, oxidative stress overload, and amino acid imbalances).[19] The following tests should be considered **mandatory.**
  - ○ **Serum copper.** Excess copper can alter synaptic activity for dopamine and norepinephrine.
  - ○ **Plasma Zinc.** Plasma zinc is usually considered the best of the several zinc tests. Zinc helps reduce oxidative stress, and zinc deficiencies can cause copper overload.
  - ○ **Methylation test.** Over 60% of people with depression, anxiety and psychosis have a serious *Methylation* (p. 54) imbalance,[1509] so testing for methylation irregularities should be considered mandatory. The best test is likely a SAM-e/SAH ratio test. (www.DoctorsData.com is one of the few labs in America that run this test). A suitable alternative is whole blood histamine.[19] (See Case Study 118, p. 281, and Case Study 119, p. 288.) People with overmethylation often thrive on vitamin B9, while people with undermethylation often improve depressive symptoms using SAM-e.
  - ○ **Urine Pyrroles.** This test can identify a pyrrole disorder (an imbalance in hemoglobin synthesis) and oxidative stress.
  - ○ **Serum ceruloplasmin.** Ceruloplasmin is a copper-binding protein. If more than 25% of copper is not bound to ceruloplasmin, a metal metabolism disorder involving oxidative stress may be present.

- o **Amino acids.** These tests look for potential amino acid abnormalities. In addition, organic acid tests can be run to provide detail on intestinal yeast and bacteria which can be helpful to determine proper gastrointestinal function. See Case Study 64 (p. 190).
- o **Liver Enzymes**. Include gamma-GT, aspartate aminotransferase, alanine aminotransferase, bilirubin, albumin, and alkaline phosphatase. Elevated enzymes, a common side effect of psychotropics, suggest that the liver is stressed—which can indicate the need to avoid high doses of vitamins B3, A, D, and E.

- **Endocrine tests.** Endocrine tests look for potential issues with the glands. Of these, the thyroid panel should be considered **mandatory** because thyroid irregularities are relatively common in those with mental distress. Detailed endocrine testing can be done based on specific situations (e.g. for treatment-resistant depression, rapid-cycling bipolar, and in cases when a woman's psychiatric symptoms seem to vary with the menstrual cycle). If needed, these are often ordered by an endocrinologist.
  - o **Thyroid Panel.** Test for T3RU, T4, and free T4. Hypothyroidism (underactive thyroid) often accompanies nutrient issues.
  - o **DHEA and DHEA-sulfate.** Test for DHEA-sulfate levels especially in patients over 40 years of age. If low, DHEA supplementation may improve depression and improve symptoms for those with schizophrenia, bipolar and dementia.
  - o **Sex-specific tests.** Women should consider tests for estrogen, progesterone, FSH, LH, and Prolactin. Men may be evaluated for free testosterone and bio-available testosterone.
  - o **ACTH test.** This test is used to diagnose adrenal insufficiency, Addison's disease, and related conditions. It can help distinguish between adrenal and pituitary issues.
  - o **Cortisol.** Cortisol is a stress hormone. A 24-hour free cortisol excretion level > 100 micrograms indicates possible Cushing's syndrome caused by endocrine tumors. CT/MRI/ultrasound scans can detect tumors. Excess cortisol is associated undermethylation and altered gene expression.[1012]
  - o **Plasma parathyroid hormone (PTH).** This tests for proper functioning of the parathyroid gland. Blood calcium levels are checked at the same time since PTH controls calcium levels.
  - o **Plasma metanephrines.** Used to determine presence of a rare pheochromocytoma tumor.

- **Allergy Tests.** Food allergies are much more common in those with mental health issues than the overall population, with gluten, soy and corn being the most common. Gluten allergy testing should be considered mandatory, especially for those with schizophrenia. A variety of testing methods are possible including elimination diets. Consider antibody tests for gluten allergy (anti-endomysial – EMA and anti-tissue transglutaminase – tTG) and sensitivity (gliadin - AGA). See *Food Allergy Tests* (p. 210).

- **Lithium.** Lithium is broadly important in mental health and may be needed for normal brain growth. It is clearly implicated in bipolar, dementia and autism. It can be assessed through hair or blood tests.
- **Heavy Metal/Toxin Tests.** These tests are often run using hair and/or blood samples. These should be considered standard in testing since toxins can be absorbed from several different sources.
- **Homocysteine.** Homocysteine levels are a strong indicator of health and high levels are associated with cognitive impairment in bipolar, schizophrenia, dementia, and depression. Deficiencies in folate, B12 and B6, and zinc nutrients can lead to an accumulation of homocysteine.
- **Broad Panel.** This includes complete blood count, glucose, serum urea, nitrogen, creatinine, calcium (assess for parathyroid issues[1510]), phosphate, iron, electrolytes, serum folate, and Vitamins B12 and D.
- **Pathogen and inflammation tests.**
  - **C-reactive protein.** C-reactive protein (CRP) is a marker of inflammation. An elevation suggests possible bacterial or viral infection.
  - **HPHPA Test.** HPHPA is a marker for the presence of Clostridia pathogens. Especially in cases of psychosis, severe depression, and autism, consider looking for elevated HPHPA. (See Clostridia difficile, p. 219 and www.GreatPlainsLaboratory.com).
  - **Autoimmune.** Psychiatric symptoms can be caused by an autoimmune dysfunction often triggered by common infections. Consider erythrocyte sedimentation rate (detects inflammation), antinuclear antibodies (present in almost all people with systemic lupus erythematosus), and serum fluorescent treponemal antibodies (diagnostic test for syphilis).
  - **Translocator proteins.** Elevated levels, a marker for brain inflammation, are associated with suicidal depression.[1466]

- **Lipid and Cholesterol Test.** Low *Cholesterol* (p. 53) is a marker of *Inflammation* and *Oxidative Stress* (p. 52) both associated with mental health issues, especially depression. Statins can adversely impact memory and cognition.[1511]
- **Cerebral spinal fluid metabolites.** A blood-brain barrier exists that inhibits the movement of certain substances from the blood to the central nervous system. Blood tests, therefore, don't necessarily give an accurate picture of the substances in the spine and brain. For more precise information, spinal fluid can be removed (a spinal tap) with a needle. A preliminary study indicates this testing may be important for treatment-resistant depression, where cerebral folate deficiency was most common imbalance discovered.[1512]

Test protocols.
- **Walsh Institute Test Protocols.** The Walsh Institute (Figure 28, p. 168) is a leader in *Nutrition Therapy* (www.WalshInstitute.org). A testing protocol overview can be found in Chapter 10 of Dr. Walsh's book *Nutrient Power*.[19]

- **Comprehensive Mental Health Panel.** Great Plains Laboratory (www.GreatPlainsLaboratory.com) offers a comprehensive set of mental health panels to consider. They can also connect you with a doctor who can order the tests and consult with you on treatment.
- **Koran Algorithm.** A baseline protocol (https://goo.gl/nBpmZK).
- **BMJ Best Practice Assessment for Psychosis.** A protocol directed toward those with psychosis. http://goo.gl/ibCU2e.
- **SpectraCell Laboratories.** www.spectracell.com.

WHAT CONSIDERATIONS SHOULD I KEEP IN MIND?

Start by finding an *Integrative Biomedical Practitioner* (p. 320) who uses comprehensive biomedical tests to help create a mental health differential diagnosis. Different combinations of tests can be run, and practitioner preferences will vary. Insurance coverage also varies. Common tests are often covered by insurance; more specialized tests may not be.

Failure to run a thorough biomedical test panel risks an important opportunity for healing. If you don't run needed tests, you face the risk of not discovering what might be a relatively straightforward path to improved mental health—keeping in mind that these test results won't automatically guarantee that an underlying disorder will be found.

Professionals and researchers in the mental health field are examining potential genetic and brain imaging solutions. Although these hold promise, they do not provide solutions today.

REAL-WORLD EXPERIENCE

Practitioner's Story 8 – Importance of Biomedical Testing
Dr. Mary Ackerley is an Integrative Physician in Tucson, Arizona, with a specialty in psychiatry. She believes that extensive biomedical tests must be run in cases of significant mental health issues, to create a quality differential diagnosis. She recognizes that this step is often not performed by psychiatrists, since medical schools historically have not focused on Biomedical Restorative Therapies and the testing that can target their use.[324]   ***Bottom Line****: To get a quality differential diagnosis, ask to have your practitioner run quality and comprehensive biomedical tests.*

Recovery Models & Tools

See the latest version of this appendix at www.OnwardMentalHealth.com (Resources).

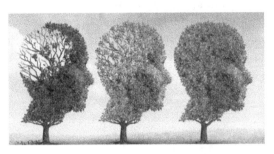

WHAT IS THE ESSENCE?

Recovery Models & Tools help us understand and take ownership of our mental health issues, which will be essential if we are to recover. Training and group interaction are part of this, as well as toolkits for goal-setting, planning, and monitoring. Recovery tools are often aligned with *recovery models*—proven wellness principles that help people regain their health.

Recovery Models & Tools emphasize the importance of *Self-Determination* (p. 87), a *Wellness Basic*. They address insufficient mental health services by encouraging people to craft and execute their own recovery plans, with guidance and a measure of independence. However, a common thread in *Recovery Models & Tools* is the need to build both a professional support system of doctors and therapists, as well as a personal support system of friends and loved-ones, so that we don't "go it alone."

Recovery is a process that requires commitment and diligence. Some tools apply to specific diagnoses; others can be used effectively by everyone, regardless of diagnosis.

Recovery Models. Recovery models are integrated frameworks for understanding and working toward recovery. They focus on the *individual/wellness* orientation, as opposed to a *doctor/illness* orientation. (See Endnote # 444 for a recovery vs. medical model discussion.)

- SAMHSA. http://goo.gl/y6S611.
- Tidal model. https://goo.gl/3g13MK.
- Mental Health Recovery Star. https://goo.gl/nH5d7u.
- Recovery Map. http://goo.gl/7ccRtd.
- Recovery Model of Mental Illness. https://goo.gl/2ISn8B.

Tools for all diagnoses.
- WRAP®. www.mentalhealthrecovery.org
- NAMI Hearts and Minds. http://www.nami.org/heartsandminds.
- Mental Health America Tools. http://goo.gl/dNKk2W.
- Wellness Self-Management. https://goo.gl/cy2isi.
- Mental Disorders Toolkit. http://goo.gl/2q92a8.
- Hafal recovery. https://goo.gl/IR5Qtt.
- BlackDog Toolkit. http://goo.gl/nHe65a.

- Here to Help Resources. https://goo.gl/5bLmB6.

Tools for specific diagnoses.
- Communication Skills and Psychosis. https://goo.gl/TvL4H9.
- University of Michigan Depression Toolkit. http://goo.gl/yMSJ6m.
- Dealing With Psychosis Toolkit. http://goo.gl/oQgJUk.
- Staying Well with Bipolar. https://goo.gl/BFUK17.
- Beating bipolar interactive course. http://www.beatingbipolar.org.
- Questions to ask your practitioners. https://goo.gl/9wvVB1.

Tools for Family Members.
- A Toolkit for Families. http://goo.gl/9G0dxF.
- ReThink Mental Illness Family training. https://goo.gl/XwsgkZ.

Mental Health Apps. These tools constantly evolve. Search the internet to evaluate current ones available. Apps can be constantly at hand, and many are based on sound clinical theory. They can be a low-cost alternative to address the shortage of therapist-based psychosocial therapies. Apps are available for:
- Cognitive Behavioral Therapy (e.g. eCBT Calm, DBT Diary Card and Skills Coach and many more)
- Post-traumatic stress disorder (e.g. PTSD Coach)
- Anxiety (e.g. Mindshift).
- Mood Tracker Apps (e.g. iMoodJournal, eMoods, T2 Mood Tracker, Optimism)
- Deep Breathing (e.g. BellyBio, Breath2Relax)
- Suicide Prevention (Operation Reach Out)
- Eating Disorders (e.g. Recovery Record)
- Substance Abuse (e.g. reSET, which is FDA approved and in initial tests has been shown to significantly improve abstinency across many substances, except opioids[1513])
- Sleep and Insomnia Apps (e.g. CBT Insomnia, Deep Sleep with Andrew Johnson, iSleepEasy)

Matrix Model. The Matrix Model is a sixteen-week outpatient treatment approach for people struggling with addictions, who want to abstain. The approach combines education (for individuals and family members), support groups, individual counseling, and urine and breath testing. A trained therapist functions as a teacher and coach whose approach is realistic and direct but not confrontational. The Matrix Model fosters self-esteem, dignity, and self-worth. The Substance Abuse and Mental Health Services Administration (SAMHSA) considers this a valuable evidence-based approach.[1514]

One study found patients treated with the Matrix Model reduced drug and alcohol use demonstrably, while improving psychological indicators.[1515] Another study found that 70% of people taking Matrix did not relapse, as compared to between 40% and 60% using other methods.[1516] In a third study, people given

Matrix treatment attended more clinical sessions, stayed in treatment longer, provided more clean urine samples, and had longer periods of abstinence— although, unfortunately, these improvements were not maintained post-treatment.[1517]

Wellness Recovery Action Plan™ (WRAP®). An evidence-based self-management program for all diagnoses, the Wellness Recovery Action Plan™ is designed to *monitor* uncomfortable feelings and behaviors, follow *planned responses*, and *reduce, modify, or eliminate* the unwanted feelings. It uses a customized "Wellness Toolbox" that offers response plans for a patient's supporters when the patients are unable to help themselves. WRAP® is the most widely used self-management therapy; over 1,500 leaders have been trained. There is a cost associated with Wrap® materials. Participants have "significant improvements in symptoms and many psychosocial outcome areas associated with recovery."[1518]

WHAT EVIDENCE SHOWS THIS IS EFFECTIVE?

Little research exists on self-management therapy, and the evidence supporting it when dealing with psychosis is inconclusive.[1519] However, many individuals claim success with self-management.

WHAT CONSIDERATIONS SHOULD I KEEP IN MIND?

The Substance Abuse & Mental Health Services Administration (SAMHSA) position is clear: *Self-determination and self-direction are the foundations for [mental health] recovery.* Self-management therapies and recovery models emphasize self-determination and self-empowerment, but we should avoid "going it alone." If you choose to use these programs, consider self-management programs that 1) engage with healthcare professionals and peers, 2) respect the value and limits of psychotropic drugs, 3) encourage *Wellness Basics*, and 4) are chosen by the person seeking recovery.

Self-management approaches are only as valuable as our commitment to use them. We must start with a small, achievable goal, then grow it as we become successful. We should attend *support groups* (p. 131). *Psychoeducation* (p. 126) offers incentives to stay on track with our self-management plan.

Onward Mental Health maintains a variety of integrative mental health resources available for free download. See *www.OnwardMentalHealth.com* → *Resources* for the latest versions.

WHAT ARE ADDITIONAL RESOURCES?

- Matrix Model. www.matrixinstitute.org.
- See Additional Resources, p. 341.

Hospital, Residential & Community Care

See the latest version of this appendix at www.OnwardMentalHealth.com (Resources).

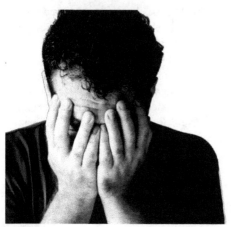

WHAT IS THE ESSENCE?

Hospital, residential, and community care are options when mental health issues become too severe to be managed by an individual and loved ones. These therapies rely heavily on psychotropics that have limited effectiveness and many risks. It may involve the agonizing choice of whether to use forced treatment.

If you or someone you love is facing a psychiatric crisis, start by calling 911, especially if the individual is either a danger to themselves or others. Safety and stabilization are the first goals. Once stabilization occurs, other therapies can be introduced.

Hospitalization. Hospitalization is generally recommended when a person in mental distress becomes a danger to themselves or others. Hospitalization targets stabilization, nearly always with psychotropic drugs; often the patient will be discharged within two weeks. Stabilization is far from wellness. A chronic shortage of hospital psychiatric beds creates pressure to release patients quickly or send patients to hospitals outside their area. Open-ward policies are noted for fewer coercive measures and medications, and less seclusion, as compared to closed wards.[1520]

Peer Respites. Peer respites (also known as crisis residential programs or crisis respites) are supportive peer-run home-like settings for psychiatric crisis. They can be an alternative to hospitalization. See *Peer Respites* (p. 132).

Residential Recovery. Residential centers are supportive living environments for those with mental health issues. Some are holistic healing communities, in which the residents learn new coping skills, independent living skills, and ways for personal fulfillment.

Assertive Community Treatment (ACT). ACT (a.k.a. Involuntary Outpatient Treatment and Assisted Outpatient Treatment) is a treatment model for people with serious mental health issues; teams consist of peer support specialists, psychiatrists, substance abuse counselors, and others. Because ACT often uses involuntary drug therapy, the model has provoked controversy and polarizing ethical dilemmas[1521] relating to how a patient's right of self-determination[1522] weighs against his/her best interests as determined by others.

Advance statement/directive. Consider writing a psychiatric advance statement or directive, a document that outlines your preferences for intervention should you become unable to communicate as result of a crisis or incapacity.

WHAT EVIDENCE SHOWS THIS IS EFFECTIVE?

Few studies are available yet to validate the effectiveness of residential therapy for adults.

Although some studies support ACT,[1523] the Cochrane Collaborative concludes that it doesn't appear to reduce health service use or improve patients' social functioning.[1524] An eight-state Rand study found no evidence that a court order is necessary for drug compliance and good outcomes.[1525] A UK study[1526] found that ACT did not significantly reduce hospital readmission rates to justify the curtailment of patients' personal liberty – a finding supported by a later meta-analysis of 5,775 people.[1527] (See endnote #100.)

WHAT CONSIDERATIONS SHOULD I KEEP IN MIND?

It is critically important for individuals or family members to give care providers a comprehensive documented medical history, especially with a record of drugs used and reactions to them. This helps avoid dead ends already tried.

Non-drug approaches are rarely considered during crisis hospitalization, so gaining access to them is nearly always an assertive effort by individuals and loved-ones that occurs after discharge.

Patients typically enter residential treatment in crisis or near-crisis situations when their needs are too severe to be managed with outpatient treatment, but not severe enough to require inpatient treatment.[1528] Residential facilities often offer psychotherapy, drug and alcohol counseling, and social skills training. If you consider a residential treatment center, ask about the history of its patients' outcomes, visit with existing patients, and do an extensive on-site evaluation. *Residential Recovery Therapy* is often very expensive.

Most important, we must look at forced treatment in raw human terms: it is an extreme choice that strips away self-determination – the basic human right so vital to recovery. It often forces on people a myriad of debilitating and life-numbing side effects. Choices here can be extremely difficult. Mightily seek effective non-coercive care, leveraging proven non-drug approaches.

WHAT ARE ADDITIONAL RESOURCES?

- Overview of crisis alternatives. https://goo.gl/pMuXXF.
- Peer respites. www.peerrespite.net, http://goo.gl/P5RcM.
- Residential facilities. www.artausa.org.
- ACT. PsychRights www.psychrights.org, SAMHSA http://goo.gl/VRwfSU.
- Advance Directives. www.nrc-pad.org, http://goo.gl/dw2oYQ.

Addiction Co-Therapy

See the latest version of this appendix at www.OnwardMentalHealth.com (Resources).

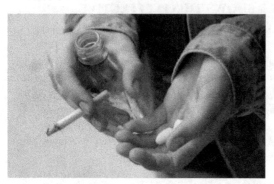

WHAT IS THE ESSENCE?

Addiction Co-therapy (dual diagnosis) helps people with simultaneously occurring mental health and substance abuse issues recover from both disorders.

About 29% of individuals with mental disorders turn to substance abuse, often as a form of self-medication; 50% of addicts have severe mental illness. Of the nearly 9 million Americans with a psychiatric and substance-abuse disorder, only 7 percent are treated for both conditions.

A major problem for those with a dual diagnosis is that parallel but separate treatment systems exist for the two disorders, so care is often fragmented and ineffective. *It is nearly impossible to solve one issue without addressing the other, so integrated treatment is vital.* Research indicates that dual-diagnosis situations require simultaneous treatment for both issues.[1529]

WHAT CAN YOU DO?

Find stable housing. Adequate and safe housing is a cornerstone for those with a dual diagnosis.[1530] (See *Housing & Security*, p. 57, for alternatives.)

Form empathetic trusting relationships. Strong, supportive, healthy relationships are vital and must be established and maintained. Trusting relationships should be a characteristic of the full treatment team.

Take a long-term staged approach. Most approaches include a four-step process. For example, stabilization → engagement/motivation → relapse prevention → rehabilitation. Different goals and different services are needed at each stage.

Assertive outreach. It is vital that patients, supporters, and practitioners stay close, usually through a combination of *intensive case management* and meetings in the client's residence. Community Mental Health Organization can often help.

Engage peer support. Clinical trials endorse dual-diagnosis peer groups as an essential component to recovery.[1531] The peer groups vary in focus, ranging from educational to behavioral skill-building to the Alcoholics Anonymous/ Narcotics Anonymous organizations.

Use Motivational Interviewing (MI). Most people with a dual diagnosis aren't ready for abstinence-oriented treatment. Many lack motivation to manage their mental health issues and achieve new goals. Motivational Interviewing (p. 126) works on patients' motivation to change substance use or other problem behaviors, by engaging them in a supportive conversation about the patients' history, stressors, and related life events. A promising treatment for patients with dual diagnosis,[1532] MI has proven as effective in reducing substance use as more extensive treatments.[1533]

Social Support and Counseling. This can include approaches to modify unhelpful thoughts and emotions with *Cognitive Behavioral Training* (p 117) or *Dialectic Behavioral Training* (p. 120). *Exposure Therapies* (p. 151) can also address trauma. The recovery path must be unique to the individual.

Nutrient Therapy. [19] Although nutrient therapy is broadly helpful in mental health recovery, typically no progress can be made with nutrient therapy when people abuse alcohol, cocaine, heroin, and other street drugs until the abusive behavior has stopped for at least six weeks. The exception to this is marijuana abuse, where progress may be made while the abuse continues.

- For *cocaine abuse*. Research suggests that *N-acetylcysteine* (p. 184) can reduce cocaine cravings.
- For *alcohol abuse*. Low zinc levels have been observed in 30% to 50% of alcoholics. Alcohol decreases the absorption of zinc and increases loss of zinc in urine.[1534]

Check cholesterol levels. Case studies have shown that low cholesterol levels are associated with marijuana craving. When cholesterol levels are brought back into range, the cravings greatly diminish.[984(a)]

Smoking cessation. There are a number of considerations:

- **Benefits.** When smoking stops, health improves and individuals reduce their risk of heart and lung diseases, many cancers, and pregnancy complications. The challenge is withdrawal, which can lead to fatigue, depression, insomnia, headaches, and nicotine craving.
- **Vitamin/Mineral deficiencies.** Smoking causes nutrient deficiencies, including calcium (causing lower bone density[1535]), Vitamin C (increasing the risk of gum disease), and Vitamin E (an important antioxidant that helps avoid infections and emphysema). Smoking also causes deficiencies in fatty acids, Vitamin B12, and Vitamin D, all associated with reduced mental health. Smokers often have a severe zinc deficiency, which compromises the immune system,[1536] so they should consider a comprehensive multivitamin and mineral formula essential to their health.[778] A high-carbohydrate diet rich in fruits and vegetables and supplemented with L-tryptophan can substantially help smokers succeed in quitting. However, when those who have recently quit use weight-loss diets, relapses are frequent.[1537]
- **Nicotine Replacement Therapy (NRT).** Chewing gum, patches, and sprays increase the chances of success in eliminating smoking by between 50% and 70%.[1538] Strong evidence shows that using a longer-acting form (patch) with

a shorter-acting form (lozenge) is more effective than using either alone, and the combination is safe.[1539]

- **Psychosocial approaches.** The most important psychosocial intervention is to follow a stop-smoking plan that offers basic information about how to quit, avoid relapse, solve problems, and develop coping skills. Group therapy significantly improves the success rate, when compared to self-help material.[1540] Studies show that a single hypnotherapy session significantly increased abstinence rates, and they were maintained at a 48-week follow-up,[1541] while three sessions of intensive hypnotherapy resulted in an 81% abstinence rate (which dropped to 48% after one year).[1542]

- **Calm Awareness Techniques.** Stress increases the urge to smoke, so minimizing stress as much as possible is critical. *Mindfulness-Based Stress Reduction* (p. 77) is one technique that, in one study, resulted in a 56% abstinence rate.[1543] *Guided Imagery* (p. 79) has been used successfully in the fight to stop smoking;[1544] one study reported a success rate of 67%.[1545]

- **Symptom Relief Techniques.** Symptom relief techniques help. An abstinence rate of 31% is achieved with *Acupuncture*[1546] (p. 159). *Aromatherapy* (p. 241) and *Massage* (p. 242) are helpful in reducing nicotine cravings by reducing anxiety.

- **It takes a village.** A good way to quit is to encourage those around you to quit. The odds improve dramatically[1547] if someone quits with a spouse (67%), friend (36%), co-worker (34%), or sibling (25%).

WHAT CONSIDERATIONS SHOULD I KEEP IN MIND?

Consider relapse prevention psychotherapy and *Mindfulness-Based Sobriety* (p. 122) to minimize cravings. See *Substance Abuse Therapies* (p. 305).

WHAT ARE ADDITIONAL RESOURCES?

- Integrated treatment for co-occurring disorders. http://goo.gl/VKBT9m.
- Mindfulness-Based Relapse Prevention. www.mindfulrp.com.
- NAMI dual diagnosis fact sheet. http://goo.gl/j6Zobl.
- Co-occurring Disorders. SAMHSA Tip 42. http://goo.gl/AH6MRh.
- Center for Science in the Public Interest. www.cspinet.org.
- Comprehensive Service Development. http://users.erols.com/ksciacca.
- How to Change Your Drinking, a Harm Reduction Guide to Alcohol, https://goo.gl/C6cJpm.

Veterans and Mental Health

See the latest version of this appendix at www.OnwardMentalHealth.com (Resources).

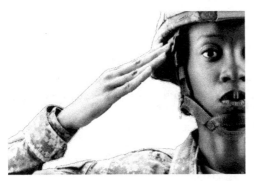

WHAT IS THE ESSENCE?

Veterans and soldiers in combat zones struggle with mental health issues. More than 100,000 combat veterans have sought help for mental illness since the war in Afghanistan started in 2001. Almost one-half of those suffered with post-traumatic stress disorder (PTSD). Mental health cases of PTSD, drug and alcohol dependency, and depression grew by 58%, to 100,580 cases, between 2006 and 2007.[1548] Over 31% of all of America's veterans have a mental health diagnosis, with the youngest group of veterans (aged 18 to 24 years) at the greatest risk.[1549]

Veterans comprise about one-third of America's homeless population. The clear majority of homeless veterans are single; most come from poor, disadvantaged communities; 45% live with a mental illness; and half have substance abuse problems. Of the homeless population of veterans, 47% served during the Vietnam era, and 56% are African American or Latino. The suicide rate for veterans is double that for the general population.[1550]

WHAT SUPPORT IS AVAILABLE TO VETERANS?

The *U.S. Department of Veterans Affairs* (VA) is dedicated to the needs of veterans. The *Veterans Health Administration* has medical centers, vet centers, and outpatient clinics offering primary and specialized care. Once veterans establish eligibility, they qualify for inpatient and outpatient care for physical and mental health needs. Services are available for anxiety, bipolar, depression, military sexual abuse, PTSD, schizophrenia, substance abuse, and suicide prevention. Treatment generally covers psychotropics and psychosocial therapies. The VA offers self-directed recovery therapies. To assist veterans in crises, emergency service is available around the clock.

Post-traumatic stress disorder. This is a common and potentially debilitating issue returning veterans face. Treatments include:

- **Mind-Body Therapies.** Mission Reconnect is a self-directed program of mind-body therapies for veterans and their partners that has been shown effective in improving physical, mental (including PTSD and depression) and relationship health.[1551]

- **Psychosocial Therapies.** *Cognitive Behavioral Therapy* (CBT, p. 117), *Cognitive Processing Therapy* (a form of CBT for trauma), and *Prolonged Exposure Therapy* (an *Exposure and Response Prevention Therapy*, p. 151) are offered. In addition, *Emotional Freedom Technique* (p. 161) is taught at some VA facilities;[1552] many case studies testify to its success.
- **Residential Treatment.** An intensive, specialized treatment for PTSD takes place within a structured 24:7 care setting.
- **Service animals for PTSD.** Veterans using dogs to help for PTSD symptoms, shows anecdotal success.[1553] Dogs can tell if a person's mood is starting to escalate into a panic attack.[1554] Unfortunately, few service dogs are available, since each costs approximately $20,000 after training, which requires between 500 and 1,500 hours. (See *Animal Therapy,* p. 138, *Equine-Assisted Therapy,* and Case Study 43, p. 140.)
- **Eye Movement Desensitization and Reprocessing** (p. 152) is under investigation as a possible psychosocial therapy for veterans.

Therapies for other diagnoses. Depending on the diagnosis, the VA may also offer *Acceptance and Commitment Therapy* (p. 121) and *Interpersonal Psychotherapy* (p. 132).

WHAT CONSIDERATIONS SHOULD I KEEP IN MIND?

To get started, contact your local VA to learn about available services. Also see the links below for the *Guide to VA Mental Health Services for Veterans & Families* (from the VA) and The *Disability Benefits for Wounded Warriors* (from the U.S. Social Security Administration).

It is important for veterans to consider non-drug treatments since one study found that vets with PTSD who took either antidepressants or antipsychotics had a significantly greater risk of later developing dementia than those who did not take these drugs.[1555]

In 2010, the VA announced new regulations, making it easier for veterans to prove their PTSD claims. Previously, to be covered, PTSD had to result from hostile military activity. For specific case studies of veterans with mental health issues, see "Veterans, Case Studies" in the index.

WHAT ARE ADDITIONAL RESOURCES?

- U.S. Department of Veterans Administration (VA) Mental Health. www.mentalhealth.va.gov.
- Guide to VA Mental Health Services. http://goo.gl/Jxb5gs.
- Disability Benefits for Wounded Warriors. https://goo.gl/ZsvVmz.
- Peace of Mind for Veterans. www.ProjectWelcomeHomeTroops.org.
- Service Dogs. www.servicedogcentral.org, www.psychdogpartners.org.

Glossary

ABIM – American Board of Internal Medicine (ABIM), which works to advance medical professionalism.

ADHD - Attention-deficit hyperactivity disorder (ADHD) is a chronic condition often diagnosed in childhood. It may include hyperactivity, impulsive behavior, and difficulty sustaining attention

Affective disorders – A set of psychiatric diagnoses, also called mood disorders. The main types of affective disorders are depression, bipolar disorder, and anxiety disorder.

APA – American Psychiatric Association or American Psychological Association. (Two different organizations)

Assisted Outpatient Treatment (AOT) – Court-ordered mental health treatment very often mandating psychotropic use. AOTs remain controversial, since they may force psychotropic drugs on individuals. See endnote # 100.

Ayurvedic – A contemporary and centuries-old medical system in India.

Biochemical Individuality – The concept that each person's body and brain have a different chemical profile and that optimum health requires a unique response based on that individual chemical profile.

Bipolar disorder - Formerly called manic depression, this mental health diagnosis brings severe high and low moods and changes in sleep, energy, thinking, and behavior.

CAM – Complementary and Alternative Medicine.

CBT – Cognitive Behavioral Therapy (p. 117) – A major category of psychosocial therapy that addresses thoughts, emotions and actions.

Clinical Laboratory Improvement Amendments (CLIA) – The Centers for Medicare & Medicaid Services approach for regulating and ensuring quality in all lab testing (except research) performed on humans in the United States.

Dopamine – One of many types of neurotransmitters in the brain essential to the central nervous system. Often psychotropic drugs target dopamine to help control symptoms of mental health issues.

DSM-5 – *Diagnostic and Statistical Manual* (DSM), currently at version 5. This U.S. practitioners' guide describes current valid mental health diagnoses and their associated symptoms. There is significant controversy *1556* over the validity and usefulness of the DSM.

Differential Diagnosis – The data gathering, testing, and evaluation used to determine a patient's specific disorder or disease.

Dual Diagnosis – A mental health diagnosis plus substance/alcohol abuse.

Epigenetic – Related to nongenetic factors not related to DNA, but to the ways genes are expressed.

Extrapyramidal Symptoms – Drug-induced movement disorders that may be irreversible, including dystonia, akathisia, Parkinsonism, and others.

EPA – United States Environmental Protection Agency

FDA – United States Food and Drug Administration, responsible for all drug approvals.

Functional Medicine – An approach to health that focuses on understanding and addressing underlying issues, not just symptoms.

GABA – Gamma-aminobutyric acid, an amino acid that serves as a vital brain neurotransmitter.

Gluten – A protein complex found in wheat, barley, rye, and triticale.

GP – General Practitioner, a medical doctor who is often a primary care physician.

HIPPA – Health Insurance Portability and Accountability Act, a United States law that sets privacy standards to safeguard patients' medical records and information available to healthcare providers.

HUD – United States Department of Housing and Urban Development.

HVN – Hearing Voices Network. (p. 150)

Iatrogenic – an unfavorable medical condition *caused by* medical intervention.

ICD-10 – The manual for the classification of Mental and Behavioral Disorders created by the World Health Organization and used widely in Europe. It is similar to the DSM (see above) used in the United States.

Longitudinal (or horizontal) study – A study that follows a population forward over time, evaluating the effects of variables on a process. If individuals are followed, it is termed a longitudinal cohort study.

MAOI - Monoamine oxidase inhibitors, an early class of antidepressants.

Meta-analysis – Statistical method contrasting and combining results from different studies to find patterns. Findings from these analyses are often considered to have a higher proof of evidence than individual studies.

Monotherapy – One therapy only is used, most typically one psychotropic.

Morbidity – A diseased state or condition. The incidence rate of a disease.

NAMI – National Alliance on Mental Illness, the largest U.S. grass-roots mental health organization.

Narcolepsy - Extreme tendency to fall asleep whenever in relaxing surroundings.

Naturopath – A primary healthcare professional who emphasizes preventive and restorative health and the individuals' self-healing processes, which includes modern and traditional scientific methods and can be used with psychiatric drugs.

Negative Symptoms – Behaviors or experiences that are normally present in the general population but are absent or diminished in a person with a mental health diagnosis. For instance, reduced social interaction and the lack of visible emotion are negative symptoms of schizophrenia. (See *Positive Symptoms*, below.)

Neuroleptic – A drug that depresses nerve functions; a major tranquilizer.

Neurotransmitter – A vital mechanism of the brain, this chemical substance is released at the end of a nerve fiber by the arrival of a nerve impulse; it diffuses across the synapse or junction.

NIMH – National Institute of Mental Health. A U.S. agency seeking the prevention and cure of mental health issues.

Norepinephrine - A hormone that is released by the adrenal medulla and by the sympathetic nerves; it functions as a neurotransmitter and is also used as a drug to raise blood pressure.

Nutraceuticals – Supplements found safe enough by the United States Food and Drug Administration for over-the-counter sales.

OCD – Obsessive compulsive disorder, characterized by unreasonable thoughts and fears (obsessions) that lead to repetitive behaviors (compulsions).

Open Label Trial - A clinical trial in which both the researchers and participants know which treatment is being administered. The "opposite" of double-blinded (see RDB / RDBPC /RPC, below).

Oppositional Defiant Disorder – A pattern of disobedient, hostile, and defiant behavior toward authority figures.

Orthomolecular Psychiatry – A discipline that conducts tests to detect influencers or root causes of mental health issues, which might be addressed with vitamins, supplements, and other approaches.

OTC – Over the counter. Therapies, supplements, and medicines that can be acquired without a prescription.

PANDAS – Pediatric Autoimmune Neuropsychiatric Disorders, conditions that seem to be associated with the strep virus. Sometimes causes OCD-like symptoms.

Positive Symptoms – behaviors or experiences that are present in those with a mental health diagnosis, but typically absent in general population. For instance, delusions and hallucinations are positive symptoms of schizophrenia. (See *Negative Symptoms*, above.)

Psychosis – A mental disorder that includes a distorted or non-existent sense of objective reality.

Psychotropics – Prescription drugs that affect the central nervous system and brain. They are differentiated from Herbs (plant-based remedies), Nutrients (essential body substances), and illegal substances (heroin, ecstasy, etc.). All four can have psychoactive properties.

PTSD – Post-traumatic stress disorder, a mental condition triggered by a terrifying event. Symptoms may include flashbacks, nightmares, severe anxiety, and uncontrollable thoughts about the event.

Pyrrole – An organic compound involved in the synthesis of the primary constituent of hemoglobin. Pyrrole Disorder is associated with elevated pyrroles in urine and severe deficiencies of zinc and Vitamin B-6.

Quantitative Electroencephalography (qEEG) – Sometimes called a "brain map", a qEEG is a report of real-time electrical brain activity. It differs from a traditional EEG in that it performs extensive computerized statistical analyses on the collected raw EEG data.

RCT / RDBT / RDBPCT / RPCT – A type of clinical trial. **R** = *randomized* (to ensure statistical accuracy by identifying a test group and control group that are as similar as possible), **P** = placebo (a pill/therapy that will have no effect), **DB** = double-blind (neither caregiver nor patient knows if they are using therapy or placebo), **C** = controlled (using a control group for comparison to a trial group), **T** = Trial. **RCT** = Randomized Controlled

Trial, considered the "gold standard," although they have flaws.[1557] (See "Gold Standard" discussion, p.42.)

Recovery – See *What is Recovery?* (p. 31).

Refractory – Cases resistant to treatment, commonly psychotropic drug treatment.

Remission – People are said to be in remission from a psychiatric disorder if their symptoms have decreased to a "significant" degree. In many trials, the measure is somewhat arbitrary, between a 50% and 60% reduction (as measured on a standardized instrument) or a reduction to a specific level of symptoms.

SAD – Seasonal Affective Disorder. See below.

SAM-e – S-adenosyl-methionine, a naturally occurring compound important to the immune system and involved in the maintenance of cell membranes and production and breakdown of neurotransmitters.

SAMHSA – Substance Abuse & Mental Health Services Administration, a U.S. agency that promotes behavioral health.

Schizophrenia – A group of disorders marked by psychosis (see above) with impaired thinking, emotions, and/or behaviors. Schizophrenic patients are typically unable to filter sensory stimuli and may have enhanced perceptions of sounds, colors, and other features of their environment.

Seasonal Affective Disorder (SAD) - A type of depression or mood disorder related to changes in seasons, typically either winter or summer. SAD begins and ends at about the same time every year.

SNRI – Serotonin Norepinephrine Re-uptake Inhibitor, a class of antidepressant drugs that suppresses the re-uptake of both serotonin and norepinephrine. SNRIs are newer than SSRIs, and may be safer than SSRIs.

SSRI – Selective Serotonin Re-uptake Inhibitor, a family of antidepressants that suppresses the re-uptake of serotonin.

TCM – Traditional Chinese Medicine.

WHO – World Health Organization.

Additional Resources

See the latest version of this appendix at www.OnwardMentalHealth.com (Resources).

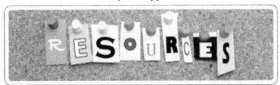

Onward Mental Health maintains a variety of integrative mental health resources available for free download including a comprehensive list of Integrative Mental Health Organizations. See *www.OnwardMentalHealth.com (Resources)* for the latest versions. Additionally, consider the resources below.

Alternative Psychiatric Treatments and Recovery Resources

- Complementary and Alternative Medicine for Mental Health, MH America, http://goo.gl/gFXz3w.
- Alternative Treatments for Extrapyramidal Symptoms, Schizophrenia, Bipolar, https://goo.gl/8VJe7X.
- Codex Alternus: Depression and Anxiety Spectrum alternative treatments, http://goo.gl/nfxVSa.
- Evidence-based Psychological Interventions in the Treatment of Mental Illness, https://goo.gl/5XS0EE.
- Clinical Naturopathy, An evidence-based guide to practice, Jerome Sarris. http://goo.gl/V6SeiJ.
- Integrative Medicine, University of Wisconsin. http://goo.gl/UdDS6E.
- Integrative Medicine for Mental Health white paper https://goo.gl/J7BZJj.
- Mad in America. www.MadInAmerica.com.
- Madness Radio www.madnessradio.net.
- Mental Health Law. See endnote #100.

Psychotropic Drug Safety and Withdrawal Resources

- Psychiatric Drug Withdrawal. Mad in America Continuing Education. https://goo.gl/DLesfj
- Early Psychosis Intervention Program Directory. https://goo.gl/wK8IEN.
- Harm Reduction Guide to Coming Off Psychiatric Drugs, Icarus Project, http://theicarusproject.net/resources/publications.
- MIND, Making Sense of Coming off Psychiatric Drugs, http://bit.ly/yPjusy.
- Addressing Non-Adherence to Antipsychotic Medication: a Harm-Reduction Approach. http://bit.ly/wbUA6A.
- Rxisk Guides for psychiatric drug withdrawal. www.rxisk.org.
- Psychiatric Drug Withdrawal: Guide for Prescribers, Therapists, Patients, and their Families, Peter Breggin.

- Over Dose, Dr. Jay Cohen, 2004. If psychotropics are used, he advocates "Start Low. Go Slow" approach.
- Psychiatric drugs and common factors: an evaluation of risks and benefits, J. Sparks, https://goo.gl/a4kpng.
- Benzodiazepine addiction, withdrawal and recovery. www.benzo.org.uk.
- Benzodiazepine Information Coalition. www.benzoinfo.com.
- Benzo support community. www.BenzoBuddies.org.
- Benzo withdrawal community. www.BenzoWithdrawalHelp.com.

Psychosis, Schizophrenia and Voices
- Hearing Voices Network, http://goo.gl/GlbkqY.
- Onward Mental Health Psychosis Resources. https://goo.gl/XwsgkZ.
- Better Sleep for Voice Hearers, http://goo.gl/HBOf3i.
- Schizophrenia Commission. 2012 report http://goo.gl/wdSjRQ, and executive summary http://goo.gl/4M0JXi.
- Ron Unger Psychosis tools. www.recoveryfromschizophrenia.org.
- Recent Advances in Understanding Mental Illness and Psychotic Experiences, http://bit.ly/fC7BGf.
- Nutrition for Schizophrenia. Overview https://goo.gl/7klKaK.
- Niacin Trials http://goo.gl/ka8sLs.
- Voices. Hearing Voices, Talking with Voices, www.rufusmay.com.
- Living with Voices, 50 Stories of Recovery, http://goo.gl/4gz653.
- Understanding Psychosis and Schizophrenia, British Psychological Society, https://goo.gl/GjoA1e.
- Dealing With Psychosis Toolkit. http://goo.gl/oQgJUk.
- Mind-Body Tools for Psychosis. https://goo.gl/Oj5Xe4.
- Living with Schizophrenia. www.LivingWithSchizophreniaUK.org.

Other tools.
- A Guide to Cooperative Communication Skills, http://goo.gl/H374Nw.
- See resources listed at the end of each therapy section of this book.
- National Mental Health Consumers' Self-Help Clearinghouse. http://goo.gl/MXoDwJ.
- WRAP. www.copelandcenter.com, www.wrapandrecoverybooks.com.

Reflections

Look Deeper

At times my vision is shallow and short-sighted as I see my loved-one
cope with the challenges we label mental illness.

At times through shallow eyes I see a *future stunted,* my loved-one's possibilities
not fully realized.
But then I look deeper.
There I see unnecessary expectations created by me, held by me, and fully
release-able by me.
There I see good in today's actualities, somewhat hidden perhaps,
but free of the prejudgment of my favored possibilities.

At times through shallow eyes I see *pain unrelenting* in the chaos of the
unexpected and unwanted.
But then I look deeper.
There I see and coalesce my strength, knowing my loved-one manages pain
and difficulties much more acute than my own.
There I see comfort in controlling what I can control, influencing what I can
influence. Knowing that can be enough.
There I see a stream of moments: each an opportunity to find contentment
in loving, even if those be the odd loves of allowing the one I cherish to
painfully fall or keeping myself at a painful distance from the one I long to
hold near.

At times through shallow eyes I see *guilt deserved* for the mistakes I made
that may have contributed to my loved-one's pain.
But then I look deeper.
There I see the natural messiness of life, where mistakes will invariably be
made.
There I see my ability to forgive myself for nothing more than garden-variety
human frailty.
There I see my resolve to do the best I know how to do now, regardless of
what has happened in the past.

At times through shallow eyes I see my loved-one as *irreparably broken.*
But then I look deeper.
There I see my loved-one whole and intact, worthy and good, sharing in my
desire for wellness.
There I see a hope in a therapy not yet tried, in a kind word not yet spoken, in
an hour not yet arrived.
There I see a beauty, not broken, not diminished, not missing, but shrouded in
a scrim of pain.

We can work together to pierce this scrim

if and only if we recognize the stunning value of what lies beneath it.

I choose to look deeper.
I choose to help my loved-one and others similarly struggling.
I choose to help, not to compensate for their weakness, but to supplement their strengths.
I choose to help, not to conform them to my ideas of recovery,
    but to liberate them to the greatest vision of wellness they can attain.
I choose to help, not because I must, but because I can.

I choose to look deeper because I choose to recognize the human treasure trove at stake.
I ask, "What do you choose?"

> --- *Craig Wagner*

Recommitment

Recommit to the goals
That you now know are true.
They provide grounding and
    direction,
And form a unique path for you.

Find joy in the small steps,
And in patience abide,
For that thousand-mile journey,
Starts with one confident stride.

Then lay aside goals,
And with great passion infuse
The doing that's required,
To gain the ends you choose.

Find joy in the process,
And the rhythms of action,
For to will yourself onward
Brings its own satisfaction.

Then lay aside passion,
And with great discernment
    embrace,
The fruits of the moment,
Whatever their race.

Find joy in that moment,
For where else can it be?
Bind joy to that moment,
By living mindfully.

So dwell on these three,
Let them commingle inside,
Aligning the vector of their
strength,
With your confident stride.

For...
The goal is the vision,
The doing is the muse,
The being in nowness
Causes the circle to fuse.

> --- *Craig Wagner*

Index

B

C

D

E

H

I

Q

R

T

U

V

References

See www.NCBI.NLM.NIH.gov/Pubmed to find studies with PMID (overview) and PMCID (full detail) numbers. "http://goo.gl..." links are case sensitive.

[1] Breggin P, Today's Greatest Mental Health Need: Psychiatric Drug Withdrawal Programs, Huffington Post, 2012, http://goo.gl/1t5IVd.

[2] Van Dahlen B, Our Shared Mission…to End Suicide, Time Magazine, 2013, http://goo.gl/VXZsQe.

[3] Cassani M, We need a smorgasbord of mental health options, Beyond Meds - Alternatives to Psychiatry, , http://goo.gl/5ZXoSk.

[4] Andrew G, Editorial: Better Options for Mental Health Treatment are Needed, 2014, http://goo.gl/fFKY2x.

[5] Bielavitz S, Effective Mental Health Consumer Education: A Preliminary Exploration, J Behav Health SR 2011, PMID: PMC3071653.

[6] **Note**: SAMHSA labels a practice "evidence-based" if a single unrandomized study shows positive results and is documented in a report (SAMHSA, SAMHSA's National Registry of Evidence-based Programs and Practices, www.nrepp.samhsa.gov). Although this definition is clear, it sacrifices signicant nuance. It is best to consider strength of evidence across a spectrum from very strong to very weak.

[7] Frese, FJ et. al, Integrating evidence-based practices and the recovery model, Psych Svcs, 2001, PMID: 11684741.

[8] Cochrane Collaboration, www.cochrane.org.

[9] American Psychological Assoc, Website on Research-Supported Psychological Treatments, http://goo.gl/EzysO2.

[10] Canadian Psychological Assoc, The Efficacy and Effectiveness of Psychological Treatments, 2013, http://goo.gl/ysJzMf.

[11] British Psychological Society Centre for Outcomes Research and Effectiveness, Treatment Choice in Psychological Therapies and Counselling, 2018, https://goo.gl/DtkX7m.

[12] Australian Psychological Association, Evidence-based Psychological Interventions in the Treatment of Mental Disorders: A Literature Review Fourth Edition, 2010, https://goo.gl/oSCaz5.

[13] World Health Organization, mhGAP Evidence Resource Centre, http://goo.gl/nveA3z.

[14] American Psychiatric Association, American Psychiatric Association Practice Guidelines, http://goo.gl/y4sgzy.

[15] Brown R et al, How to Use Herbs, Nutrients and Yoga in Mental Health Care, WW Norton & Co, 2009, http://goo.gl/cWlG0g.

[16] Lake J MD and Spiegel D MD, Complementary and Alternative Treatments in Mental Health Care, American Psychiatric Publishing, 2007, http://goo.gl/viTvLs.

[17] Lake J, Textbook of Integrative Mental Health Care, Thieme Medical Publishers, 2007.

[18] Lake J, Book series "The Integrative Mental Health Solution", 2015, Includes: a) Dementia and mild cognitive impairment, b) Alcohol and Drug Abuse, c) Psychosis, d) Insomnia, e) Post-traumatic Stress Distorder (PTSD), f) Anxiety, g) Bipolar disorder and h) Depression.

[19] Walsh W, Nutrient Power Heal Your Biochemistry and Heal your Brain, Skyhorse Publishing, 2014, http://goo.gl/DxolvQ.

[20] Stradford D et al, Complementary and Alternative Medicine Treatments in Psychiatry, 2012, http://goo.gl/sC856.

[21] Sarris J, Herbal medicine for depression, anxiety and insomnia: A review of psychopharmacology and clinical evidence, European Neuropsychopharmacology , 2011. PMID: 21601431, http://goo.gl/v2CSm4.

[22] Zessin D, Codex Alternus : Treatment of Schizophrenia, BipolarDisorder and Drug-induced Side Effects, 2015, www.alternativementalhealth.com.

[23] Zessin D, Codex Alternus: Alternative Treatments for Depression and Anxiety - A Comprehensive Review of Scientific Studies Since 1950, 2014.

[24] Mental Health America, Complementary & Alternative Medicine for Mental Health, 2013, http://goo.gl/fTQIAo.

[25] Dixon L, The 2009 Schizophrenia PORT Psychosocial Treatment Recommendations and Summary Statements, Schizophrenia Bulletin, 2010, http://goo.gl/Jf6vKw.

[26] Lake J, Integrative Treatment of Bipolar Disorder: A Review of the Evidence and Recommendations, Psych Times, 2013, http://goo.gl/7IGU7U.

[27] Van Etten M, Comparative Efficacy of Treatments for Post-traumatic Stress Disorder: A Meta-Analysis, Clinl Psychology and Psychoth, 1998, http://goo.gl/QSs5Gx.

[28] Pūras D, United Nations General Assembly, Report of the Special Rapporteur on the right of everyone to the enjoyment of the highest attainable standard of physical and mental health, 2017, https://goo.gl/R5LbPJ.

[29] Bellack A et al, Scientific and Consumer Models of Recovery in Schizophrenia: Concordance, Contrasts, and Implications, Schiz Bulletin, 2006, PMID: 16461575, http://goo.gl/cB2Ydg.

[30] American Psychiatric Publishing, DSM-5 Handbook of Differential Diagnosis, Chapter 1. Differential Diagnosis Step by Step, copied 6/2/15 http://goo.gl/KrebGV.

[31] First M, Essentials of Making an Accurate Psychiatric Diagnosis, Video from online Psychiatric Times, 2014, http://goo.gl/bvtPuF.

[32] **Note**: The DSM-V includes a Cultural Formulation Interview (http://goo.gl/MKq5W5) for assessing potential psychosocial stressors.

[33] LeBano L, Six Steps to Better DSM-5 Differential Diagnosis, Psych Congress Network, 2014, http://goo.gl/sUuXXg.

[34] American Psychiatric Publishing, Textbook of Psychiatry, 6th Edition, Chapter 4, http://goo.gl/Y2tAkU.

[35] Sarris J et al, International Society for Nutritional Psychiatry Research consensus position statement: nutritional medicine in modern psychiatry, World Psychiatry. 2015, PMCID: PMC4592666.

[36] **Note**: The American Psychiatric Association has formed the "APA Caucus on Complementary, Alternative and Integrative Medicine", www.intpsychiatry.com.

[37] American Psychiatric Association, Integrative Medicine, http://goo.gl/cPcHua.

[38] NAMI, Family-to-Family Education Program: 2013, p.6.2.

[39] Sullivan, WP, A lo, ng and winding road: The process of recovery from severe mental illness, 1997 In L. Spaniol C et al, Psychological and social aspects of psychiatric disability. Boston: Center for Psychiatric Rehabilitation. http://goo.gl/WoirOv.

[40] National Alliance on Mental Illness, Treatment and Services, http://goo.gl/oiwKPm. copied 10/31/2013.

[41] Trevidi MH et al, Sequenced Treatment Alternatives to Resolve Depression, Am J Psych, 2006, PMID: 15061154.

[42] Kirsch I et al, Initial Severity and Antidepressant Benefits: A Meta-Analysis of Data Submitted to the Food and Drug Admin, PLoS Med. 2008, PMCID: PMC2253608.

[43] Jakobsen JC et al, Selective serotonin reuptake inhibitors versus placebo in patients with major depressive disorder. A systematic review with meta-analysis and Trial Sequential Analysis, 2017, BMC Psych, https://goo.gl/D2Y97G.

[44] Laughren T, Treating Depression: Is there a placebo effect?, CBS News, 60 Minutes broadcast, 2012, https://goo.gl/ug78Av.

[45] Lieberman JA et al, Effectiveness of Antipsychotic Drugs in Patients with Chronic Schizophrenia, NEJM, PMID: 16172203, http://goo.gl/SkDQs8.

[46] Alenius M, Treatment Response in Psychotic Patients in a Naturalistic Setting, Uppsala Universitet, http://goo.gl/9EIPHf.

[47] **Note**: Medication side effects are a major reason for medication noncompliance (Balon R, Psychiatric Times, 2014, http://goo.gl/ooNawD). Over 70% of patients on antipsychotics describe weight gain from antipsychotic use as extremely distressing (Weiden P et al, PMID: 14693352, http://goo.gl/c5gZI3). 62.5% of men and 38.5% of women felt that their psychiatric medications were causing sexual side-effects, especially important since mental health issues typically hit young adults during their most sexually active years (Rosenberg KP et al. PMID: 14504017. In a 57-clinic study of antipsychotics, 64-82% of patients stopped taking the drugs (Lieberman JA et al, , PMID: 16172203, http://goo.gl/SkDQs8. There are many other side effects including lethargy, tremors and increased risk of suicide.

[48] Read J et al, Adverse emotional and interpersonal effects reported by 1829 New Zealanders while taking antidepressants, Psychiatry Res. 2014, PMID: 24534123.

[49] Reefhuis J et al, Specific SSRIs and birth defects: bayesian analysis to interpret new data in the context of previous reports, BMJ 2015, http://goo.gl/YY071b.

[50] Nat'l Institute of Health, Antidepressant Medications for Children and Adolescents: Information for Parents and Caregivers, copied 1/5/17 https://goo.gl/nicPm8.

[51] Yan J, FDA Extends Black-Box Warning to All Antipsychotics, Psychiatric News, 2008, https://goo.gl/IGy7o6.

[52] Insel T, National Inst of Mental Health Director's Blog: Antipsychotics: Taking the Long View, Aug 2013, http://goo.gl/LFmP0V.

[53] Wunderink L et al, Recovery in Remitted First-Episode Psychosis at 7 Years of Follow-up of an Early Dose Reduction/Discontinuation or Maintenance Treatment Strategy: Long-term Follow-up of a 2-Year Randomized Clinical Trial. JAMA Psychiatry 2013 PMID: 23824214.

[54] Harrow M, Does Long-term treatment of Schizophrenia With Antipsychotic Medications Facilitate Recovery? Schiz Bulletin 2013, Advance Access publication 3/19/13 2013, PMID: 23512950, https://goo.gl/pOVxoo.

[55] Harrow M, Does treatment of schizophrenia with antipsychotic medications eliminate or reduce psychosis? A 20-year multi-follow-up study, 2014, Psych Med, PMID: 25066792, http://goo.gl/ovhNJR.

[56] Fusar-Poli P et al, Progressive brain changes in schizophrenia related to antipsychotic treatment? A meta-analysis of longitudinal MRI studies, Neurosci Biobehav Rev. 2013, PMCID: PMC3964856; Beng-Choon H, Long-term Antipsychotic Treatment and Brain Volumes A Longitudinal Study of First-Episode Schiz., Arch Gen Psych, 2011, PMID: 21300943, http://goo.gl/fSS4eC. J Moncrieff, Antipsychotics and brain shrinkage: an update, 2013, http://goo.gl/M7pj1U.

[57] Citizens commission on human rights® international, The side effects of common psychiatric drugs, http://goo.gl/YSI0RL.

[58] Trehani MF et al, Second Generation Antipsychotic-Induced Obsessive-Compulsive Symptoms in Schizophrenia: A Review of the Experimental Literature, Current Psych Rep, 2014, PMID: 25256097.

[59] Science Daily, Benzodiazepines ineffective in treating anxiety disorders may increase dementia risk, 2015, http://goo.gl/IZylXR.

[60] Martin A, Age Effects on Antidepressant-Induced Manic Conversion, Archives of Pediatric Adolescent Medicine, 2004, PMID: :15289250, https://goo.gl/G8yxLl.

[61] Koranyi EK et al, Physical illnesses underlying psychiatric symptoms, Psycho Psychosom. 1992, PMID: 1488499, http://goo.gl/V9Wi23.

[62] Koran L, MEDICAL EVALUATION FIELD MANUAL, 1991, http://goo.gl/TPNL9t, copied 10/30/2013.

[63] Hall RC, Physical illness manifesting as psychiatric disease. II. Analysis of a state hospital inpatient population, Arch Gen Psychiatry. 1980, PMID: 7416911.

[64] Mahler A, Efficacy and Comparative Effectiveness of Atypical Antipsychotic Medications for Off-Label Use in Adults, JAMA, 2011, PMID: 21954480, http://goo.gl/D28W6X. Also see Consumer Reports, Off-label drug prescribing: What does it mean for you?, 2012, http://goo.gl/OE7TVA.

[65] Alexander G, Increasing off-label use of antipsychotic medications in the United States, Pharmaco Drug Saf. 2011, PMCID: 3069498.

[66] **Note**: Therrien, F et al, Selective serotonin reuptake inhibitors and withdrawal symptoms: A review of the literature, 1997, Human Psychopharmacology: Clinical and Experimental, http://goo.gl/07o5i9; Gardos G, Withdrawal syndromes associated with antipsychotic drugs, Am J Psychiatry, 1978. Criteria for SSRI Discontinuation Syndrome are being defined and the withdrawal difficulty clinically proven (Michelson D, PMID: 10827885).

[67] Frances A, Interview from the film, Crazywise, an advanced preview, 2017, https://crazywisefilm.com.

[68] Icarus Project & Freedom Center, Harm Reduction Guide to Coming Off Psychiatric Drugs, http://goo.gl/62q20b.

[69] Pétursson H, The benzodiazepine withdrawal syndrome, Addiction. 1994, PMID: 7841856.

[70] Datta V, Withdrawing From Psychiatric Drugs: What Psychiatrists Don't Learn, Mad In America, 2013, http://goo.gl/IBQccJ.

[71] Brogan K, Stop the Madness: Coming off Psych Meds, 2015, http://goo.gl/zT6q2n, copied 3/15/16.

[72] Stonecipher A, Psychotropic discontinuation symptoms: a case of withdrawal neuroleptic malignant syndrome, 2006, PMID: 17088172.

[73] Duckworth K, The Sensible Use of Psychiatric Medications, NAMI Advocate, Winter 2013.

[74] National Alliance on Mental Illness, Family-to-Family Teacher Manual, 2014.

[75] **Note on Antidepressants**: [1] Martin A, Age Effects on Antidepressant-Induced Manic Conversion, Archives of Pediatric Adolescent Medicine, 2004, PMID: :15289250, https://goo.gl/G8yxLl; [2] Kirsh Antidepressants and the Placebo Effect, 2014, PMCID: PMC4172306; [3] National Institute of Health, Antidepressant Medications for Children and Adolescents: Information for Parents and Caregivers, copied 1/5/17 from https://goo.gl/nicPm8; [4] Turner EH et al, Selective publication of antidepressant trials and its influence on apparent efficacy, N Engl J Med. 2008, PMID: 18199864; [5] Read J et al, Adverse emotional and interpersonal effects reported by 1829 New Zealanders while taking antidepressants, Psychiatry Res. 2014, PMID: 24534123; [6] Khan, A et al, Antidepressants versus placebo in major depression: an overview. World Psychiatry, 2015, PMCID: PMC4592645.

[76] Farah WH et al, Non-pharmacological treatment of depression: a systematic review and evidence map, Evid Based Med. 2016, PMID: 27836921; Vaswani A, Non-Pharmacological Treatments (NPTs) for Depression Are Effective, Mad in America, https://goo.gl/Zrlvjh.

[77] Zayfert C, Exposure utilization and completion of cognitive behavioral therapy for PTSD in a real world clinical practice, J Trauma Stress. 2005, PMID: 16382429.

[78] **Note on Antipsychotics**: [1] Citrome L et al, Schizophrenia, Clinical Antipsychotic Trials of Intervention Effectiveness (CATIE) and number needed to treat: how can CATIE inform clinicians, Int J Clin Pract. 2006, PMID: 16893436, https://goo.gl/iQXmVa. Lieberman J et al, Effectiveness of Antipsychotic Drugs in Patients with Chronic Schizophrenia, N Engl J Med. 2005, PMID: 16172203, https://goo.gl/hQeWv5; [2] Zhu Y et al, How well do patients with a first episode of schizophrenia respond to antipsychotics: A systematic review and meta-analysis, 2017, European Neuropsychopharm, https://goo.gl/xJTmZ; [3] Leucht S et al, Sixty Years of Placebo-Controlled Antipsychotic Drug Trials in Acute Schizophrenia: Systematic Review, Bayesian Meta-Analysis, and Meta-Regression of Efficacy Predictors, 2017, Amer Jof Psychiatry, https://goo.gl/bndxBq; [4] Leucht S et al, How effective are second-generation antipsychotic drugs? A meta-analysis of placebo-controlled trials, Molecular Psychiatry, 2009, PMID: 18180760, https://goo.gl/nhMXx2. (58% = 24% placebo response rate / 41% antipsychotic response rate); [5] Lindström E et al, Patient-rated versus clinician-rated side effects of drug treatment in schizophrenia. Clinical validation of a self-rating version of the UKU Side Effect Rating Scale (UKU-SERS-Pat), Nord J Psychiatry. 2001, PMID: 11860666; [6] Ucok, Sexual dysfunction in patients with schizophrenia on antipsychotic medication, Eur Psych, 2007, PMID: 17344032. Young SL et al, "First do no harm." A systematic review of the prevalence and management of antipsychotic adverse effects, PMID: 25516373, https://goo.gl/on3k62; [7] Diva N et al, Second-Generation Antipsychotics and Extrapyramidal Adverse Effects, BJPsych Open. 2018, PMC6060488; [8] Fusar-Poli P et al, Progressive brain changes in schizophrenia related to antipsychotic treatment? A meta-analysis of longitudinal MRI studies, Neurosci Biobehav Rev. 2013, PMCID: PMC3964856; [9] Waddington JL, Mortality in schizophrenia. Antipsychotic polypharmacy and absence of adjunctive anticholinergics over the course of a 10-year prospective study, Br J Psychiatry 1998, PMID: 9926037. Joukamaa M et al, Schizophrenia, neuroleptic medication and mortality. Br J Psychiatry, 2006, PMID: 16449697. Ito H et al, Polypharmacy and excessive dosing: psychiatrists' perceptions of antipsychotic drug prescription. Br J Psychiatry. 2005, PMID: 16135861; [10] Rajkumar, AP et al, Endogenous and antipsychotic-related risks for diabetes mellitus in young people with schizophrenia: a Danish population-based cohort study, Am J Psychiatry. 2017, PMID: 28103712; [11] Xiang Y et al, Almost All Antipsychotics Result in Weight Gain: A Meta-Analysis, 2014, PMCID: PMC3998960; [12] Harrow M et al, A 20-Year multi-followup longitudinal study assessing whether antipsychotic medications contribute to work functioning in schizophrenia, 2017, Psychiatry Research, PMID: 28651219; [13] Harrow M, Do all schizophrenia patients need antipsychotic treatment continuously throughout their lifetime? A 20-year longitudinal study, Psychological Medicine, 2012, PMID: 22340278, https://goo.gl/HwU0j8 ; Wunderink et al, Recovery in remitted first-episode psychosis at 7 years of follow-up of an early dose reduction/discontinuation or maintenance treatment strategy: long-term follow-up of a 2-year randomized clinical trial, JAMA Psychiatry. 2013, PMID: 23824214; [14] Ray et al, Atypical Antipsychotic Drugs and the Risk of Sudden Cardiac Death, NE J Med 2009, PMID: PMC2713724.

[79] NAMI, Family-to-Family 2014 Teacher Manual, 5th Edition, Edited by Terri Brister, Ph.D.

[80] Duckworth K, The Sensible Use of Psychiatric Medications, NAMI Advocate Magazine, Winter 2013, https://goo.gl/GMIuSU.

[81] Duckworth K,Science Meets the Human Experience Integrating the Medical and Recovery Models, NAMI Advocate Magazine, Winter 2014, https://goo.gl/iF6EWy.

[82] Reyers C,Different Strokes: Whole Health, CAM and Lifestyle When It Comes to Recovery, Many Approaches Can Help, NAMI Advocate Magazine, Winter 2014, https://goo.gl/SCBMX9.

[83] **Note on Benzodiazepines**: [1] American Addiction Centers, 6 of the Hardest Drugs to Quit, copied 1/29/17 from https://goo.gl/jpeVbG. Pétursson H, The benzodiazepine withdrawal syndrome, Addiction. 1994, PMID: 7841856.[2] Ashton H, Guidelines for the rational use of benzodiazepines. When and what to use, Drugs 1994, PMID: 7525193. Dell'Osso B et al, Bridging the gap between education and appropriate use of benzodiazepines in psychiatric clinical practice, Neuropsychiatr Dis Treat. 2015, PMC4525786.[3] Mehdi T, Benzodiazepines Revisited, BJMP.org, 2012, copied 1/27/17. [4] Wang P et al, Hazardous Benzodiazepine Regimens in the Elderly: Effects of Half-Life, Dosage, and Duration on Risk of Hip Fracture, Am J Psych, 2001, PMID: 11384896. [5] Connor KM et al, Discontinuation of clonazepam in the treatment of social phobia. Journal of clinical psychopharmacology. 1998, PMID: 9790154; Higgitt AC et al, Clinical management of benzodiazepine dependence, Br Med J (Clin Res Ed), 1985, PMC1416639; Pétursson H, The benzodiazepine withdrawal syndrome, Addiction, 1994, PMID: 7841856. [6] Maust, D et al, No End in Sight: Benzodiazepine Use in Older Adults in the United States, 2016, J of the Amer Geriatrics Society, PMID: 27879984; Lembke, A et al, Our Other Prescription Drug Problem, New England Journal of Medicine, 2018, PMID: 2946616, https://goo.gl/vwAbhb. [7] Dodds TJ, Prescribed Benzodiazepines and Suicide Risk: A Review of the Literature, Prim Care Companion CNS Disord. 2017, PMID: 28257172. [8] Dasgupta N et al, Cohort Study of the Impact of High-Dose Opioid Analgesics on Overdose Mortality, Pain Med Malden Mass, 2016, PMID: 26333030. [9] Tannenbaum et al, A systematic review of amnestic and non-amnestic mild cognitive impairment induced by anticholinergic, antihistamine, GABAergic and opioid drugs, Drugs Aging. 2012, PMID: 22812538..

[84] World Health Organization, Guide to Good Prescribing, 1994, http://goo.gl/9BPdmj.

[85] Harris G, Talk Doesn't Pay, So Psychiatry Turns Instead to Drug Therapy, 2011, http://goo.gl/N7gbfL.

[86] Brown H, Looking for Evidence That Therapy Works, Mar 2013, The New York Times, http://goo.gl/kexU17.

[87] Ohio Department of Mental Health Office of Program Evaluation & Research, Toward Best Practices: Top Ten Findings from the Longitudinal Consumer Outcomes Study, 1999, http://goo.gl/cULzSM.

[88] **Note**: The pipeline for new psychotropic drugs is slowing.. Many psychotropics are of the "me too" variety –similar to existing drugs.. The probability of failure of introducing new drugs, the long drug development cycle (averaging 18 years), the complexity of the brain and the profit erosion by generic drug all contribute to very high psychotropic drug development costs (http://goo.gl/duIU7Q). It is becoming increasingly difficult for drug companies to justify placing scarce research dollars on mental health efforts.Pharmaceutical companies have reduced research funding for new psychotropics (http://goo.gl/ITYv6d).

[89] Merick K, The New York Times and all that..., Mad in America, 2012, http://goo.gl/bqaeyT.

[90] Rethink Mental Illness, Caring for Yourself - Recovery and Hope, 2012, http://goo.gl/MVVwUP.

[91] Schrank B et al, Recovery in psychiatry, Psychiatric Bulletin, 20 07, http://goo.gl/5H405d.

[92] White W et al, Recovery from Addictions and From Mental Illness: Shared and Contrasting Lessons, From *Recovery in Mental Illness: Broadening our understand of wellness*, APA, http://goo.gl/kexQ7B.

[93] Freese FJ, Integrating Evidence-based Practices and the Recovery Model, Psych Svc, 2001, PMID: 11684741, http://goo.gl/iUoksC.

[94] Kirkpatrick H et al, How people with schizophrenia build their hope, J of Psychosocial Nursing, 2001, PMID: 11197995.

[95] Lehigh University, Self-rating mental health as 'good' predicts positive future mental health, Science Daily, 2018, https://goo.gl/nk6yfv.

[96] Andresen, R et.al, Stages of recovery instrument: development of a measure of recovery from serious mental illness, Australian and New Zealand Journal of Psychiatry, 2006, PMID: 17054565. http://goo.gl/Xr9a15.

[97] **Note**: See James Prochaska's book *Changing for Good* (William Morrow and Company, 1994); "transtheoretical model of change" by Leamy (next endnote); and the 4-step mental health recovery process by Mark Ragins in *Road to Recovery*, http://goo.gl/WxbuJA.

[98] Leamy M, Conceptual framework for personal recovery in mental health: systematic review and narrative synthesis, 2011,BJ Psych, PMID: 22130746, http://goo.gl/w7blRb.

[99] Meyer B et al., Treatment expectancies, patient alliance and outcome: Further analyses from the National Institute of Mental Health Treatment of Depression Collaborative Research Program, Journal of Consulting and Clinical Psychology, 2002, PMID: 12182269.

[100] **Note**: Assisted/involuntary treatment presents a contentious ethical dilemma (See *Hospital, Residential and Community Therapy* and associated endnotes). Those who favor AOTs cite studies that show statistically relevant reductions in hospitalization rates, the ability to help those who may otherwise be unreachable, reduced overall cost and other realities seen in places where AOT laws are enacted. Others, particularly those who have experienced assisted/involuntary drug treatment, are sometimes strongly against AOT laws citing the sometimes debilitating effects of psychotropics, increased risk of suicide, studies that show that AOTs offer little/no value, lack of emphasis on recovery, the loss of their right of self-determination and other realities. The UN Committee on the Rights of Persons with Disabilities adopted a General Comment that states that nonconsensual psychiatric interventions must be eliminated (http://goo.gl/FH75xI).

[101] Allen MH, What do consumers say they want and need during a psychiatric emergency?, J Psychiatr Pract. 2003, PMID: 15985914, http://goo.gl/gxvR52.

[102] Corrigan, PW, How stigma interferes with mental health care. American Psychologist, 2004.

[103] Cornwall M, Responding To People In Extreme States With Loving Receptivity, Dabney Alix interview, 2015, http://goo.gl/Fok8TT, and www.MichaelCornwall.com.

[104] Cooke N (editor), Understanding Psychosis and Schizophrenia, British Psychol Society, 2014, http://goo.gl/b1t322.

[105] Tomes N, The Patient As A Policy Factor: A Historical Case Study Of The Consumer/Survivor Movement In Mental Health, Health Aff May 2006, PMID: 16684736, http://goo.gl/KQ763r.

[106] Xie H, Strengths-Based Approach for Mental Health Recovery, Iran J Psychiatry Behav Sci. 2013, PMCID: PMC3939995.

[107] **Note**: Many thanks to my good friend Bob Nassauer for this grounding phrase, "Mistakes will be made".. It has served me and many others very well.

[108] Knox D et al, Use and Avoidance of Seclusion and Restraint: Consensus Statement of the American Association for Emergency Psychiatry Project BETA Seclusion and Restraint Workgroup, West J Emerg Med. 2012, PMC3298214.

[109] NAMI, Psychiatric Advance Directives: An Overview, copied Dec 2014, http://goo.gl/J8ym1y.

[110] Sarris J, Integrative Mental Healthcare White Paper: Establishing a new paradigm through research, education, and clinical guidelines, Advances in Integrative Medicine, 2014, http://goo.gl/qfhXdT.

[111] Malenka R, Moving Beyond 'Chemical Imbalance' Theory of Depression, 2012, Brain and Behavior Res Found, http://goo.gl/F0fsRp.

[112] Kendler K, Toward a Philosophical Structure for Psychiatry, Am J Psychiatry. 2005, PMID: 15741457.

[113] Ples R, Nuances, Narratives, and the "Chemical Imbalance" Debate, Psychiatric Times, 2014, http://goo.gl/ILG6aZ.

[114] Johnstone L, Publication of the Power Threat Meaning Framework, Mad In America, 2017, https://goo.gl/fFhJs7.

[115] **Note**: Statements regarding severity tended to be vague (e.g. 'most adverse effects were mild to moderate') and it was frequently unclear how different degrees of severity had been defined. Authors typically failed to state whether investigators attributed adverse effects to the study drug, dosage or other factors. Pope A, PMID: 20592438, http://bjp.rcpsych.com/content/197/1/67.full. P Rothwell notes "Reporting of adverse effects of treatment in RCTs and systematic reviews is often poor", Factors That Can Affect the External Validity of Randomised Controlled Trials, PLoS Clin Trials. 2006, PMCID: PMC1488890.

[116] Grohol J, Withdrawal from Psychiatric Meds Can Be Painful, Lengthy, Psychcentral, 2013, http://goo.gl/P6EGZh.

[117] Stonecipher A, Psychotropic discontinuation symptoms: a case of withdrawal neuroleptic malignant syndrome, GHPJournal, 2006, PMID: 1708817, http://goo.gl/aA35Ic.

[118] LaMatinna J, Pharma Controls Clinical Trials Of Their Drugs. Is This Hazardous To Your Health?, Forbes, 2013, http://goo.gl/B9ySfQ.

[119] Turner E et al, Selective Publication of Antidepressant Trials and Its Influence on Apparent Efficacy, N Engl J Med 2008, PMID: 18199864, http://goo.gl/acVv2n.

[120] Riveros C et al, Timing and Completeness of Trial Results Posted at ClinicalTrials.gov and Published in Journals, PLOS Medicine, 2013, PMCID: 3849189.

[121] US House of Representatives, The Fair Access to Clinical Trials Act HR 5252.

[122] World Health Organization, WHO Statement on Public Disclosure of Clinical Trial Results, 2015, http://goo.gl/oh7o6Q.

[123] Black N, Why we need observational studies to evaluate the effectiveness of health care, BMJ, 1996, PMCID: 2350940.

[124] Hunt N, Methodological Limitations of the RCT in Determining the Efficacy of Psychological Therapy for Trauma, Journal of Traumatic Stress Disorders & Treatment, 2012, http://goo.gl/65WBi9.

[125] Clay R, More than one way to measure, American Psychological Association, 2010, http://goo.gl/dDDC5b.

[126] Hunsley J et al, Research-informed benchmarks for psychological treatments: Efficacy studies, effectiveness studies, and beyond, Professional Psychology: Research and Practice, 2007.

[127] Lehman A, Practice Guideline for the Treatment of Patients With Schizophrenia Second Edition, http://goo.gl/WQCdJx.

[128] Frank R, Mental Health Policy and Psychotropic Drugs, Milbank Quarterly, 2005, http://goo.gl/BWKJxb.

[129] Simon G, Long-term Effectiveness and Cost of a Systematic Care Program for Bipolar Disorder, JAMA Psychiatry, 2006, PMID: 16651507, http://goo.gl/8JWT2f.

[130] Citizens commission on human rights® international, Psychiatric Drugs–Just the Facts, copied Dec 2014, http://goo.gl/Og13cl.

[131] Arehart-Treichel J, Several Medications Linked to Violent Acts, Ameri Psych Assoc, 2010, http://goo.gl/ED27RH.

[132] US Food and Drug Admin, Public Health Advisory: Deaths with Antipsychotics in Elderly Patients with Behavioral Disturbances, 2013, http://goo.gl/LHCSoV.

[133] Brownlee, Nutraceuticals Move In, Modern Drug Discovery, American Chemical Society, 2002, http://goo.gl/sVI9G9.

[134] FDA, How Drugs are Developed and Approved, 2014, http://goo.gl/IG5mD5.

[135] Khouri A, 4 big retailers accused of selling herbal formulas containing no herbs, Los Angeles Times, 2015.

[136] BC Partners for Mental Health and Addictions Info, Family Self-Care and Recovery From Mental Illness, 2008, http://goo.gl/Q1K8oB.

[137] **Note**: Katz D et al, Preventive Medicine, Integrative Medicine & Health of the Public, Commissioned for the US Institute of Medicine Summit on Integrative Medicine and the Health of the Public, 2009, http://goo.gl/RWOPrb. Over-care avoidance is an addition by: European Union of General Practitioners/Family Physicians, UEMO position on Disease Mongering / Quaternary Prevention, 2011, http://goo.gl/usrpEC. "Preventive", "restorative", "symptom relief" and "over-care avoidance" are more descriptive terms and used in place of "primary", "secondary", "tertiary" and "quaternary" used in these references.

[138] Institute of Functional Medicine, What is Functional Medicine?, https://goo.gl/LASFUm.

[139] Makary M et al, Medical error–the third leading cause of death in the US, BMJ 2016, http://goo.gl/VAaZfA.

[140] **Note**: SAMHSA indicates, "Trauma can occur from a variety of causes, including maltreatment, separation, abuse, criminal victimization, physical and sexual abuse, natural and manmade disasters, war, and sickness… many (people) suffer a variety of negative physical and psychological effects (from this trauma). Trauma exposure has been linked to later … mental illness." (SAMHSA, Leading Change: A plan for SAMHSA's roles and actions 2011-2014, http://goo.gl/n5uRqZ). Varese F, Childhood Adversities Increase the Risk of Psychosis: A Meta-analysis of Patient-Control, Prospective- and Cross-sectional Cohort Studies, 2012, Schizophrenia Bulletin, PMCID: 3406538). Etain B, Childhood trauma is associated with severe clinical characteristics of bipolar disorders, 2013, J Clin Psychiatry, PMID: 24229750). Investigating and addressing previous trauma may be vital for mental health recovery. The primary therapeutic response for trauma is a *Psychosocial Restorative* response with EMDR and Emotion Freedom Technique among the most effective.

[141] Walsh R, Lifestyle and Mental Health, American Psychologies, 2011, http://goo.gl/xjrrDa.

[142] Harvard mental health letter. Sleep and Mental Health, July 2009. copied 10/30/2013, http://goo.gl/SFCguv.

[143] Fuller ET et al, Adjunct Treatments for Schizophrenia and Bipolar Disorder: What to Try When You Are Out of Ideas, Clinical Schizophrenia & Related Psychoses January 2012, PMID: 22182458, http://goo.gl/yOFzTr.

[144] Dickerson F et al, Elevated serum levels of C-reactive protein are associated with mania symptoms in outpatients with bipolar disorder. Prog Neuropsychopharmacol Biol Psychiatry, 2007, PMID: 17391822.

[145] Goldstein BI et al, Inflammation and the phenomenology, pathophysiology, comorbidity, and treatment of bipolar disorder: a systematic review of the literature. J Clin Psychiatry, 2009, PMID: 19497250.

[146] Köhler O et al, Effect of Anti-inflammatory Treatment on Depression, Depressive Symptoms, and Adverse Effects A Systematic Review and Meta-analysis of Randomized Clinical Trials, AMA, 2014, PMID: 25322082, http://goo.gl/VsFDHU.

[147] Ford E et al, Depression and C-Reactive Protein in US Adults Data From the Third National Health and Nutrition Examination Survey, JAMA 2004, PMID: 15136311, http://goo.gl/9juCei.

[148] Copeland W et al, Generalized Anxiety and C-Reactive Protein Levels: A Prospective, Longitudinal Analysis, 2012, Psychol Med, PMCID: PMC2763246.

[149] Sommer IE, Efficacy of anti-inflammatory agents to improve symptoms in patients with schizophrenia: an update, Schizophr Bull. 2014, PMCID: PMC3885306.

[150] Laan W et al, Adjuvant aspirin therapy reduces symptoms of schizophrenia spectrum disorders: results from a randomized, double-blind, placebo-controlled trial. J Clin Psych, 2010. PMID: 20492850.

[151] NG F et al, Oxidative stress in psychiatric disorders: evidence base and therapeutic implications, Intl J Neuropsychopharma, 2008, PMID: 18205981, http://goo.gl/iInMGk.

[152] Lake J, Cholesterol and Mood: What's the Link?, Psychiatric Times, 2010, https://goo.gl/nQV14k.

[153] Marie-Laure A et al, Gender and genotype modulation of the association between lipid levels and depressive symptomatology in community-dwelling elderly (The ESPRIT Study), Biol Psychiatry. 2010, PMID: 20537614.

[154] Bird A, Perceptions of epigenetics, Nature, 2007.

[155] SAMHSA, SAMHSA's WORKING DEFINITION OF RECOVERY, http://goo.gl/pmIp5w.

[156] Rios-Ellis B, Critical Disparities in Latino Mental Health: Transforming Research into Action, Nat'l Council of La Raza, 2005, http://goo.gl/67o87x.

[157] Stephen EH, Health of the foreign-born population: United States, 1989-90, Adv Data. 1994, PMID: 10132138.

[158] NAMI, The Latino Paradox: Mental Health Appears to Not Be an Exception, 2013, http://goo.gl/RhsySv.

[159] Sussner K, The Influence of Immigrant Status and Acculturation on the Development of Overweight in Latino Families: A Qualitative Study, J Immigr Minor Health, 2008, PMCID: 3090681.

[160] Lara, M et al, "ACCULTURATION AND LATINO HEALTH IN THE UNITED STATES: A Review of the Literature and its Sociopolitical Context". Annual Review of Public Health. PMID: 15760294.

[161] NAMI, Treatment and Services, http://goo.gl/IHgfTm.

[162] NSW Health, Food Security Options Paper: A planning framework and menu of options for policy and practice interventions, NSW DoH 2003, http://goo.gl/G24hyD.

[163] Jones A, Food Insecurity and Mental Health Status: A Global Analysis of 149 Countries, Univ of Michigan, Am J Prev Med, 2017, https://goo.gl/0xrx26.

[164] NAMI, Social Security Benefits, copied 2/16/14, http://goo.gl/mro L0v.

[165] National Center for Family Homelessness, Homelessness and Traumatic Stress Training package, http://goo.gl/CMFBjC.

[166] Pevalin DJ et al, The impact of persistent poor housing conditions on mental health: A longitudinal population-based study, Prev Med. 2017, PMID: 28963007.

[167] University College London, Psychosis incidence highly variable internationally, ScienceDaily, 2017, https://goo.gl/SU5Bw9.

[168] Teplin L et al, Crime Victimization in Adults With Severe Mental Illness, Arch Gen Psych, 2005, PMCID: 1389234.

[169] Evans G, Housing and Mental Health: A Review of the Evidence and a Methodological and Conceptual Critique, J of Social Issues, 2003, http://goo.gl/DUQbfW.

[170] Faris, REL et al, Mental disorders in urban areas, 1939, Chicago: University of Chicago Press. Molarius et al, Mental health symptoms in relation to socio-economic conditions and lifestyle factors – a population-based study in Sweden, BMC Public Health, 2009, PMCID: PMC2736164.

[171] Hudson, C.G., Socioeconomic Status and Mental Illness: Tests of the Social Causation and Selection Hypotheses, Amer J of Orthopsychiatry, PMID: 15709846, http://goo.gl/vEWnyC.

[172] Yeich, Susan et al, The Case for a Supported Housing Approach: A Study of Consumer Housing and Support Preferences" Psychosocial Rehabilitation J, 1994 http://goo.gl/bhKfuO.

[173] Brazelon Center for Mental Health Law, SUPPORTIVE HOUSING: The Most Effective and Integrated Housing for People with Mental Disabilities, http://goo.gl/IDbWLl.

[174] Coalition for the Homeless, Proven Solutions to the Problem of Homelessness, http://goo.gl/zZS1wt.

[175] Watson D et al, Understanding the Critical Ingredients for Facilitating Consumer Change in Housing First Programming: A Case Study Approach, J Behav Health Serv Res. 2013, PMCID: 3642235.

[176] Padgett P et al, Substance Use Outcomes Among Homeless Clients with Serious Mental Illness: Comparing Housing First with Treatment First Programs, Comm Ment Hlth J. 2011, PMCID: 2916946.

[177] National Coalition for the Homeless, Mental Illness and Homelessness, July 2009, http://goo.gl/eoAeBi.

[178] Firth J et al, Diet as a hot topic in psychiatry: a population-scale study of nutritional intake and inflammatory potential in severe mental illness, World Psych, 2018, PMC6127755.

[179] Shivappa N et al, Designing and developing a literature-derived, population-based dietary inflammatory index, Public Health Nutr. 2014, PMC3925198.

[180] Pataracchia R, Orthomolecular Treatment for Depression, Anxiety & Behavior Disorders, Naturopathic Med Research Clinic, 2008. http://goo.gl/q26VUR.

[181] Emsley R et al, Clinical potential of omega-3 fatty acids in the treatment of schizophrenia, CNS Drugs, 2003, PMID: 14661986.

[182] Rogers PJ, A healthy body, a healthy mind: long-term impact of diet on mood and cognitive function, Proc Nutr Soc, 2001, PMID: 11310419.

[183] Kiecolt-Glaser JK et al, Depressive symptoms, omega-6:omega-3 fatty acids, and inflammation in older adults, Psychosom Med. 2007, PMID: 17401057.

[184] Jacka FN, The association between habitual diet quality and the common mental disorders in community-dwelling adults: the Hordaland Health study, Psychosom Med, 2011, PMID: 21715296, http://goo.gl/H7sehR.

[185] NAMI, Eating Healthy, http://goo.gl/BQ4q7s, copied 11/4/2013.

[186] Silvers KM et al, Fish consumption and self-reported physical and mental health status, Public Health Nutr, 2002, PMID: 12003654.

[187] Hibbeln JR, Fish consumption and major depression, Lancet 1998, PMID: 9643729.

[188] Peet M, International variations in the outcome of schizophrenia and the prevalence of depression in relation to national dietary practices: an ecological analysis, 2004, PMID: 15123503.

[189] Palmer C, Ketogenic diet in the treatment of schizoaffective disorder: Two case studies, Schizophr Res. 2017, PMID: 28162810.

[190] Noaghiul S et al, Cross-national comparisons of seafood consumption and rates of bipolar disorders, Am J Psych, 2003, PMID: 14638594.

[191] Phelps JR et al, The ketogenic diet for type II bipolar disorder, Neurocase. 2013, PMID: 23030231.

[192] Bowman G, Nutrient biomarker patterns, cognitive function, and MRI measures of brain aging, Neurology, 2012, PMCID: 3280054.

[193] Christensen L, The effect of carbohydrates on affect, Nutrition, 1997, PMID: 9263230.

[194] Dinan TG et al, Gut Instincts: microbiota as a key regulator of brain development, ageing and neurodegeneration, J Physiol. 2016, PMID: 27641441.

[195] Côté C et al, Hormonal Signaling in the Gut, J Biol Chem. 2014, PMC4002074.

[196] Maguen S, Association of mental health problems with gastrointestinal disorders in Iraq and Afghanistan Veterans, Depression and Anxiety, PMID: 23494973.

[197] Harvard Health Publications, The gut-brain connection, 2012, copied from http://goo.gl/ZkkaJv.

[198] Burnet, PW et al, Psychobiotics highlight the pathways to happiness, Biological Psychiatry, 2013, PMID: 24144322.

[199] Divan TG et al, Psychobiotics: A novel class of psychotropic, Biological Psychiatry, 2013, PMID: 23759244.

[200] Messaoudi M et al, Assessment of psychotropic-like properties of a probiotic formulation (Lactobacillus helveticus R0052 and Bifidobacterium longum R0175)in rats and human subjects, British Journal of Nutrition (2011), PMID: 20974015, http://goo.gl/mlDzBE.

[201] Proceedings of the National Academy of Sciences 2011, http://goo.gl/LaqLFk.

[202] Steenbergen L et al, A randomized controlled trial to test the effect of multispecies probiotics on cognitive reactivity to sad mood, Brain, Behavior, and Immunity, published online 2015, http://goo.gl/keaWTn.

[203] Logan AC, Major depressive disorder: probiotics may be an adjuvant therapy, Med Hypotheses 2005, PMID: 15617861.

[204] Shaw W, Increased Urinary Excretion of a 3-(3-Hydroxyphenyl)-3-Hydroxypropionic Acid (HPHPA), An Abnormal Phenylalanine Metabolite of Clostridia Spp. in the Gastrointestinal Tract, in Urine Samples from Patients with Autism and Schizophrenia, Nutritional Neurosci, 2010, PMID: 20423563.

[205] Medical News Today, Gut microbes important for serotonin production, April 2015, http://goo.gl/SNMsVp.

[206] Hussin NM et al, Efficacy of fasting and calorie restriction (FCR) on mood and depression among ageing men, J Nutr Health Aging. 2013, PMID: 24097021.

[207] Boehme, DH, "Preplanned Fasting in the Treatment of Mental Disease: Survey of Current Soviet Literature, Schiz Bull, 1977, PMID: 887908, http://goo.gl/cDjmDZ.

[208] Cott A, Controlled Fasting Treatment of Schizophrenia in the U.S.S.R., Schizophrenia, http://goo.gl/Wup3mY.

[209] Suzuki J et al, Fasting therapy for psychosomatic diseases with special reference to its indication and therapeutic mechanism, Tohuku J Exp Med, 1976, PMID: 964029.

[210] Polishchuk Lul, Fasting-diet therapy of elderly patients with borderline mental disorders, Zhurnal Nevropatologii i Psikhiatrii Imeni S.S. Korsakova, 1991, PMID: 1650075.

[211] Yamamoto H et al, Psychophysiological study on fasting therapy, Psychother Psychosom. 1979. PMID: 550177.

[212] Zargar AH, Ramadan and Diabetes Care, JP Medical Ltd, 2013.

[213] NAMI, Dual Diagnosis fact sheet, http://goo.gl/j6Zobl.

[214] Bruce MS et al, Caffeine abstention in the management of anxiety disorders, Psychol Med, 1989, PMID: 2727208.
[215] Hollingworth HL, The influence of caffeine on mental and motor efficiency, Arch Psychol, 1912.
[216] UK Medicines Information, Smoking and Drug Interaction, 2007, http://goo.gl/UnVQXK.
[217] Cavazos-Rehg PA et al, Smoking cessation is associated with lower rates of mood/anxiety and alcohol use disorders, Psycholog Med, 2014, http://goo.gl/f84M54.
[218] Holford P, Optimum Nutrition for the Mind, Laguna Beach Ca: Basic Health Publications, 2004.
[219] McClernon FJ et al, The effects of foods, beverages and other factors on cigarette palatability, Nicotine Tob Res, 2007, PMID: 17454706.
[220] Parletta N et al, A Mediterranean-style dietary intervention supplemented with fish oil improves diet quality and mental health in people with depression: A randomized controlled trial (HELFIMED), Nutr Neurosci. 2017, PMID: 29215971.
[221] Hibbeln J et al, Vegetarian diets and depressive symptoms among men, J Affective Disord, 2018, https://goo.gl/DFUvbt.
[222] Conner TS et al, Let them eat fruit! The effect of fruit and vegetable consumption on psychological well-being in young adults: a randomized controlled trial. PLoS One. 2017, PMCID: PMC5291486.
[223] Severance EG, Gastrointestinal inflammation and associated immune activation in schizophrenia, Schizophr Res. 2012, Epub 2012, PMID: 22446142.
[224] MedlinePlus, Malabsorption, http://goo.gl/hwRVUz.
[225] Nagamin T et al, Probiotics Reduce Negative Symptoms of Schizophrenia: A Case Report, Int'l Medical J, 2012, http://goo.gl/52Jc1T.
[226] Greenblatt J, Examining the gut-brain connection and its implications for Trichotillomania treatment, Great Plains Laboratory, 2016, https://goo.gl/Qw2TVz.
[227] Kraft, Bryan D., et al., "Schizophrenia, Gluten, and Low-Carbohydrate, Ketogenic Diets: A Case Report and Review of the Literature, Nutrition & Metabolism, 2009 BIOMED CENTRAL LTD, PMID: 19245705.
[228] Landers DM, The influence of exercise on mental health. President's Council on Physical Fitness & Sport Res Dig, 1997.
[229] Fox KR. The influence of physical activity on mental well-being, Pub Hlth Nutr, 1999, PMID: 10610081.
[230] Deslandes A et al. Exercise and mental health: many reasons to move. Neuropsychobiology 2009, PMID: 19521110.
[231] Richardson CR, Integrating physical activity into mental health services for persons with serious mental illness, Psych Serv. 2005, PMID: 15746508.
[232] Dunn AL et al, Physical activity dose-response effects on outcomes of depression and anxiety, Med Sci Sports Exerc, 2001, PMID: 11427783.
[233] Paluska SA et al, Physical activity and mental health: current concepts, Sports Med, 2000, PMID: 10739267.
[234] Atlantis E et al, An effective exercise-based intervention for improving mental health and quality of life measures: a randomized controlled trial. Prev Med 2004, PMID: 15226056.
[235] US Dept Health and Human Services, Physical Activity abnd Health, a report of the Surgeon General, Centers for Disease Control and Prevention, 1996.
[236] Craft LL et al, The effect of exercise on clinical depression and depression resulting from mental illness: a meta-analysis, J of Sport and Exercise Psychology, 1998.
[237] Bhui K et al, Common mood and anxiety states: gender difference in the protective effective of physical activity. Soc Psychiatry Psychiatr Epidemio, 2000.
[238] Laurin D et al, Physical activity and risk of cognitive impairment and dementia in elderly persons, Arch Neurol, 2001.
[239] Hassmén P, Physical exercise and psychological well-being: a population study in Finland, Prev Med 2000, PMID: 10642456.
[240] Paluska SA et al, Physical activity and mental health: Current concepts. Sports Med 2000, http://goo.gl/i6zHs9.
[241] Cooney GM et al, Exercise for depression, Cochrane Database Syst Rev. 2013, PMID: 24026850.
[242] Babyak M, Exercise Treatment for Major Depression: Maintenance of Therapeutic Benefit at 10 Months, Psychosomatic Medicine, 2000, PMID: 11020092.
[243] Samuel H et al, Exercise and the Prevention of Depression: Results of the HUNT Cohort Study, Am J of Psychiatry, 2017.
[244] Brooks A et al, Comparison of aerobic exercise, clomipramine, and placebo in the treatment of panic disorder, Am J Psych, 1998, PMID: 9585709.
[245] Abrantes AM, Acute changes in obsessions and compulsions following moderate-intensity aerobic exercise among patients with obsessive-compulsive disorder, J Anxiety Disord. 2009 , PMID: 19616916.
[246] Medical News today, Study reveals structured exercise helps PTSD recovery, 2014, http://goo.gl/BG3Jgk.
[247] Firth J, Aerobic Exercise Improves Cognitive Functioning in People With Schizophrenia: A Systematic Review and Meta-Analysis, Schiz Bulletin, 2016, https://goo.gl/9xOKOl.
[248] Yoon S et al, Preliminary Effectiveness and Sustainability of Group Aerobic Exercise Program in Patients with Schizophrenia, J Nerv Mental Dis, 2016, PMID: 2721822.
[249] Teri L et al, Exercise plus behavioral management in patients with Alzheimer's disease, JAMA, 2003.
[250] Harvard Health, Sleep and Mental Health, July 2009, http://goo.gl/1oWWsH.
[251] Ohavon MM, The effects of breathing-related sleep disorders on mood disturbances in the general population, J Clin Psych. 2003, PMID: 14658968.
[252] Shinba T et al, Alcohol Consumption and insomnia in a sample of Japanese alcoholics. Addiction, 2004, PMID: 8044125.
[253] Salzer HM, Relative hypoglycemia as a cause of neuropsychiatric illness, Journal of the National Med Assoc, 1966, PMID: 2611193.
[254] Gradisar M et al, The Sleep and Technology Use of Americans: Findings from the National Sleep Foundation's 2011 Sleep in America Poll, Journal of Clin Sleep Medicine, 2013, http://goo.gl/3LzUqj.
[255] Stevens RG et al, Adverse health effects of nighttime lighting: comments on American Medical Association policy statement, Am J Prev Med. 2013, http://goo.gl/1kXnAs.
[256] Neckelmann D et al, Chronic insomnia as a risk factor for developing anxiety and depression, Sleep, 2007, PMID: 17682658.
[257] Wirz-Justice A et al, Chronotherapeutics for Affective Disorders: A Clinician's Manual for Light and Wake Therapy. Basel, Switzerland: S Karger AG; 2009.
[258] Riemann D et al, How to preserve the antidepressive effect of sleep deprivation:A comparison of sleep phase advance and sleep phase delay, Eur Arch Psychiatry Clin Neurosci, 1999, PMID: 10591988, https://goo.gl/nZsq4s.
[259] Benedetti F et al, Combined total sleep deprivation and light therapy in the treatment of drug-resistant bipolar depression: acute response and long-term remission rates. J Clin Psychiatry. 2005, PMID: 16401154.
[260] Life Lessons, Course Material, Michigan Heart and Vascular, St. Joseph's Mercy Hospital, Ann Arbor Michigan. 1998.
[261] National Commission on Sleep Disorders Research: Wake up America: A National Sleep Alert, Executive Summary, Nat'l Heart, Lung and Blood Institute, 1993.
[262] Myles H et al, How long will we sleep on obstructive sleep apnoea in schizophrenia, Aust N Z J Psychiatry, 2016, PMID: 27535956.
[263] Youngstedt SD et al, The effects of acute exercise on sleep: a quantitative synthesis, Sleep, 1997.
[264] NAMI, The quest for sleep by Milly Dawson, http://goo.gl/6KKGEq, copied 11/3/2013.
[265] Gramprie, Dr. James, Neurologist, University of Michigan Health Systems, personal conversation, 2014.
[266] Morin CM et al, Behavioral and pharmacological therapies for late-life insomnia: a randomized controlled trial, Journal of the American Medical Assoc, 1999.
[267] Safe Harbor, Recovery from psychosis, mania, anxiety, and other symptoms, http://goo.gl/cqN2pB.
[268] Searle A et al, Patients' views of physical activity as treatment for depression: a qualitative stud, Br J Gen Pract. 2011, PMCID: PMC3063043.
[269] Davis M et al, The relaxation and stress reduction workbook, 2nd edition, Oakland CA, New Harbinger Press.
[270] Smith C, A randomised comparative trial of yoga and relaxation to reduce stress and anxiety, Complementary Therapies in Med, 2007, http://goo.gl/EYWZDV.
[271] Chen, Wen-Chun, Efficacy of Progressive Muscle Relaxation Training in Reducing Anxiety in Patients with Acute Schizophrenia, J of Clin Nursing, 2009, PMID: 19583651.
[272] Nicassio P et al, A comparison of progressive relaxation and autogenic training as treatments for insomnia, J of Abnormal Psychology, 1974, PMID: 4844912.
[273] Shibata J. "Clinical Evaluation with Psychological Tests of Schizophrenic Patients Treated with Autogenic Training." The American J of Clinical Hypnosis, 1967.
[274] WebMD, Autogenic Training - Topic Overview, copied 4/28/15, http://goo.gl/ZV3jH3.
[275] Stetter et al, Autogenic training: a meta-analysis of clinical outcome studies, 2002, Appl Psychophysiol Biofeedback. 2002, PMID: 12001885.
[276] Philippot, P et al, Respiratory feedback in the generation of emotion, 2010, Cognition and Emotion, https://goo.gl/m4o3al.
[277] Elliot S, The new science of breath, Cohrence press, 2005, http://goo.gl/EKB9eV.
[278] Brown RP et al, Sudarshan kriya yogic breathing in the treatment of stress, anxiety, and depression: part II-clinical applications and guidelines, J Altern Complement Med 2005.
[279] Greater Good Science Center, What Is Mindfulness?, University of California, Berkeley, copied 10/3/2016, https://goo.gl/3BwFdb.
[280] Weinzweig A Zingerman's Guide to Good Leading, Part 3: A lapsed Anarchist's Approach to Managing Ourselves, 2013.
[281] Neurotech Coaching, see http://yourbraintraining.com/what-is-mindfulness.html.
[282] Mind Fitness Training Institute, www.mind-fitness-training.org.
[283] Prison-Ashram Project, http://www.humankindness.org/prison-ashram-project/.
[284] Borchard T, Non-Judging, Non-Striving and the Pillars of Mindfulness Practice, PsychCentral, 2015, copied Sep 2015, http://goo.gl/mZThfM.
[285] Khoury B et al, Mindfulness-based therapy: a comprehensive meta-analysis, Clin Psychol Rev. 2013, http://goo.gl/ewYcH4.
[286] US Dept. of Veterans Affairs, Health Services Research & Development, Management Brief no. 88, Evidence Map of Mindfulness, 2015, http://goo.gl/2bCJVc.
[287] Grossman P, Mindfulness-based stress reduction and health benefits A meta-analysis, Journal of Psychosomatic Research, 2004, http://goo.gl/IVsIQS.
[288] Stefan Hofmann, professor of psychology at Boston University's Center for Anxiety and Related Disorders. as quoted in the Los Angeles Times, Mindfulness therapy is no fad, experts say, copied 10/29/2013. http://goo.gl/psTxlR.

[289] Kabat-Zinn et al, Effectiveness of a meditation-based stress reduction program in the treatment of anxiety disorders, American Journal of Psychiatry, 1992.
[290] Keefer L et al, The effects of relaxation response meditation on the symptoms of irritable bowel syndrome: Results of a controlled treatment study, Behavior Research and Therapy, 2001.
[291] Chien, WT et al, Effects of a mindfulness-based psychoeducation programme for Chinese patients with schizophrenia: 2-year follow-up, British Journal of Psychiatry, 2014, PMID: 24809397.
[292] Black D et al, Mindfulness Meditation and imoprovement in sleep quality and daytime impairment among older adults with sleep disturbances, JAMA Intern Med, 2015, http://goo.gl/mu9Wgj.
[293] Sundquist J et al, The effect of mindfulness group therapy on a broad range of psychiatric symptoms: A randomised controlled trial in primary health care, Eur Psychiatry. 2017, PMID: 28365464.
[294] Brown KW et al, Mindfulness: Theoretical foundations and evidence for its salutary effects, 2007, Psychological Inquiry, http://goo.gl/y13U3z.
[295] Stanley E et. al, Mindfulness-based Mind Fitness Training: A Case Study of a High-Stress Predeployment Military Cohort, Cognitive and Behavioral Practice 18, 2011, http://goo.gl/BwmwlO.
[296] Reibel DK et al, Mindfulness-based stress reduction and health-related quality of life in a heterogeneous patient population, Gen Hosp Psychiat 2001, http://goo.gl/sPqBMZ.
[297] Price CJ et al, Mindful awareness in body-oriented therapy as an adjunct to women's substance use disorder treatment: a pilot feasibility study, J Subst Abuse Treat. 2012, PMCID: PMC3290748.
[298] Price CJ et al, Mindful Awareness in Body-oriented therapy for female veterans with Post-Traumatic Stress Disorder taking prescription analgesics for chronic pain: A feasibility Study, Altern Ther Health Med, 2011, PMCID: PMC3037268.
[299] Buddhanet, An Overview of Loving-Kindness Meditation, http://goo.gl/zFYWR.
[300] Chodren P, The Practice of Tonglen, copied 3/17/16 https://goo.gl/NBxXMc.
[301] Helgason C, Mind-Body Medicine for Schizophrenia and Psychotic Disorders: A Review of the Evidence, CLINICAL SCHIZOPHRENIA & RELATED PSYCHOSES, 2013, http://goo.gl/qFejpG.
[302] Johnson, David P. "A Pilot Study of Loving-Kindness Meditation for the Negative Symptoms of Schizophrenia." Schizophrenia Research, 2011, ELSEVIER.
[303] Johnson DP et al. A pilot study of loving-kindness meditation for the negative symptoms of schizophrenia. Schizophr Res 2011, PMID: 21385664, http://goo.gl/04T2UU.
[304] Arias AJ, Steinberg K, Banga A, Trestman RL . .J Altern Complement Med 2006;12:817-32.
[305] Segal Z et al, Antidepressant Monotherapy vs Sequential Pharmacotherapy and Mindfulness-Based Cognitive Therapy, or Placebo, for Relapse Prophylaxis in Recurrent Depression, Arch Gen Psychiatry. 2010, http://goo.gl/Q0pu6p.
[306] Rubia K, The neurobiology of Meditation and its clinical effectiveness in psychiatric disorders, Biological Psychology 82 (2009), http://goo.gl/0TB6eU.
[307] Shannahof-Khalsa D et al, Randomized Controlled Trial of Yogic Meditation Techniques for Patients with Obsessive-Compulsive Disorder, CNS Spectr. 1999, PMID: 18311106.
[308] Danforth K et al, Reduced Trauma Symptoms and Perceived Stress in Male Prison Inmates through the Transcendental Meditation Program: A Randomized Controlled Trial, Perm J 2016, https://goo.gl/HuxbBV.
[309] Nidich S et al, Non-trauma-focused meditation versus exposure therapy in veterans with post-traumatic stress disorder: a randomised controlled trial, Lancet, 2018, https://goo.gl/ktgXwM.
[310] Davidson RJ, et al. Alterations in brain and immune function produced by mindfulness meditation. Psychosom Med 2003, http://goo.gl/updpn7.
[311] Bormann JE et al, Efficacy of frequent mantram repetition on stress, quality of life, and spiritual well-being in veterans: a pilot study, J Holist Nurs. 2005, PMID: 16251489.
[312] NAMI, Family-to-Family course material, 2013, p. 8.15.
[313] Amaresha A et al, Expressed Emotion in Schizophrenia: An Overview, Indian J Psychol Med, 2012, http://goo.gl/HZeBsZ.
[314] Hogarty GE, Anderson CM, Reiss DJ, Kornblith SJ, Greenwald DE, Janva CD, et al. Family psychoeducation, social skills training, and maintenance chemotherapy in the aftercare treatment of schizophrenia. Arch Gen Psychiatry. 198.6, http://goo.gl/0uTPxQ.
[315] Brown GW et al, Influence of family life on the course of schizophrenia disorder, Br J Psych. 1972, http://goo.gl/n715zi.
[316] Kavanagh DJ. Recent developments in expressed emotion and schizophrenia. Br J Psych. 1992, http://goo.gl/jHirms.
[317] Achterberg J, Imagery in healing: Shaminism and modern medicine, Boston, New Science Library, 1985.
[318] Achterberg J et al, Rituals of healing: Using imagery for health and wellness, New York Bantam Books, 1985.
[319] Titlebaum HM, Relaxation, Alternative Health Practitioner, 1998.
[320] Federman R, Facing Bipolar, New Harbinger Publishers, 2010, as extracted from BPHope.com, http://goo.gl/nQuwpA.
[321] Ananda Sangha, The Energization Exercises of Paramhansa Yogananda, http://goo.gl/b8nShG.
[322] Nancy L. Sin et al, Affective Reactivity to Daily Stressors Is Associated With Elevated Inflammation, Health Psychology, 2015, http://goo.gl/eZcZZW.
[323] Frankl V, The Will to Meaning Foundations and Applications of Logotherapy, Meridian Penguin, 1988.
[324] Bragdon E, 15 Psychiatrists Transforming Psychiatry: When Psych Meds are No Longer #1 (courseware), Integrative Mental Health for You, 2015, www.imhu.org.
[325] Ong J et al, A Mindfulness-Based Approach to the Treatment of Insomnia, J Clin Psychol. 2010, http://goo.gl/HQO4x9.
[326] Baumeister R, Some key differences between a happy life and a meaningful life, J Positive Psychol, 2013, http://goo.gl/isYRO9m.
[327] **Note**: There are a variety of examples in philosophy, psychology and religion. One can be found in Raja Yoga as found in Yogananda, Paramahansa, Man's Eternal Quest, "The Desire that Satisfies All Desires", Self-Realization Fellowship, 1982.
[328] Davidson L, Sense of self in recovery from severe mental illness, British Journ of Med Psych, 1992, http://goo.gl/vAzdxW.
[329] Petty D et al, The Search for Identity and Meaning in the recovery process, Psych Rehab Journ, 1999.
[330] Jopling DA, Self-knowledge and the Self, New York, Routledge, 2000.
[331] Neff K et al, Self-Compassion: What it is, what it does, and how it relates to mindfulness, University of Texas at Austin, pre-publish, http://goo.gl/hQmHz9.
[332] Blatt, S J, The destructiveness of perfectionism: Implications for the treatment of depression. Amer psychologist,1995.
[333] BARNARD, LK et al, The relationship of clergy burnout to self-compassion and other personality dimensions. Pastoral Psychology, 2012.
[334] Heffernan, M et al, Self-compassion and emotional intelligence in nurses. International J of Nursing Practice, 2010.
[335] Neff KD, Self-compaassion, Self-Esteem and Well-Being, Social and Personality Psychology, 2011, http://goo.gl/hVooiG.
[336] Germer C et al, Self-Compassion inClinicalPractice, JOURNAL OF CLINICAL PSYCH: IN SESSION, 2013, http://goo.gl/JWQxMW.
[337] Leary, M. R. Making sense of self-esteem. Current Directions in Psychological Science, 1999.
[338] Aberson, C. et al, Ingroup bias and self-esteem: A meta-analysis, Personality & Social Psychol Rvw, 2000.
[339] Hogg, MA et.al., Social identifications: A social psychology of intergroup relations and group processes, 1988, London: Routledge.
[340] Heine S, Is There a Universal Need for Positive Regard? Psychological Review, 1999, http://goo.gl/FTcJMv.
[341] Gecas V, The Social Psychology of Self-Efficacy, Annual Review of Sociology, 1989, https://goo.gl/fsijln.
[342] Peck M. Scott, The Road Less Traveled, Simon & Schuster Publishers, 1978.
[343] Flores P, Group Psychotherapy with Addicted Populations: An Integration of Twelve-Step & Psychodynamic Theory, Routledge, 2013.
[344] World Health Organization European Office, User Empowerment in Mental Health, 2010, http://goo.gl/n6hQll.
[345] Lawn S et al, Control in chronic condition self-care management: how it occurs in the health worker-client relationship and implications for client empowerment, J Adv Nurs. 2014, PMID: 23834649.
[346] Alenius M, Treatment Response in Psychotic Patients in a Naturalistic Setting, 2009, Uppsala Universitet, https://goo.gl/T7a6EP.
[347] Ulemann and M, Effects o f Covert an d Overt Modeling on the Development of Empathy, Canadian J Counselling, 1989.
[348] Wolpe J, The Practice of Behavior Therapy, Elmsford: Pergamon Press, 1969.
[349] Budzynski T, "Tuning in on the Twilight Zone", Psychology Today, 1977.
[350] Taylor S et al, Cognitive restructuring in the treatment of social phobia. Behavior Mod, 1997, PMID: 9337603.
[351] Brooks AW, Get Excited: Reappraising Pre-Performance Anxiety as Excitement, J of Exper Psychol, 2013, http://goo.gl/iLwb1P.
[352] Richins M, A consumer values orientation for materialism and its measurement: Scale development and validation, J of Consumer Res, 1992, http://goo.gl/jPOGyc.
[353] Kasser T, A dark side of the American dream: Correlates of financial success as a central life aspiration, J of Personality and Social Psychol, 1993, http://goo.gl/9buxs8.
[354] Myers DG, The funds, friends and faith of happy people, American Psychologist, 2000, http://goo.gl/9tuofc.
[355] Brown W, Narratives of Mental Health Recovery, Social Alternatives, 2008, http://goo.gl/LufBcR.
[356] Ashcraft L et al, META Peer Employment Training Workbook, http://goo.gl/kDHxRG.

[357] Esso L, How I perceive and Manage My Illness, Schizophrenia Bulletin, 1989, http://goo.gl/5p5WM7.
[358] Geer J et al, Treatment of a Recurrent Nightmare by Behavior-modification Procedures: A Case Study, J of Abnormal Psychol, 1967, http://goo.gl/dzO6RQ.
[359] Castagnaro L, Advice on Coping With Voices, Mad In America, 2016, http://goo.gl/ifVkpB.
[360] Frankl V, Man's Search for Meaning, an introduction to Logotherapy, Beacon Press, 1992.
[361] Mauss I et al, Can Seeking Happiness Make People Happy? Paradoxical Effects of Valuing Happiness, Emotion. 2011, PMCID: PMC3160511.
[362] Cassels C, Sense of Purpose Predicts Mental Health Outcomes Following Severe Trauma, Medscape, 2008, http://goo.gl/4MuEiK.
[363] Bonab BG et al, Hope, Purpose in Life and Mental Health in College Students, International Journal of the Humanities, Vol 5 Issue 5.
[364] Boyle P, Effect of a Purpose in Life on Risk of Incident Alzheimer Disease and Mild Cognitive Impairment in Community-Dwelling Older Persons, JAMA Psychiatry, 2010, http://goo.gl/e7HJHM.
[365] Boyle P, Purpose in Life Is Associated With Mortality Among Community-Dwelling Older Persons, Psychosomatic Medicine, 2009, http://goo.gl/kn0DMJ.
[366] Boyle P, Effect of Purpose in Life on the Relation Between Alzheimer Disease Pathologic Changes on Cognitive Function in Advanced Age, JAMA Psychiatry, 2012, http://goo.gl/7tK3Zh.
[367] Carlson M et al, Impact of the Baltimore Experience Corps Trial on cortical and hippocampal volumes, Alzheimer's & Dementia, March 2015, http://goo.gl/vgZLCQ.
[368] Johns Hopkins Bloomberg School of Public Health, Civic engagement may stave off brain atrophy, improve memory, 2015, http://goo.gl/4qmfJ3.
[369] Fredrickson B et al, A functional genomic perspective on human well-being, PNAS, 2013, http://goo.gl/dObKMk.
[370] Smith EE, Meaning Is Healthier Than Happiness, The Atlantic, 2013, http://goo.gl/mxTj4O.
[371] Ricoeur P, Time and Narrative, Chicago: University of Chicago Press, 1984.
[372] Fallot R, Spiritual and Religious Dimensions of Mental Health Recovery Narratives, New Directions for Mental Hlth Svcs, 1998.
[373] Lysaker PH et al, Changes in narrativestructure and content in schizophrenia in long term individual psychotherapy: a single case study. Clin Psychol Psychother, 2005.
[374] Yanos P, The Impact of Illness Identity on Recovery from Severe Mental Illness, Am J Psychiatr Rehabil, 2010, http://goo.gl/bdkozm.
[375] Kobau R, Well-Being Assessment: An Evaluation of Well-Being Scales for Public Health and Population Estimates of Well-Being among US Adults, Center for Disease Control, 2010, http://goo.gl/bAOGjb.
[376] Holstein A, Tough Grace, Fellowship for International Community, Mar 7 2011, Community Magazine, http://goo.gl/sWgKdY.
[377] Carey B, Finding Purpose in Life with Delusion, International New York Times, 11/25/2011, http://goo.gl/70YQ9N.
[378] Hasiam A, Social groups alleviate depression, preliminary from Science Daily, 2014, http://goo.gl/lkbQnG.
[379] Garfield C, Seven Keys to a Good Death, Greater Good Science Center, 2014, copied 1/25/17, https://goo.gl/MPN2SO.
[380] Connell J et al, Qualityof life of people with mental health problems: a synthesis of qualitative research, BioMed Central, 2012, http://goo.gl/1x1XkU.
[381] Economic and Social Research Council, Mental Health and Social Relationships, 2013, http://goo.gl/umi6Cu.
[382] Fuller-Thomson E et al, Flourishing after depression: Factors associated with achieving complete mental health among those with a history of depression, Psychiatry Res. 2016, PMID: 27267442.
[383] Jones KC, HAWMC Day 6 - Emotional Safety, 2015, http://goo.gl/qqjdl0O.
[384] Henri Nouwen, Henri Nouwen and Soul Care: A Ministry of Integration, http://www.henrinouwen.org/
[385] Davidson L, Recovery from psychosis: What's love got to do with it?, Psychosis, 2011, https://goo.gl/iPujYp.
[386] World Health Organization, Promoting Mental Health - Concepts, Emerging Evidence, Practice, 2005, http://goo.gl/LBV99u.
[387] Bjornestad J et al, "Everyone Needs a Friend Sometimes" - Social Predictors of Long-Term Remission In First Episode Psychosis, Front. Psych, 2016, PMC5047905.
[388] National Research Council (US) Committee on Aging Frontiers in Social Psychology, Personality, and Adult Developmental Psychology; Carstensen LL editor. When I'm 64. Washington (DC): National Academies Press, 2006, http://goo.gl/VfwOYb.
[389] Cacioppo, JT, Loneliness as a specific risk factor for depressive symptoms: Cross-sectional and longitudinal analyses, Psychology and Aging, 2006, http://goo.gl/20DqFS.
[390] Holt-Lunstad J et al, Loneliness and Social isolation as Risk Factors for Mortality: A meta-analytic Review, Perspectives on Psychol Science, 2015, http://goo.gl/iI13Lq.
[391] Link B, On Stigma and Its Consequences: Evidence from a Longitudinal Study of Men with Dual Diagnoses of Mental Illness and Substance Abuse, Journal of Health and Social Behavior 1997.
[392] Link B et al, Stigma as a Barrier to Recovery: The Consequences of Stigma for the Self-Esteem of People With Mental Illnesses, http://goo.gl/n84wW9.
[393] Markowitz F, The Effects of Stigma on the Psychological Well-being and Life Satisfaction of Persons with Mental Illness, J of Health and Social Behavior, 1998.
[394] Medical News Today, Older adults who volunteer are more likely to be happier and healthier, 2014, http://goo.gl/lLaKlw.
[395] Tabassum F, Association of volunteering with mental well-being: a lifecourse analysis of a national population-based longitudinal study in the UK, BMJ Open 2016, https://goo.gl/0DGAMS.
[396] Piliavin JA, Health Benefits of Volunteering in the Wisconsin Longitudinal Study, Journal of Health and Social Behavior, 2007, http://goo.gl/nCtQoN.
[397] Mental Health America, http://goo.gl/HCxV0s, copied March 2015.
[398] Rohner R et al, Worldwide Mental Health Correlates of Parental Acceptance-Rejection: Review of Cross-Cultural and Intracultural Evidence, J Child Neurology, 2015, http://goo.gl/ONF2Aj.
[399] Gold S, THE PLACE OF COMFORT: HAMAKOM, http://goo.gl/c8uTRj, copied Oct 2015.
[400] Wagner L, Personal conversation, 2015.
[401] Kivelä SL, Effects of Garden Visits on Long-term Care Residents as Related to Depression, HortTechnology, 2005, http://goo.gl/ROMqVE.
[402] Pergams O et al, Evidence for a fundamental and pervasive shift away from nature-based recreation, PNAS, 2007, http://goo.gl/XR21yD.
[403] Jerrett M et al, Nature Exposure Gets a Boost From a Cluster Randomized Trial on the Mental Health Benefits of Greening Vacant Lots, JAMA Network Open. 2018, https://goo.gl/2kx1dQ.
[404] Bezold C et al, The relationship between surrounding greenness in childhood and adolescence and depressive symptoms in adolescence and early adulthood, Ann Epidemiol. 2018, PMID: 29426730.
[405] Bratman G et al, Nature experience reduces rumination and subgenual prefrontal cortex activation, Proc Natl Acad Sci 2015, PMCID: PMC4507237.
[406] Shanahan D et al, Health Benefits from Nature Experiences Depend on Dose, Scientific Reports, 2016, PMCID: PMC4917833.
[407] Sundquist K et al, Urbanisation and incidence of psychosis and depression: follow-up study of 4.4 million women and men in Sweden, Br J Psychiatry. 2004, PMID: 15056572.
[408] Miyazaki Y et al, Preventive medical effects of nature therapy, Nihon Eiseigaku Zasshi. 2011, PMID: 21996763.
[409] Faber Taylor A et al, Could exposure to everyday green spaces help treat ADHD? Evidence from children's play settings. Appl Psychol Health Well-being, 2011.
[410] Minding Our Bodies, copied 10/29/2013, http://goo.gl/GaAwRB.
[411] Van Den Berg AE et al, Green space as a buffer between stressful life events and health. Soc Sci Med 2010, PMID: 20163905.
[412] Fisher D, Dialogical Recovery from Monological Medicine, www.MadinAmerica.com, 2012, http://goo.gl/VTlack.
[413] VAUGHAN-CLARK,F. Transpersonal perspectives in psychotherapy.J. Humanistic Psychology, Spring 1977.
[414] Mooney E, Excursions with Kierkegaard: Others, Goods, Death, and Final Faith, Bloomsbury, 2013.
[415] Vaughan F, Transpersonal Psychotherapy: Context, Content and Process, J TranspersonalPsychol,1979, http://goo.gl/4cGpQA.
[416] Gallup Polls, Religious Awakenings Bolster Americans' Faith, Religious and Social Trends, January 2003, http://goo.gl/CBx264.
[417] Lukoff D, From Spiritual Emergency to Spiritual Problem: The Transpersonal Roots of the New DSM-IV Category, Journal of Humanistic Psychology, 1998, http://goo.gl/n2tnfy.
[418] Fallot RD, Spirituality and religion in psychiatric rehabilitation and recovery from mental illness, International Review of Psychiatry 2001, http://goo.gl/BdkCER.
[419] Keonig H, Religion, Spirituality, and Medicine: Research Findings and Implications for Clinical Practice, Southern Med Assoc, 2004, http://goo.gl/jWxVS1.
[420] Rosmarin D, A test of faith in God and treatment: The relationship of belief in God to psychiatric treatment outcomes, Journal of Affective Disorders, 2013, http://goo.gl/NKw9wU.
[421] Corrigan P, McCorkle B, Schell B, Kidder K, Religion and Spirituality in the Lives of People with Serious Mental Illness, Community Mental Health Journal, 2003.
[422] Levin J, Religion and Mental Health: Theory and Research, International Journal of Applied Psychoanalytic Studies Int. J. Appl. Psychoanal. Studies, 2010, http://goo.gl/qMfdLl.
[423] Deegan P, Recovery and the Conspiracy of Hope, 1996, https://goo.gl/gDGPUJ.
[424] Luther L, Expectancies of success as a predictor of negative symptoms reduction over 18 months in individuals with schizophrenia, Psychiatry Res, 2015, http://goo.gl/O0HeBr.
[425] Fisher D, An Empowerment Model of Recovery From Severe Mental Illness: An Expert Interview With Daniel B. Fisher, MD, PhD, Medscape Multispecialty, http://www.medscape.com/viewarticle/496394.
[426] Tepper L, The Prevalence of Religious Coping Among Persons With Persistent Mental Illness, Psychiatric Svcs 2001.
[427] Koenig H, Research on Religion, Spirituality and Mental Health: A Review, Canadian J of Psychiatry, 2008.

[428] Zhang R et al, Perceived Primal Threat of Mental Illness and Recovery: The Mediating Role of Self-Stigma and Self-Empowerment, Am J Orthopsychiatry, 2016, https://goo.gl/xjBEqa.
[429] Grant PM et al, Asocial beliefs as predictors of asocial behavior in schizophrenia, Psychiatry Res. 2010, PMID: 20163875.
[430] Assagioli R, Psychosynthesis, A collection of Basic Writings, Esalen Publishing, 1965, 1993.
[431] Bhagavad-Gita, Chapter 2 verse 47, http://goo.gl/1I2ToV.
[432] Cloninger CR, The science of well-being: an integrated approach to mental health and its disorders, World Psychiatry. 2006, PMCID: PMC1525119.
[433] Ellermann CR, Self-transcendence and depression in middle-age adults, West J Nurs Res. 2001, PMID: 11675796.
[434] Cloninger CR et al, Personality and the perception of health and happiness, J of Affective Disorders, 2011, PMID: 20580435, http://goo.gl/kvTSjF
[435] Firmin RL, Self-Initiated Helping Behaviors and Recovery in Severe Mental Illness: Implications for Work, Volunteerism, and Peer Support, Psychiatric Rehabilitation J, 2015, PMID: 26053530.
[436] Emmons RA et al, Why Gratitude Enhances Well-Being: What We Know, What We Need to Know, first proof, 2010, https://goo.gl/A2gBrp.
[437] Lambert N et al, A changed perspective: How gratitude can affect sense of coherence through positive reframing, J Pos Psych, 2009, https://goo.gl/12It1O.
[438] Emmons RA et al, Counting blessings versus burdens: an experimental investigation of gratitude and subjective well-being in daily life, J Pers Soc Psychol. 2003, PMID: 12585811.
[439] Culliford L, Spirituality and clinical care, BMJ, 2002 Dec 21, http://goo.gl/4aCA0p.d
[440] WebMD, Schizophrenia Health Center, http://goo.gl/bi7qMh.
[441] NIH, Medline Plus, Schizophrenia, http://goo.gl/8COVGK.
[442] Corrigan P et al, Self-stigma and the "why try" effect: impact on life goals and evidence-based practices, World Psychiatry. 2009, PMCID: PMC2694098.
[443] Harris K et al, Religious Involvement and the Use of Mental Health Care, Health Serv Res 2006.
[444] **Note**: The "recovery model" is a counterpoint to the "medical model" found in historic psychiatric treatment. The medical model focuses primarily on brain biology and psychoactive drugs. It is often includes a somewhat passive patient involvement where medication compliance is the major responsibility. The recovery model has many variants (see *Recovery Models & Tools*) that share a theme of self-directedness and self-determination by the person with diagnosis. Recovery models also often embrace a wellness orientation as opposed to disease recovery orientation and a much larger array of therapeutic options beyond psychotropics. There is often strident controversy between medical model and recovery model proponents. Adopting elements of the recovery model is becoming increasingly prevalent (see National Assoc of Social Workers, NASW Practice Snapshot: The Mental Health Recovery Model, 2006, http://goo.gl/IZOUJc).
[445] Deegan P, Recovery: The lived experience of rehabilitation, Psychosocial Rehab J, 1988, http://goo.gl/DM8EIY.
[446] Ruiz B, Hope, Hopelessness and Hearing Voices Groups, Mad in America, 2017, https://goo.gl/5wGms9.
[447] University of California Television, Amy's Mental Health Recovery Story, https://goo.gl/eakklQ.
[448] Knutson S, 72 Hour Hold for Inalienable Personhood, Mad in America, 2017, https://goo.gl/E3kU9K.
[449] Loupos, John. Inside Tai Chi.YMAA Publication Center, Boston, MA. 2002.
[450] Miller JJ et al, Three-year follow-up and clinical implications of a mindfulness-based stress reduction intervention in the treatment of anxiety diosrders, Gen Hosp Psychiatry, 1995.
[451] Kirkwood G, Yoga for anxiety: a systematic review of the research evidence, Br J Sports Med 2005, http://goo.gl/Rkedlc.
[452] Woolery A et al, A yoga intervention for young adults with elevated symptoms of depression, Alternative Therapy and Health Medicine, 2004.
[453] Shapiro D et al, Yoga as a complementary treatment of depression: effects of traits and moods on treatment outcome, Oxfound University Press, 2007.
[454] Chaudhary AK et al, Comparative study of the effect of drugs and relaxation exercise (yoga shavasan) in hypertension, J of the Assoc of Physicians in India, 1988.
[455] Shannahoff-Khalsa DS, Kundalini yoga meditation techniques for the treatment of obsessive-compulsive and OC spectrum disorders. Grief Treatment and Crisis Intervention, 2003.
[456] Descilo T et al, Comparison of a yoga breath-based program and a client-centered exposure therapy for relief of PTSD and depression in survivors of tsunami disaster, Proceedings World Conference Expanding Paradigms: Science Consciousness and Spirituality, 2006.
[457] Seppälä EM, Breathing-based meditation decreases posttraumatic stress disorder symptoms in U.S. military veterans: a randomized controlled longitudinal study, J Trauma Stress. 2014, http://goo.gl/9sKQpL.
[458] Medical News Today, Benefits, risks of yoga for bipolar disorder: survey results, Sep 2014, http://goo.gl/XTPnDN.
[459] Bangalore N Gangadhar, Yoga therapy for Schizophrenia, Int J Yoga. 2012, http://goo.gl/dfrmBz.
[460] Duraiswamy, G, Yoga Therapy as an Add-on Treatment in the Management of Patients with Schizophrenia--a Randomized Controlled Trial, Acta Psychiatrica Scandinavica, 2007.
[461] Bhatia T, Adjunctive Cognitive Remediation for Schizophrenia Using Yoga: An Open, Non-Randomized Trial, Acta Neuropsychiatrica, 2012.
[462] Sageman S, Breathing through the despair: spiritually oriented group therapy as a means of healing women with severe mental illness, J Am Acad Psychoanl Dyn Psychiatry, 2004.
[463] Walsh R, Roche L. Precipitation of acute psychotic episodes by intensive meditation in individuals with a history of schizophrenia. Am J Psychiatry, http://goo.gl/Bkl8mG.
[464] Cohen L et al, Psychological adjustment and sleep quality in a randomized trial of the effects of a Tibetan yoga intervention in patients with lymphoma, Cancer, 2004.
[465] Vedamurthachar A et al, Antidepressant efficacy and hormonal effects of Sudarshana Kriya Yoga (SKY) in alcohol dependent individuals, Journal of Affective Disorders, 2006, PMID: 16740317.
[466] Lavey R, The effects of yoga on mood in psychiatric inpatients. Psychiatr Rehabil J 2005, http://goo.gl/SsDqgq.
[467] Tang C, et al, T'aiChi on psychological well-being: systematic review and meta-analysis, BMC Complementary and Alternative Medicine 2010, http://goo.gl/KqOvtG.
[468] Mortimer JA, Changes in brain volume and cognition in a randomized trial of exercise and social interaction in a community-based sample of non-demented Chinese elders, J Alzheimer's Dis., 2012, http://goo.gl/7O5y3F.
[469] Abbott R et al, Tai Chi and Qigong for the Treatment and Prevention of Mental Disorders, Psychiatr Clin North Am. 2013, http://goo.gl/LDE7vy.
[470] Tang C, et al, Effects of qigong and Taijiquan on reversal of aging process and some psychological functions, Third Nat'l Acad Conference on Qigong, 1990.
[471] Li L et al, A comparative study of quigong and biofeedback therapy, 2nd International Conference on Qigong, 1989.
[472] Janke R et al, A Comprehensive Review of Health Benefits of Qigong and Tai Chi, Am J Health Promot, 2010, http://goo.gl/w4Hduk.
[473] Li M et al, Use of qigong therapy in the detoxification of heroin addicts. Alternative Therapy and Health Medicine, 2002. PMID: 11795622.
[474] Korn L, Integrative Medicine for Posttraumatic Stress and Complex Trauma, 2018.
[475] NAMI, Psychosocial Treatments, http://goo.gl/WrAag5
[476] Barton R, Psychosocial Rehabilitation Services in Community Support Systems: A Review of Outcomes and Policy Recommendations, 1999, Psychiatric Services, http://goo.gl/QCE5Xq.
[477] Cook A (editor), Understanding Psychosis and Schizophrenia, British Psychol Society, 2014,http://goo.gl.b1t322.
[478] MAPS, Phase 3 Trials: FDA Grants Breakthrough Therapy Designation for MDMA-Assisted Psychotherapy for PTSD, Agrees on Special Protocol Assessment, 2018. http://www.maps.org/research/mdma.
[479] Hayes S et al, The third wave of cognitive behavioral therapy and the rise of process-based care, World Psychiatry. 2017, PMC5608815.
[480] Vivyan C, An Introductory Self-Help Course in Cognitive Behaviour Therapy, 2009-2013, http://goo.gl/MPkLPx.
[481] Smith L, Cognitive Behavioral Therapy for Psychotic Symptoms: A Therapist's manual, Center for Clinical Interventions: Psychotherapy, Research and Training, 2003, http://goo.gl/TqYP33.
[482] National Institute for Clinical Excellence, Schizophrenia: Core interventions in the treatment and management of schizophrenia in primary and secondary care (update), 2009.
[483] Jauhar S, et al, Cognitive-behavioural therapy for the symptoms of schizophrenia: systematic review and meta-analysis with examination of potential bias, British Journal of Psychiatry, 2014, PMID: 24385461, http://goo.gl/YYBmSu.
[484] Kråkvik B et al, Cognitive Behaviour Therapy for Psychotic Symptoms: A Randomized Controlled Effectiveness Trial, Behav Cogn Psychother. 2013, PMC3775151.
[485] Turner DT, Psychological Interventions for Psychosis: A Meta-Analysis of Comparative Outcome Studies, Am Journal of Psych, Feb 2014, PMID: 24525715.
[486] Penn DL et al, A randomized controlled trial of group cognitive-behavioral therapy vs. enhanced supportive therapy for auditory hallucinations, Schizophrenia Research, 2009, PMID: 19176275.
[487] Rathod S, et al, Cognitive-behavioral therapy for medication-resistant schizophrenia: a review, Journal of Psychiatric Practice, 2008, PMID: 18212600.
[488] National Institute for Health and Care Excellence (2014). Psychosis and schizophrenia in adults: treatment and management. NICE clinical guidelines. London: National Institute for Hlth and Care Excellence, http://goo.gl/M8IbbD.
[489] Harvey AG et al, Cognitive behaviour therapy for primary insomnia: Can we rest yet?, Sleep Medicine Reviews, 2003, PMID: 12927123.

[490] Wu JQ et al, Cognitive Behavioral Therapy for Insomnia Comorbid With Psychiatric and Medical Conditions: A Meta-analysis, JAMA Intern Med. 2015, PMID: 26147487.

[491] Siversten B et al, Cognitive behavioral therapy vs zopiclone for treatment of chronic primary insomnia in older adults: a randomized controlled trial, JAMA, 2006, PMID: 16804151.

[492] Hunot V et al, Psychological therapies for generalized anxiety disorder, Cochrane Database of System Rvws, 2010.

[493] Mitte K et al, A meta-analysis of the efficacy of psycho- and pharmacotherapy in panic disorder with and without agoraphobia, Journal of Affective Disorder, 2005, PMID: 16005982.

[494] Gava I, et al, Psychological treatments versus treatment as usual for obsessive compulsive disorder (OCD), Cochrane Database of Systematic Reviews, 2007.

[495] Mahli GS et.al., Clinical practice recommendations for bipolar disorder, Acta Psychiatrica Scandinavia, 2009, PMID: 19356155.

[496] Szentagotai A et.al., The efficacy of cognitive-behavioral therapy in bipolar disorder: A quantitative meta-analysis. J of Clinical Psychiatry, 2010, PMID: 19852904.

[497] National Institute for Health and Care Excellence, Computerised cognitive behaviour therapy for depression and anxiety: Review of Technology Appraisal 51, 2006, http://goo.gl/rZ1cvT.

[498] Brand BL et al, A review of dissociative disorders treatment studies, J of Nervous and Mental Disease, 2009, PMID: 19752643.

[499] Australian Centre for Posttraumatic Mental Health, Australian guidelines for the treatment of adults with acute stress disorder and posttraumatic stress disorder, 2007.

[500] Grant PM et al, Randomized Trial to Evaluate the Efficacy of Cognitive Therapy for Low-Functioning Patients With Schizophrenia, Arch Gen Psychiatry. 2012, PMID: 21969420, http://goo.gl/D1Ur20.

[501] Hodge D, Spiritually Modified Cognitive Therapy : A review of Literature, Social Work; 2006, http://goo.gl/yvv9lv.

[502] McCoullough ME, Research on religion-accomodated counseling: Review and meta-analysis, Journ Counsel Psychology, 1999.

[503] Andrews G, Computer Therapy for the Anxiety and Depressive Disorders Is Effective, Acceptable and Practical Health Care: A Meta-Analysis, 2010, PMC2954140.

[504] Mitchell N, Attitudes Towards Computerized CBT for Depression Amongst a Student Population, Behav and Cognitive Psychother, 2007, http://goo.gl/Zu9EOX.

[505] Andersson G, Internet-Based and Other Computerized Psychological Treatments for Adult Depression: A Meta-Analysis, Cogn Behav Ther. 2009, PMID: 20183695.

[506] Andersson G et al, Guided Internet-based vs. face-to-face cognitive behavior therapy for psychiatric and somatic disorders: a systematic review and meta-analysis, World Psychiatry, 2014, PMCID: PMC4219070.

[507] Carlbring P, Benefits were also observed regarding anxiety symptoms and quality of life, BJ Psych 2007, http://goo.gl/aVyA35.

[508] Lynch TR et al, Dialectical behaviour therapy for borderline personality disorder. Annual Review of Clinical Psychology, 2007.

[509] Chapman A, Dialectical Behavior Therapy, Psychiatry (Edgmont) 2006, http://goo.gl/6y3LR5.

[510] McMain S et al, Advances in psychotherapy of personality disorders: a research update, Cur Psychiatry Rep 2007.

[511] DeVylder JE, Dialectical Behavior Therapy for the Treatment of Borderline Personality Disorder: An Evaluation of the Evidence, 2010, International Journal of Psychosocial Rehabilitation, http://goo.gl/JxtpCb.

[512] Lynch TR et al, Dialectical behavior therapy for depressed older adults, International Jof Geriatric Psychiatry, 2003.

[513] Smout M, The empirically supported status of acceptance and commitment therapy: An update, Australian Psychological Society, 2012, http://goo.gl/QnXOdC.

[514] Forman EM et al, A randomized controlled effectiveness trial of acceptance and commitment therapy and cognitive therapy for anxiety and depression, Behavior Modification, 2007, PMID: 17932235.

[515] Derbyshire D, Should we be mindful of mindfulness?, The Guardian, 2014, http://goo.gl/tl69GW.

[516] Stange J et al, Mindfulness-Based Cognitive Therapy for Bipolar Disorder: Effects on Cognitive Functioning, J Psychiatr Pract. 2011, PMCID: PMC3277324.

[517] Parswani M et al, Mindfulness-based stress reduction program in coronary heart disease: A randomized control trial, Int'l J of Yoga, 2013, PMCID: PMC3734636.

[518] Williams JM et al, Mindfulness-based cognitive therapy (MBCT) in bipolar disorder: Preliminary evaluation of immediate effects on between-episode functioning, J of Affective Disorders, 2007, PMCID: PMC2881943.

[519] Ives-Deliperi VL et al, The effects of mindfulness-based cognitive therapy in patients with bipolar disorder: A controlled functional MRI investigation, J of Affective Disord, 2013, PMID: 23790741.

[520] Segal ZV et al, Mindfulness-based cognitive therapy for depression Washington, D.C., Amer Psychol Assoc, 2005.

[521] Chiesa A et al, A systematic review of neurobiological and clinical features of mindfulness meditations, Psychological Medicine, 2010, PMID: 19941676.

[522] Centre for Suicide Research, University of Oxford, Mindfulness Based Cognitive Therapy and the prevention of relapse in depression, http://goo.gl/Kn4vij.

[523] Lu S, Mindfulness holds promise for treating depression, Amer Psychological Assoc, 2015, http://goo.gl/AyWV7V.

[524] Knouse LE et al, Recent developments in the psychosocial treatment of adult ADHD, Expert Rvw of Neurotherapeutics, 2008.

[525] Albert Ellis Institute, FAQs of REBT, www.rebt.org/public/rebt.html.

[526] Sturmey P, Behavioral activation is an evidence-based treatment for depression, Behav Modif. 2009, PMID: 19933444.

[527] Richards D et al, Cost and Outcome of Behavioural Activation versus Cognitive Behavioural Therapy for Depression (COBRA): a randomised, controlled, non-inferiority trial, Lancet, 2016, http://goo.gl/yTbu2o.

[528] Satterfield J, Cognitive-Behavioral Therapy for Depression in an Older Gay Man: A Clinical Case Study, Cogn Behav Pract. 2010, PMCID: PMC3494402.

[529] Cribbet MR et al, Cognitive Behavioral Therapy for Insomnia Case Study and Commentary, JCOM 2013, http://goo.gl/BNbzyp.

[530] University of Exeter. "Depression Treatment: Mindfulness-based Cognitive Therapy As Effective As Anti-depressant Medication, Study Suggests." ScienceDaily, 2 December 2008., http://goo.gl/Da1ma6.

[531] Grant PM et al, Successfully breaking a 20-year cycle of hospitalizations with recovery-oriented cognitive therapy for schizophrenia, Psychological Services, 2014, PMID: 24079355.

[532] NAMI, www.nami.org, Personal Stories, 31 Stories, 31 Days; (a): Nathan Scruggs, May 29, 2015, http://goo.gl/nUKB4B, (b) Herb Cotner, 5/19/2015, http://goo.gl/bhpKuA, (c) Yashi's Story 11/26/13, https://goo.gl/49RPjx, (d) Recovering from Schizophrenia and OCD 4/24/15 https://goo.gl/WUVFPN, (e) Personal Stories - How To Love Someone With A Mental Illness, 3/4/15, https://goo.gl/Eiy3lp, (f) Eric's Story, 12/3/13, https://goo.gl/RQcyYY.

[533] NAMI, Peer-to-Peer training overview, http://goo.gl/OrM8sw.

[534] See www.NAMI.org.

[535] Dalgard O, A randomized controlled trial of a psychoeducational group program for unipolar depression in adults in Norway, Clinical Practice and Epidemiology in Mental Health, 2006, PMCID: PMC1538590.

[536] Miller W, Tip 35: Enhancing Motivation for Change in Substance Abuse Treatment: Treatment Improvement Protocol (TIP) Series 35, US Dept of Health and Human Services, 1999, http://goo.gl/7IVUvF.

[537] Noonan WC et al, Motivational interviewing, J of Substance Misuse. 1997, http://goo.gl/xeu7Kj.

[538] Rusch N et al, Movitational Interviewing to Improve Insight and Treatment Adherence in Schizophrenia, Psychiatr Rehabil J. 2002, PMID: 12171279, http://goo.gl/TbFvHD.

[539] Westra H et al, Adding a Motivational Interviewing Pretreatment to Cognitive Behavioral Therapy for Generalized Anxiety Disorder: A Preliminary Randomized Controlled Trial, J Anxiety Disord. 2009, PMCID: PMC2760690.

[540] Westra H et al, Integrating Motivational Interviewing With Cognitive-Behavioral Therapy for Severe Generalized Anxiety Disorder: An Allegiance-Controlled Randomized Clinical Trial, J of Consulting and Clinical Psychology, 2016, https://goo.gl/xljZxQ.

[541] Bruke B, The Efficacy of Motivational Interviewing: A Meta-Analysis of Controlled Clinical Trials, Journal of Consulting and Clinical Psychology, 2003, PMID: 14516234, http://goo.gl/V2kGOB.

[542] Knekt P et al, Randomized trial on the differences of long and short-term psychodynamic psychotherapy and solution-focused therapy on psychiatric symptoms during a 3-year follow-up, Psychological Med, 2006.

[543] Jakes SC, The effect of different components of psychological therapy on people with delusions: Five experimental single cases, Clinical Psychology and Psychotherapy, 2003, http://goo.gl/gyCQdA.

[544] Shedler J, The Efficacy of Psychodynamic Psychotherapy, American Psychologist, 2010, http://goo.gl/4iYw7B.

[545] Leichsenring F et al, Short-term psychodynamic psychotherapy and cognitive-behavioural therapy in generalised anxiety disorder: A randomised, controlled trial, American Journal of Psychiatry, 2009.

[546] Driessen E et al, The efficacy of short-term psychodynamic psychotherapy for depression: A meta-analysis, Clin Psychol Rev. 2010, PMID: 19766369.

[547] Maina G et al, Brief dynamic therapy combined with pharmacotherapy in the treatment of major depressive disorder: Long-term results, Journal of Affective Disorders, 2009, PMID: 18728001.

[548] National Institute for Clinical Excellence, Clinical guidelines for the management of anxiety: Panic disorder (with or without agoraphobia) and generalised anxiety disorder, 2004.

[549] Izquierdo de Santiago A., Hypnosis for schizophrenia, Cochrane Database of Systematic Reviews, 2007.

[550] Izquierdo de Santiago A, Hypnosis for schizophrenia, Cochrane Collaboration, http://goo.gl/sHq2kD.

[551] Sturt J et al, Neurolinguistic programming: a systematic review of the effects on health outcomes, Br J Gen Pract. 2012, PMCID: PMC3481516.

552 Genser_Medlitsch M, et al, Does Neuro-Linguistic psychotherapy have effect? TZ-NLP, Wiederhofergasse, Wien, Austria, 1997.
553 Karunaratne M, Neuro-linguistic programming and application in treatment of phobias, Complementary Therapies in Clinical Practice, 2010, http://goo.gl/NyBUci.
554 Muss D, A new technique for treating post-traumatic stress disorder, British J Clin Psychol, 1991, PMID: 2021791.
555 Allen K, An investigation of the effectiveness of neuro linguistic programming procedures in treating snake phobias, Dissertation Abstracts International, 1982.
556 Lawn S et al, Working effectively with patients with comorbid mental illness and substance abuse: a case study using a structured motivational behavioural approach, BMJ Case Rep. 2009, PMCID: PMC3027853.
557 Ross K, Case Study Overcoming Depression with NLP, Fresh Ways Forward, http://goo.gl/ERu7SL, copied 9/3/15.
558 Howard P, A case study involving the use of Hypnotherapy for Anxiety, Surrey Institute of Clinical Hypnotherapy, 2011, http://goo.gl/yeDpAQ, copied 9/3/15.
559 Wikipedia, Peer Support Specialists, http://en.wikipedia.org/wiki/Peer_support_specialist.
560 Campbell, COSP Preliminary Findings 2004, as quoted in EVIDENCE-BASED SUPPORT FORTHE USE OF PEER SPECIALISTS, http://goo.gl/zAfGbd.
561 SAMHSA National consensus statement on mental health recovery, U.S. Department of Health and Human Services, Substance Abuse and Mental Health Services, 2004. Administration; Center for Mental Health Services, www.samhsa.gov.
562 Sells D et al, The treatment relationship in peer-based and regular case management services for clients with severe mental illness. Psychiatric Services, 2006.
563 Lloyd-Evans B et al, A systematic review and meta-analysis of randomised controlled trials of peer support for people with severe mental illness, BMC Psychiatry 2014, PMCID: 3933205.
564 Toseland RW et al, When to recommend group treatment: a review of the clinical and the research literature, Int'l J of Group Psychother, 1986, PMID: 3733290.
565 McDermut W et al, The efficacy of group psychotherapy for depression: a meta-analysis and review of the empirical research, 2001, Clinical Psychology: Science and Practice, http://goo.gl/1WflPa.
566 Davidson L et al, Peer support among persons with severe mental illnesses: a review of evidence and experience, World Psychiatry. 2012, PMCID: PMC3363389.
567 Houston, TK et al, Internet support groups for depression: a 1-year prospective cohort study. Amer J of Psychiatry, 2002, PMID: 12450957.
568 Andersson G, Internet-based self-help for depression: randomised controlled trial, BJ Psych, 2005, PMID: 16260822.
569 Medical News Today, Crisis Residential Facilities Healthier Than Psychiatric Hospitals? - Study Finds More Mental Health Improvements At Consumer-Managed Program, 2008, copied April 2014, http://goo.gl/wTr6AP.
570 Nusslock R, Interpersonal Social Rhythm Therapy (IPSRT) for Bipolar Disorder Review and Case Conceptualization, 2011, http://goo.gl/cSaL6p.
571 IPSRT.org, Current Research, copied 4/8/15 from https://www.ipsrt.org/currentResearch.
572 National Institute for Clinical Excellence, London: Author, Depression: The treatment and management of depression in adults NICE clinical guideline 90, 2009.
573 Feijo de Mello M et al, A systematic review of research findings on the efficacy of interpersonal therapy for depressive disorders, Eur Arch Psychiatry Clin Neurosci, 2005, PMID: 15812600, http://goo.gl/Hx2rPo.
574 Clark J, Improving care for people with serious mental illness, American Psychological Association, 2009, quoting Shirley M. Glynn, http://goo.gl/f9IsUD.
575 Miklowitz, as quoted in Family-Focused Therapy: Involving Families in Treatment Aids Bipolar Patients, Grinnell R, Psych Central, http://goo.gl/E7B3HF.
576 Miklowitz DJ, et al. Integrated family and individual therapy for bipolar disorder: results of a treatment development study. J of Clin Psych. 2003, PMID: 12633127.
577 Fiorentine R, After Drug Treatment: Are 12-Step Programs Effective in Maintaining Abstinence?, American J of Drug and Alcohol Abuse, 1999, PMID: 10078980.
578 Jacobs Y, What the Research Has Told Us About Peer-Run Respite Houses: The Second Story Story, Mad in America, 2015, https://goo.gl/GLJFPb.
579 Health Workforce Australia, Mental Health Peer Workforce Study, 2014, https://goo.gl/Qe28bX.
580 Bipolar UK, Bipolar Awareness Day, https://goo.gl/xTJc9h.
581 United Way of Central Indiana, FRIDAY SUCCESS STORY: HENDRICKS COUNTY RESIDENT MANAGES DEPRESSION, 2014, http://goo.gl/klmcED.
582 McGurk S et al, A Meta-Analysis of Cognitive Remediation in Schizophrenia, Am J Psych, 2007, PMCID: PMC3634703.
583 Hogarty G, Cognitive Enhancement Therapy for Schizophrenia Effects of a 2-Year Randomized Trial on Cognition and Behavior, JAMA Psych, 2004, PMID: 15351765.
584 Eack S, Cognitive enhancement therapy for early-course schizophrenia: effects of a two-year randomized controlled trial. Psychiatric Svcs, 2009, PMC3693549.
585 Hogarty G, A Memorial Tribute: Durability and Mechanism of Effects of Cognitive Enhancement Therapy, Psychiatric Services, 2006, http://goo.gl/9CxvDi.
586 Eack S, Cognitive Enhancement Therapy Protects Against Gray Matter Loss in Early Schizophrenia: Results From a Two-Year Randomized Controlled Trial, Arch General Psych, 2010, PMCID: PMC3741671.
587 Gonzalez R as quoted in "Improving Cognition in Schizophrenia" by Hisaho Blair, NAMI Advocate, 2013, http://goo.gl/ttB1QD.
588 McLean Hospital, Brain training shows promise for patients with bipolar disorder, ScienceDaily. ScienceDaily, 2017, https://goo.gl/bceFFj.
589 Center for Cognition and Recovery, web introduction, copied 2/15/2014 from http://goo.gl/oec8JJ.
590 American Music Therapy Association, Music Therapy in Mental Health– Evidence-Based Practice Support, http://www.musictherapy.org, copied 10/29/2013.
591 Talwar N et al, Music therapy for inpatients with schizophrenia: an exploratory, randomized, controlled trial. Br J Psychiatry 2006.
592 Van der Steen T et al, Music-based therapeutic interventions for people with dementia, Chochrane Library, 2017, http://goo.gl/6wVFka.
593 Maratos A et al, Music therapy for depression. Cochrane Database of Systematic Reviews 2008, http://goo.gl/fUUM9L.
594 Fancourt D et al, Effects of Group Drumming Interventions on Anxiety, Depression, Social Resilience and Inflammatory Immune Response among Mental Health Service Users, PLoS One. 2016, PMCID: PMC4790847.
595 Queen's University, Music therapy reduces depression in children, adolescents, ScienceDaily. 2014, http://goo.gl/Qmb0UB.
596 Crawford M, For people with bipolar disorder and other mental illnesses, evidence suggests the visual and performing arts can help enhance mental health, BMJ 2012, www.bmj.com/content/344/bmj.e846.
597 Pfennig A, The Diagnosis and Treatment of Bipolar Disorder, Dtsch Arztebl Int. Feb 110(6) 92-100.
598 Collingwood J, The Link Between Bipolar Disorder and Creativity, Psych Central, http://goo.gl/yKkm25.
599 Heenan D, Art as therapy: an effective way of promoting positive mental health?, Disability & Society, 2006, http://goo.gl/evtGEX.
600 Fanner D et al, Bibliotherapy for mental health service users Part 1: a systematic review, Health Information & Libraries Journal, 2008, http://goo.gl/jDTekd.
601 Largo-Marsh L et al, The effects of writing therapy in comparison to EMD/R on traumatic stress: The relationship between hypnotizability and client expectancy to outcome, Professional psychology, research and practice , 2002, http://goo.gl/CSxxIT.
602 Apodaca TR, A meta-analysis of the effectiveness of bibliotherapy for alcohol problems, Journal of Clinical Psychology, 2003, http://goo.gl/WLVaHc.
603 Ullrich P et al, Journaling about Stressful Events: Effects of Cognitive Processing and Emotional Events, University of Iowa, 2002.
604 Stone M, Journaling with clients, Journal of Individual Psychology, 1998.
605 Canada KE, Military veterans: Therapeutic journaling in a veterans treatment court, J of Poetry Therapy, 2015, http://goo.gl/o8shmj.
606 Bird K, Peer Outdoor Support Therapy (POST) for Australian Contemporary Veterans: A Review of the Literature, J Military and Vet Health, http://goo.gl/X7IlMT.
607 Scheinfeld D et al, Outward Bound Veterans, The therapeutic impact of Outward Bound for Veterans, http://goo.gl/xaMIGb.
608 Wikipedia, topic "Psychiatric Service Dogs", http://en.wikipedia.org/wiki/Psychiatric_service_dog.
609 Helpguide.org, The Therapeutic and Health Benefits of Pets, http://goo.gl/crZDL, copied 2/16/14.
610 Hundley J (1991), Pet Project: The use of pet facilitated therapy among the chronically mentally ill. J Psychosoc Nurs Ment Health Serv, PMID: 1920191.
611 Margariti A. An application of the Primitive Expression form of dance therapy in a psychiatric population. The Arts in Psychotherapy, 2012, http://goo.gl/prR8tD.
612 Pinniger R et al, Argentine tango dance compared to mindfulness meditation and a waiting-list control: A randomised trial for treating depression, Complementary Therapies in Medicine, 2012, PMID: 23131367.
613 Takahashi H. Effects of sports participation on psychiatric symptoms and brain activations during sports observation in schizophrenia, T Psyc, 2012, PMC3316153.
614 Xia J et al, Dance therapy for schizophrenia. Cochrane DataB Syst Rev, 2009, PMID: 24092546.
615 Grisolia C, Warrior Horses, Kentucky Monthly, October 10, 2012, http://goo.gl/HhRmvo.
616 Lipe A, Music Therapy in Alzheimer's Disease, American Music Therapy Association, http://goo.gl/gq7IPG.
617 NAMI, ADHD information, copied from http://goo.gl/ewOAKY, 4/8/15.
618 Listen and Learn Centre, http://goo.gl/oCAi90.
619 Yasuma F, Respiratory sinus arrhythmia: why does the heartbeat synchronize with respiratory rhythm?, Chest. 2004, PMID: 14769752.
620 Lehrer P, Heart rate variability biofeedback: how and why does it work?, Front Psychol. 2014, PMCID: PMC4104909.
621 Lofthouse N, A review of neurofeedback treatment for pediatric ADHD, J Atten Disord, 2012, PMID: 22090396.
622 Van Dongen-Boomsma M et al, A randomized placebo-controlled trial of electroencephalographic (EEG) neurofeedback in children with attention-deficit/hyperactivity disorder. J Clin Psychiatry, 2013, PMID: 24021501.
623 Arnold LE et al, EEG Neurofeedback for ADHD Double-Blind Sham-Controlled Randomized Pilot Feasibility Trial, J Atten Disord. 2013, PMID: 22617866.
624 Roome J et al, Reducing anxiety in gifted children by inducing relaxation, Roeper Review, 1985.
625 Fehring RJ, Effects of biofeedback-aided relaxation on the psychological stress symptoms of college students, Nursing Research, 1983, PMID: 6387631.

[626] Scott WC et al, Effects of an EEG biofeedback protocol on a mixed substance abusing population. Am J Drug Alcohol Abuse 2005, PMID: 16161729.
[627] Surmeli T, Schizophrenia and efficacy of qEEG-guided neurofeedback treatment, Clin EEG Neuro 2012, PMID: 22715481.
[628] Bolea AS. Neurofeedback Treatment of Cronic Inpatient Schizophrenia. Journal of Neurotherapy: Investigations in Neuromodulation, Neurofeedback and Applied Neuroscience, 2010, http://goo.gl/MxLI1R.
[629] Rocha N, Neurofeedback treatment to enhance cognitive performance in Schizophrenia. Porto, 2011.
[630] Pharr, O. M. The Use and Utility of EMG Biofeedback with Chronic Schizophrenic Patients. Biofeedback and Self-Regulation, 1989, PLENUM PRESS.
[631] Ghaziri J, Neurofeedback Training Induces Changes in White and Gray Matter, Clinical EEG and Neuroscience, 2013, http://goo.gl/Z7u5LC.
[632] Nauert R, Neurofeedback Trains Brain Waves, Restores Brain Function, Psych Central, 2012, http://goo.gl/QWH9SO.
[633] Larsen S et al, The LENS (Low Energy Neurofeedback System): A clinical outcomes study of one hundred patients at Stone Mountain Center, New York. Journal of Neurotherapy, 2006, https://goo.gl/xg1OH9.
[634] Nelson DV, Neurotherapy of Traumatic Brain Injury/Post-Traumatic Stress Symptoms in Vietnam Veterans, Mil Med. 2015, PMID: 26444476.
[635] DC Hammond, LENS Neurofeedback Treatment of Anger: Preliminary Reports, Journal of Neurotherapy, 2010, http://goo.gl/fwIWA1.
[636] Siepmann M et al, A Pilot Study on the Effects of Heart Rate Variability Biofeedback in Patients with Depression and in Healthy Subjects, Appl Psychophysiol Biofeedback, 2008, PMID: 18807175, http://goo.gl/xZopWf.
[637] Gevirtz R et al, Psychophysiologic treatment of chronic low back pain. Prof. Psychol. Res. Pract, 1996.
[638] Gevirtz R et al, Heart Rate Variability Biofeedback in the Treatment of Trauma Symptoms, Biofeedback, https://goo.gl/vaKclh.
[639] Thomas J, Treatment of Chronic Anxiety Disorder with Neurotherapy: A Case Study, Journal of Neurotherapy, 1997.
[640] McLay R et al, Use of a Portable Biofeedback Device to Improve Insomnia in a Combat Zone, a Case Report, Appl Psychophyysiol Biofeedback, 2009, PMID: 19655243, https://goo.gl/KYPO9v.
[641] Cripe CT, Effective Use of LENS Unit as an Adjunct to Cognitive Neuro-Developmental Training, J or Neurotherapy, 2008, http://goo.gl/9ecnOl.
[642] Integral Health, Accuracy of nurses' perceptions of voice hearing and psychiatric symptoms, Journal of Advanced Nursing, 2007, http://goo.gl/udRzdt.
[643] [1] Read J et al, Child Maltreatment and Psychosis: A Return to a Genuinely Integrated Bio-Psycho-Social Model. Clinical, 2008, Clinical Schizophrenia, https://goo.gl/nMLrx4; [2] Shevlin et al, Cumulative Traumas and Psychosis: an Analysis of the National Comorbidity Survey and the British Psychiatric Morbidity Survey, Schizophr Bull. 2008, PMCID: PMC2632373; [3] Read J, 2013, Childhood Adversity and Psychosis: From Heresy to Certainty, https://goo.gl/5LYCQA; [4] Read J, Childhood trauma, psychosis and schizophrenia: a literature review with theoretical and clinical implications, Acta Psychiatr Scand. 2005, PMID: 16223421.
[644] Dykshoorn K, Trauma-related obsessive-compulsive disorder: a review, Health Psychol Behav Med. 2014, PMCID: PMC4346088.
[645] Corstens, D., May, R. & Longden, E. (2011). Talking with voices. Copied Dec 2014 from http://goo.gl/EtDkfX.
[646] Corstens D et al, Talking with voices: Exploring what is expressed by the voices people hear, Psychosis: Psychological, Social and Integrative Approaches. Advance online publication, 2011.
[647] Seikkula J, The Open Dialog Approach to Acute Psychosis Its Poetics and Micropolitics, Fam Proc, 2003, PMID: 14606203.
[648] Dialog Practice, www.dialogicpractice.net/open-dialogue%E2%84%A0/, copied 10/29/2013.
[649] SEIKKULA J et al, Five-year experience of first-episode nonaffective psychosis in open-dialogue approach: Treatment principles, follow-up outcomes, and two case studies, Psychotherapy Research, 2006, https://goo.gl/7g4N56.
[650] Steingard S, Antipsychotics: Short and Long-Term Effects, Mad In America Education, video #3, copied 1/27/17, https://goo.gl/Iix6s4.
[651] Gordon C et al, Adapting Open Dialogue for Early-Onset Psychosis Into the U.S. Health Care Environment: A Feasibility Study, Psychiatry Online, 2016, https://goo.gl/L6yGQB.
[652] Mosher L, Soteria and Other Alternatives to Acute Psychiatric Hospitalization A Personal and Professional Review, 1999, THE JOURNAL OF NERVOUS AND MENTAL DISEASE, PMID: 10086470, https://goo.gl/jyvje1.
[653] Shergill SS et al, Auditory Hallucinations: a review of psychological treatments, Schizophr Res, 1998, PMID: 9720119.
[654] Sokolov, A.N. Inner Speech and Thought. New York: Plenum Press, 1972
[655] Pitner R, Inner Speech during silent reading, Psychol New, 1913.
[656] Bick PA et al, Auditory hallucinations and subvocal speech in schizophrenic patients, Am J Psych, 1987, PMID: 3812794.
[657] Green MF, Subvocal Activity and Auditory Halluinations: Clues for Behavioral Treatments?,Schizophrenia Bulletin, 1990, PMID: 2077639, http://goo.gl/2j2oHr.
[658] Romme AJ et . al., Hearing Voices, Schizophrenia Bulletin, 1989, http://goo.gl/fqr7M1.
[659] Kaneko Y. Two cases of intractable auditory hallucination successfully treated with sound therapy, International Tinnitus Journal 2010, PMID: 21609910.
[660] Johnston O, The efficacy of using a personal stereo to treat auditory hallucinations. Behav Modif 2002, PMID: 12205826.
[661] Mallya AR, Radio in the treatment of auditory hallucinations. Am J Psychiatry 1983, PMID: 6614254.
[662] Bagul C et al, Effects of Coping Strategies on Chronic Drug Resistant Auditory Hallucinations in Schizophrenia: A Cross Over Study, Indian Journal of Occupational Therapy, 2012, http://goo.gl/FaE6T1.
[663] Ng Petrus, Recovering from Hallucinations: A Qualitative Study of Coping with Voices Hearing of People with Schizophrenia in Hong Kong, The Scientific World Journal, 2012, http://goo.gl/FRzTXl.
[664] Haddock G et al, A comparison of the long-term effectiveness of distraction and focusing in the treatment of auditory hallucinations, Br J Med Psychol, 1998, PMID: 9733427.
[665] Brauser D, Novel 'Avatar Therapy' May Silence Voices in Schizophrenia, Medscape Med News, 2014, http://goo.gl/e3QHoN.
[666] Leff J, Avatar therapy for persecutory auditory hallucinations: What is it and how does it work?, Psychosis: Psychological, Social and Integrative Approaches, 2014, PMCID: PMC4066885.
[667] Leff J et al, Computer-assisted therapy for medication-resistant auditory hallucinations: proof-of-concept study, British J of Psychiatry Jun 2013, PMID: 23429202.
[668] Pinto MD et al, Avatar-Based Depression Self-Management Technology: Promising Approach to Improve Depressive Symptoms Among Young Adults, Appl Nurs Res. 2013, PMCID: PMC3551988.
[669] Burton C, Pilot randomised controlled trial of Help4Mood, an embodied virtual agent-based system to support treatment of depression, J OF TELEMEDICINE AND TELECARE, 2015, https://goo.gl/AXjKFI.
[670] Ness T, Compassion and the Voice of the Tormentor, Mad in America, 2015, http://goo.gl/ehKYQ2.
[671] Longden E et al, Assessing the impact and effectiveness of Hearing Voices Network self-help groups, CMH Journal, 2017, PMID: 28638952.
[672] Waters F, Auditory Hallucinations in Psychiatric Illness, Psychiatric Times, 2010, http://goo.gl/L0qNWR.
[673] Coffey M et al, 'You don't talk about the voices': voice hearers and community mental health nurses talk about responding to voice hearing experiences, Journal of Clinical Nursing, 2008, PMID: 18482121.
[674] Lysaker, PH et al, Narrative enrichment in the psychotherapy for persons with schizophrenia: A single case study. Issues in Mental Health Nursing, 2006, PMID: 16484168.
[675] Favrod, J et al, Improving insight into delusions: A pilot study of metacognitive training for patients with schizophrenia, Journal of Advanced Nursing, 2011, PMID: 20955184.
[676] Jørgensen R et al, Effects on cognitive and clinical insight with the use of Guided Self-Determination in outpatients with schizophrenia: A randomized open trial, Eur Psychiatry. 2015, PMID: 25601635.
[677] Gavie J, The future of lucid dreaming treatment Commentary on "The neurobiology of consciousness: Lucid dreaming wakes up" by J. Allan Hobson, nternational Journal of Dream Research, 2010, https://goo.gl/rU34cg.
[678] EUROPEAN SCIENCE FOUNDATION, New links between lucid dreaming and psychosis could revive dream therapy in psychiatry, 2009, http://goo.gl/1xc6GE.
[679] Bourke P et al, Spontaneous lucid dreaming frequency and waking insight, Dreaming, 2014, http://goo.gl/pYmRgw.
[680] Brylowski A, Lucid dreaming as a treatment for nightmares in posttraumatic stress of Vietna combat veterans, presented at the Southern Association for Research in Psychiatry meeting, Tampa, FL, 1991.
[681] Khodarahimi, S, Satiation therapy and exposure response prevention in the treatment of obsessive compulsive disorder, J of Contemporary Psychotherapy. 2009, http://goo.gl/n8D7eY.
[682] Simpson HD et al, A randomized controlled trial of cognitive-behavioral therapy for augmenting pharmacotherapy in obsessive-compulsive disorder, Amer J of Psychiatry, 2008, PMCID: PMC3945728.
[683] Foa E, et al, Effective Treatments for PTSD. NY: The Guilford Press; 2000.
[684] Foa, EB et al, Treatment of posttraumatic stress disorder in rape victims: A comparison between cognitive-behavioral procedure and counseling, Journal of Consulting and Clinical Psychology, 1991.
[685] Davis JL, Treating Post-Trauma Nightmares: A Cognitive Behavioral Approach, Springer Publishing Co.
[686] Davis JL, Physiological Predictors of Response to Exposure, Relaxation, and Rescripting Therapy for Chronic Nightmares in a Randomized Clinical Trial, J Clin Sleep Med. 2011, PMCID: PMC3227708.

[687] Rizzo A et al, Virtual Reality Applications to Address the Wounds of War, Psychiatric Annals, 2013.

[688] Rizzo A et al, Virtual Iraq/Afghanistan: development and early evaluation of a virtual reality exposure therapy system for combat-related PTSD. Ann N Y Acad Sci. 2010.

[689] Emmelkamp P et al, Virtual reality treatment in acrophobia: A comparison with exposure in vivo, Cyberpsychology Behav, 2001, PMID: 11710257.

[690] Vincelli M et al, Experiential cognitive therapy in the treatment of panic disorders with agoraphobia: a controlled study, Cyberpsychology and Behav, 2003, PMID: 12855090.

[691] EMDR Institute, Inc., What is EMDR?, http://www.emdr.com/general-information/what-is-emdr.html.

[692] Bisson, J, Psychological treatment of post-traumatic stress disorder (PTSD), 2005, Cochrane DB Sys Rev, http://goo.gl/aMvhCi.

[693] Seidler GH, Comparing the efficacy of EMDR and trauma-focused cognitive-behavioral therapy in the treatment of PTSD: a meta-analytic study, Psychol Med, 2006, PMID: 16740177.

[694] Van den Berg DP et al, Treating trauma in psychosis with EMDR: a pilot study, J Behav Ther Exp Psychiatry. 2012, PMID: 21963888.

[695] Brom D et al, Somatic Experiencing for Posttraumatic Stress Disorder: A Randomized Controlled Outcome Study, J Trauma Stress. 2017, PMCID: PMC5518443.

[696] Kingdon D et al, Schizophrenia and Borderline Personality Disorder Similarities and Differences in the Experience of Auditory Hallucinations, Paranoia, and Childhood Trauma, Journal of Nervous and Mental Disease, 2010, PMID: 20531117, http://goo.gl/JwRwQ0.

[697] Larkin W, Childhood trauma and psychosis: evidence, pathways, and implications, J Postgrad Med. 2008, PMID: 18953148.

[698] Goff DC et al, Self-reports of childhood abuse in chronically psychotic patients, Psychiatry Res. 1991, PMID: 1862163.

[699] Read J, Hallucinations, delusions, and thought disorder among adult psychiatric inpatients with a history of child abuse, Psychiatr Serv. 1999, PMID: 10543857.

[700] Andrew EM et al, The relationship between trauma and beliefs about hearing voices: a study of psychiatric and non-psychiatric voice hearers. Psychol Med, 2008, PMID: 18177529.

[701] Cutajar MC, Schizophrenia and Other Psychotic Disorders in a Cohort of Sexually Abused Children, Arch Gen Psychiatry. 2010, PMID: 21041612, http://goo.gl/EWj2BV.

[702] Read J, Childhood trauma, psychosis and schizophrenia: a literature review with theoretical and clinical implications, Acta Psychiatr Scand. 2005, PMID: 16223421.

[703] Read J et al, Psychological trauma and psychosis: another reason why people diagnosed schizophrenic must be offered psychological therapies, J Am Acad Psychoanal Dyn Psychiatry. 2003, http://goo.gl/49L6E8.

[704] Ragins M, Talking About Psychosis, Part 1: Why Do It?, www.MadInAmerica.com, 2014, http://goo.gl/P5u5pG.

[705] Hilpern K, How I tamed the voices in my head, Intervoice, 2007, https://goo.gl/IdJQHg.

[706] Science Daily, Voices in people's heads more complex than previously thought, 2015, http://goo.gl/19dikO.

[707] Wesson M et al, Intervening Early With EMDR on Military Operations, Journal of EMDR Practice and Research, 2009, http://goo.gl/rMvVSG.

[708] Rizzo A et al, Virtual Reality Exposure Therapy for Combat-Related PTSD, in the book Post-Traumatic Stress Disorder, 2009, http://goo.gl/YBSCxQ.

[709] Jørgensen R et al, Changes in Persistent Delusions in Schizophrenia Using Guided Self-Determination: A Single Case Study, Issues in Mental Health Nursing,2012, PMID: 22545636, http://goo.gl/FLMVyo.

[710] Haverkos H, Acupuncture treatment for drug abuse: a technical review, JOURNAL OF SUBSTANCE ABUSE TREATMENT, 1993, PMID: 8308942.

[711] Luo H et al, Electroacupuncture vs. amitriptyline in the treatment of depressive states, J Tradit Med, 1985.

[712] Mischoulon D. A pilot study of acupuncture monotherapy in patients with major depressive disorder. J Affect Disord 2012, PMID: 22521855.

[713] Cheng J, Electro-acupuncture versus sham electro-acupuncture for auditory hallucinations in patients with schizophrenia: a randomized controlled trial, 2009, PMID: 19470551.

[714] Shi ZX, Observation on the curative effect of 120 cases of auditory hallucination treated with auricular acupuncture, 1989, PMID: 2615449.

[715] Lee MS, Acupuncture for schizophrenia: a systematic review and meta-analysis, Intl J Clinical Prac, 2009, PMID: 19832819, http://goo.gl/tvsse7.

[716] Lio ZZ et al, Therapeutic effect of He-Ne laser irraqditation of point erman in schizophrenic auditory hallucination – a clinical assessment, Journal of Traditional Chinese Medicine, 1986.

[717] Jia YK t al, A study on the treatment of schizophrenia with He-Ne laser irradiation of acupoint, J of Traditional Chinese Med, 1987.

[718] Engel CC et al, Randomized effectiveness trial of a brief course of acupuncture for post-traumatic stress disorder, Med Care, 2014, PMID: 25397825.

[719] Agelink MW et al, Does acupuncture influence the cardiac autonomic nerous system in patients with minor depression or anxiety disorders? Fortschr Neurol Psychiatr, 2003.

[720] Arranz L et al, Effect of acupuncture treatment on the immune function impairment found in anxious women, Am J Chin Med. 2007, PMID: 17265549.

[721] Samuels N et al, Acupuncture for psychiatric illness: a literature review Behav Med. 2008, PMID: 18682338.

[722] Xu G, Forty-five cases of insomnia treated by acupuncture, Shanghai J of Acupuncture and Moxibustion, 1997.

[723] Cao H et al, Acupuncture for Treatment of Insomnia: A Systematic Review of Randomized Controlled Trials, J Altern Complement Med. 2009, PMC3156618.

[724] Shi ZX, Tan MZ, An analysis of the therapeutic effect of acupuncture treatment in 500 cases of schizophrenia, J Tradit Chin Med. 1986, PMID: 3773564.

[725] Spence et al, Acupuncture Increases Nocturnal Melatonin Secretion and Reduces Insomnia and Anxiety:A Preliminary Report, J Neuropsychiatry Clin Neurosci. 2004, PMID: 14990755.

[726] Bullock, M.L., Culliton, P.D., & Olander, R.T. (1989). Controlled trial of acupuncture for severe recidivist alcoholism. The Lancet, PMID: 2567439.

[727] Avants SK et al, A randomized controlled trial of auricular acupuncture for cocaine dependence. Arch Intern Med. 2000, PMID: 10927727.

[728] Behere RV et al, Complementary and alternative medicine in the treatment of substance use disorders–a review of the evidence, DRUG AND ALCOHOL REVIEW, 2009, PMID: 21462415.

[729] Astin J et al, A review of the incorporation of complementary and alternative medicine by mainstream physicians, Arch Intern Med, 1998, PMID: 9827781.

[730] Shore, AG, Long term effects of energetic healing on symptoms of psychological depression and self-perceived stress. Alternative Therapies in Health and Medicine, 2004, PMID: 15154152.

[731] Diaz-Rodriguez L et al, Immediate effects of Reiki on heart rate variability, cortisol levels, and body temperature in health care professionals with burnout. Biol Res Nurs, 2011. Retrieved June 23, 2012, from http://www.centerforreikiresearch.org.

[732] Bier D, Reiki Healing and Mental Health: What the Research Shows, Psych Central, copied 4/9/15 from http://goo.gl/vbpyyi.

[733] Baldwin AL et al, Reiki improves heart rate homeostasis in laboratory rats, Journal of Alternative and Complementary Medicine, 2008, Retrieved June 23, 2012, from http://www.centerforreikiresearch.org.

[734] Jain S et al, Healing Touch with Guided Imagery for PTSD in returning active duty military: a randomized controlled trial, Mil Med. 2012, PMID: 23025129.

[735] Church D, Psychological trauma symptom improvement in veterans using emotional freedom techniques: a randomized controlled trial, J Nerv Ment Dis, 2013, PMID: 23364126.

[736] Karatzias T, A controlled comparison of the effectiveness and efficiency of two psychological therapies for posttraumatic stress disorder, J Nerv Ment Dis, 2011, PMID: 21629014.

[737] Church D et al, Epigenetic Effects of PTSD Remediation in Veterans Using Clinical Emotional Freedom Techniques A Randomized Controlled Pilot Study, Am J Health Promot. 2016, PMID: 27520015.

[738] Sakai CS et al, Treatment of PTSD in Rwandan genocide survivors using Thought Field Therapy. Int J Emergency MH, 2010, https://goo.gl/i8ESYT.

[739] Feinstein D, Acupoint stimulation in treating psychological disorders: evidence of efficacy, Review Gen Psychology, 2012, https://goo.gl/8VeySy.

[740] Church D et al, The effect of emotional freedom techniques on stress biochemistry: a randomized controlled trial, J Nerv Ment Dis. 2012, PMID: 22986277.

[741] McCaslin D, A review of efficacy claims of energy therapy, Psychotherapy: Theory, Research, Practice, Training, 2009, https://goo.gl/eTW6Rr.

[742] Merrell WC et al, Homeopathy, Med Clin North Am, 2002.

[743] Ullman D, Homeopathic Family Medicine: Integrating the Science and Art of Natural Health Care, Homeopathic Educational Services, 2002.

[744] Bonne O et al, A randomized double-blind placebo controlled study of classical homeopathy in generalized anxiety disorder, J Clin Psych, 2003, PMID: 12716269.

[745] Mathie RT et al, Outcomes from homeopathic prescribing in medical practice: a prospective, research-targeted, pilot study. Homeopathy. 2006, PMID: 17015190.

[746] Faculty of Homeopathy, RANDOMISED CONTROLLED TRIALS, http://goo.gl/UirW2e.

[747] Bragdon E, Spiritism and Mental Health, Singing Dragon, 2011, http://goo.gl/K9Saqb.

[748] Lucchetti G et al, Spiritist Psychiatric Hospitals in Brazil: Integration of Conventional Psychiatric Treatment and Spiritual Complementary Therapy, Cult Med Psychiatry, 2011, http://goo.gl/uUKMkU.

[749] Herve I MD et al, 2003, referenced by Emma Bragdon in 10 Ways to Add Spirituality to Mental Health Care and Why, 2014, www.imhu.org.

[750] Miller T et al, Measure of Significance of Holotropic Breathwork in the Development of Self-Awareness, J Altern Complement Med. 2015, PMCID: PMC4677109.

[751] McCaslin DL, A review of efficacy claims in energy psychology. Psychotherapy, PMID: 22122622.

[752] Veterans Stress Project, http://stressproject.org/.

[753] Nicosia, G. (2008) World Trade Center Tower 2 Survivor: EP Treatment of Long-term PTSD: A case study. Presented at the ACEP Association for Comprehensive Energy Psychology conference, Baltimore, May. Gregory J. Nicosia, PhD

[754] Bosch P, A case study on acupuncture in the treatment of schizophrenia, Acupunct Med. 2014, PMID: 24614531.

[755] Acupuncture Without Borders, Military Stress Recovery (Veterans Project), http://goo.gl/wgcqAP.

[756] Golden G, The Lasting Effects of Using Auricular Acupuncture to Treat Combat-related PTSD: A Case Study American Acupuncturist Summer 2012, http://goo.gl/RQCjov.

[757] Bragdon E, Spiritism and Mental Health, Singing Dragon, 2012.

[758] Awad AG, The Thyroid and the Mind and Emotions/Thyroid Dysfunction and Mental Disorders, Thyrobulletin, 2000, http://goo.gl/iPkUsh.

[759] Wittenborn JR et al, Niacin in the long term treatment of schizophrenia, Arch Gen Psychiatry, 1973, PMID: 4569673, http://goo.gl/uet77j.

[760] Walsh Institute, www.walshinstitute.org, bio at http://www.walshinstitute.org/william-j-walsh-phd.html.

[761] **Note**: Mensah A, Shizophrenia: an Orthomolecular Approach to rebalancing brain and body chemistry, a presentation from a video, copied 2014, http://www.mensahmedical.com/videolibrary.html. Dana Zingrone of Mensah Medical indicates in a 10/28/2014 email, "Our physicians rely on the extensive clinical research conducted by William J. Walsh, PhD, at the Walsh Research Institute (Naperville, IL). Dr. Walsh's schizophrenia open-label outcome study included more than 3,600 patients diagnosed with schizophrenia. These schizophrenic patients were being treated at the Pfeiffer Treatment Center (now closed) by founder and president Dr. William J. Walsh. Drs. Mensah and Bowman served as physicians at the Pfeiffer Treatment Center… ". Also see Walsh's book, Nutrient Power.

[762] Glugston R et al, The Adverse Effects of Alcohol on Vitamin A Metabolism, Nutrients. 2012, PMCID: PMC3367262.

[763] Pfeiffer C, Nutrition and Mental Illness, an Orthomolecular approach to balancing body chemistry, Healing Arts Press, 1987.

[764] Mayo-Smith MF et al, Management of Alcohol Withdrawal Delirium An Evidence-Based Practice Guideline, Arch Intern Med. 2004, PMID: 15249349, http://goo.gl/BWTFLD.

[765] George S et al, A 3 year case study of alcohol related psychotic disorders at Hospital Seremban, Medical J of Malaysia, 1998, PMID: 10968157.

[766] Miyake Y et al, Maternal and Child Health Study Group. Dietary folate and vitamins B12, B6 and B2 intake and the risk of postpartum depression in Japan: the Osaka maternal and child health study, J Affect Disord, 2006, PMID: 16815556.

[767] Walsh W, Advanced Nutrient Therapies for Bipolar Disorders with Dr. Walsh, Natural Treatments for Bipolar, video, https://goo.gl/l6h8Y5.

[768] Kleijnen J et al, Niacin and vitamin B6 in mental functioning: a review of controlled trials in humans, Biological Psychiatry, 1991, PMID: 1828703.

[769] Hawkins DR et al, Orthomolecular psychiatry: niacin and megavitamin therapy. Psychosomatics 1970, PMID: 5470684.

[770] Hoffer A, Negative and Positive Side Effects of Vitamin B3, Journal of Orthomolecular Medicine, 2003, http://goo.gl/n40RbX.

[771] Morris MC et al, Dietary niacin and the risk of incident Alzheimer's disease and of cognitive decline. J Neurol Neurosur Ps 2004, PMCID: PMC1739176.

[772] Smith RF, A five-year field trial of massive nicotinic acid therapy of alcoholics in Michigan, J Orthomolec Psych, 1974

[773] Prousky J, Niacinamide's Potent role in Alleviating Anxiety with its Benzodiazepine-like Properties: A Case Report, J Orthomolecular Medicine, 2004, http://goo.gl/AkCjOL

[774] Birkmayer JG, Coenzyme nicotinamide adenine dinucleotide: New therapeutic approach for improving dementia of the Alzheimer type, Ann Clin Lab, 1006, PMID: 8834355.

[775] Wyatt KM et al, Efficacy of vitamin B-6 in the treatment of premenstrual syndrome: systematic review. Bmj. 1999 May, PMCID: PMC27878.

[776] Bucci L, Pyridoxine and schizophrenia, Br J Psychiatry, 1973, PMID: 4714839.

[777] Sandyk R et al, Pyridoxine improves drug-induced parkinsonism and psychosis in a schizophrenic patient, Int J Neurosci, 1990, PMID: 2269609.

[778] Fredricks, R, Healing & Wholeness Complementary and Alternative Therapies for Mental Health, All Things Well Publications, 2008.

[779] Miller JW et al, Homocysteine, vitamin B6 and vascular disease in AD patients, Neurology, 2002, PMID: 12034781.

[780] Sun Y et al, Efficacy of multivitamin supplementation containing vitamins B6 and B12 and folic acid as adjunctive treatment with a cholinesterase inhibitor in Alzheimer's disease: a 26-week, randomized double-blind, placebo-controlled study in Taiwanese patients, Clin Ther, 2007, PMID: 18042476.

[781] Mock DM et al, Marginal biotin deficiency during normal pregnancy, Am J Clin Nutr, 2002, PMCID: PMC1426254.

[782] Chengappa KN. Inositol as add-on treatment for bipolar depression. Bipolar Disord , 2000, http://goo.gl/9ANNnb. Also see http://goo.gl/wRgWKY for a broader Inositol discussion.

[783] Benjamin J et al, Inositol treatment in psychiatry. Psychopharmacol Bull. 1995, PMID: 7675981.

[784] Levine J. Double-blind, controlled trial of inositol treatment of depression. Am J Psychiatry 1995, PMID: 7726322.

[785] Levine B et al, Double-blind, Placebo-controlled, Crossover Study of Inositol Treatment for Panic Disorder, American Journal of Psychiatry, 1995.

[786] Benjamin J et al, 1995. Double-blind, placebo-controlled, crossover trial of inositol treatment of panic disorder. Am J Psych.

[787] Fux M. Inositol treatment of obsessive-compulsive disorder. Am J Psychiatry 1996, PMID: 8780431.

[788] Palatnik, A. et al., Double-blind, controlled, crossover trial of inositol versus fluvoxamine for the treatment of panic disorder. J Clin Psychopharmacol, 2001, PMID: 11386498.

[789] Belmaker RH et al, Inositol in the Treatment of Psychiatric Disorders, in Natural Medications for Psychiatric Disorders: Considering the Alternatives, Lippincott, Williams and Wilkins, Philadelphia 2002/2008.

[790] Ding Y et al, Association of Folate Level in Blood with the Risk of Schizophrenia, Comb Chem High Throughput Screen. 2017, PMID: 28124599.

[791] Hill M et al, Folate supplementation in schizophrenia: a possible role for MTHFR genotype. Schizophr Res 2011, PMID: 21334854.

[792] Godfrey PS et al, Enhancement of recovery from psychiatric illness by methylfolate. Lancet. 1990, PMID: 1974941.

[793] Papakostas G, Serum Folate, Vitamin B12, and Homocysteine in Major Depressive Disorder, Part 2: Predictors of Relapse During the Continuation Phase of Pharmacotherapy, J Clin Psychiatry, 2004, PMID: 15323595.

[794] Procter A, Enhancement of recovery from psychiatric illness by methylfolate, Br J Psych, 1991, PMID: 1773245.

[795] Papakostas GI. L-methylfolate as adjunctive therapy for SSRI-resistant major depression: results of two randomized, double-blind, parallel-sequential trials. Am J Psychiatry 2012, PMID: 23212058.

[796] Venkatasubramanian R. A randomized double-blind comparison of fluoxetine augmentation by high and low dosage folic acid in patients with depressive episodes. J Affective Disord 2013, PMID: 23507369.

[797] Hasanah CI et al, Reduced red-cell folate in mania. J Affect Disord. 1997, PMID: 9479613.

[798] Coppen A et al, Folic acid enhances lithium prophylaxis. J Affect Disord. 1986, PMID: 2939126.

[799] Weir DG et al, Microvascular disease and dementia in the elderly: are they related to hyperhomocysteinemia? Am J Cli9n Nutr, 2000, PMID: 10731489.

[800] Luchsinger JA et al, Relation of higher folate intake to lower risk of Alzheinmer's disease in the elderly, Arch Neurol, PMID: 17210813.

[801] Shen H et al, Dietary Folate Intake and Lung Cancer Risk in Former Smokers, Cancer Epidemiology Biomarkers & Prevention, 2003, PMID: 14578132.

[802] Edelman E, Natural Healing for Bipolar Disorder, Borage Books, 2009.

[803] Gilbody S et al, Methylenetetrahydrofolate reductase (MTHFR) genetic polymorphisms and psychiatric disorders: a HuGE review. Am J Epidemiol 2007, PMID: 17074966.

[804] Valizadeh M et al, Obsessive Compulsive Disorder as Early Manifestation of B12 Deficiency, Indian J Psychol Med. 2011, PMCID: PMC327150.

[805] Stabler SP et al, Megoblastic anemias. Cecil Textbook of Medicine. 22nd ed. 2004, as reference in Evatt M et al, Why Vitamin B12 Deficiency Should Be on Your Radar Screen.

[806] Syed EU. Vitamin B12 supplementation in treating major depressive disorder: a randomized controlled trial. Open Neuro J. 2013, PMCID: PMC3856388.

[807] Zhang Y et al, Decreased Brain Levels of Vitamin B12 in Aging, Autism and Schizophrenia, PLoS One. 2016, PMCID: PMC4723262.

[808] Brown HE et al, Vitamin Supplementation in the Treatment of Schizophrenia, CNS Drugs. 2014 PMCID: PMC4083629.

[809] Greenblatt J, Integrative Medicine for the Treatment of Obsessive Compulsive Disorder, Great Plains Laboratory, 2015, https://goo.gl/6HrqYW.

[810] Goggans FC, A case of mania secondary to vitamin B12 deficiency, Amer J of Psychiatry, 1984. PMID: 6691503.

[811] Ohta T et al, Treatment of persistent sleep-wak schedule disorders in adolescents and vitamin B12, Jpn J Psychiatr Neurol, 1991., PMID: 1759094.

[812] Chang HY et al, Effects of intravenously administered vitamin B12 on sleep in the rat, Physiol Behav , 1995, PMID: 7652019.

[813] Chase B, How B Vitamins Affect Your Sleep, Progressive Health, http://goo.gl/AJ5we3.

[814] Skarupski KA. 2010. Longitudinal association of vitamin B-6, folate, and vitamin B-12 with depressive symptoms among older adults over time. Amer J of Clinical Nutrition, 2010. PMCID: PMC2904034.

[815] Firth J et al, The effects of vitamin and mineral supplementation on symptoms of schizophrenia: a systematic review and meta-analysis. Psychological Med, 2017, https://goo.gl/NHe90Y.

[816] Amr M. Efficacy of vitamin C as an adjunct to fluoxetine therapy in pediatric major depressive disorder: a randomized, double-blind, placebo-controlled study. Nutr J 2013, PMCID: PMC3599706.

[817] Dakhale GN, Supplementation of Vitamin C with Atypical Antipsychotics Reduces Oxidative Stress and Improves the Outcome of Schizophrenia, Psychopharmacology 2005 SPRINGER-VERLAG, PMID: 16133138.

[818] Arvindakshan M et al, Supplementation with a combination ofN-3 fatty acidsand antioxidants (vitamins E and C) improvesthe outcome of schizophrenia, Schiz Res, 2003, https://goo.gl/AVtjwu.

[819] Beauclair L et al, An adjunctive role for ascorbic acid in the treatment of schizophrenia?, J Clin Psychopharmacol, 1987, PMID: 3624518.

[820] Naylor GJ, Vanadium and manic depressive psychosis, Nutr Health, 1984, PMID: 6443582.

[821] Naylor GJ et al, A possible aetiological factor in manic depressive illness, Psychol Med, 1981, PMID: 6791192.

[822] Kerr D et al, Associations between vitamin D levels and depressive symptoms in healthy young adult women, Psychiatry Res. 2015, PMID: 25791903.

[823] Shivakumar V et al, Serum vitamin D and hippocampal gray matter volume in schizophrenia, Psychiatry Res. 2015, PMID: 26163386.

[824] Hedelin M, et al. Dietary intake of fish, omega-3, omega-6 polyunsaturated fatty acids and vitamin D and the prevalence of psychotic-like symptoms in a cohort of 33,000 women from the general population. BMC Psychiatry. 2010, PMID: 20504323.

[825] McGrath, John, "Vitamin D Supplementation during the First Year of Life and Risk of Schizophrenia: A Finnish Birth Cohort Study" Schizo Res, 2004, PMID: 14984883.

[826] Zhu DM, High levels of vitamin D in relation to reduced risk of schizophrenia with elevated C-reavice protein, Psychiatry Res, 2015, PMID: 26106052.

[827] Parker G et al, 'D' for depression: any role for vitamin D? Acta Psychiatritrica Scandinavica, 2011, https://goo.gl/JmSNwM.

[828] Jorde R. Effects of vitamin D supplementation on symptoms of depression in overweight and obese subjects: randomized double blind trial. J Intern Med 2008, PMID: 18793245.

[829] Penckofer S, Vitamin D and Depression: Where is all the Sunshine?,Issues Ment Health Nurs. 2010, PMCID: PMC2908269.

[830] Mokry LE et al, Genetically decreased vitamin D and risk of Alzheimer disease, Neurology, 2016, https://goo.gl/MYRgEp.

[831] Humble M et al, Low serum levels of 25-hydroxyvitamin D (25-OHD) among psychiatric out-patients in Sweden: Relations with season, age, ethnic origin and psychiatric diagnosis. J Steroid Biochem Mol Biol. 2010, PMID: 20214992.

[832] Berkeley Wellness, Vitamin D: What's the Latest?, 2015, https://goo.gl/A3GzJL.

[833] Greenblatt J, Psychological Consequences of Vitamin D Deficiency, Psychology Today, https://goo.gl/5v5xVr.

[834] Maes M et al, Lower serum vitamin E concentrations in major depression, J Affective Disord, 2000, PMID: 10802134.

[835] Sano M et al, A controlled trial of selegiline, alpha-tocopherol or both as treatment for Alzheimer's Disease, N Engl J Med, 1997, PMID: 9110909.

[836] Lohr J, Vitamin E in the Treatment of Tardive Dyskinesia: The Possible Involvement of Free Radical Mechanisms, Schizophrenia Bulletin, 1988, PMID: 2904696.

[837] Fioravanti M et al, Cytidinediphosphocholine (CDP Choline) for Cognitive and Behavioural Disturbances Associated with Chronic Cerebral Disorders in the Elderly, Cochrane Database Syst. Rev, 2005, PMID: 15846601.

[838] Stoll AL et al, Choline in the treatment of rapid-cycling bipolar disorder: clinical and neurochemical findings in lithium-treated patients. Biol Psychiatry. 1996, PMID: 8874839.

[839] Cotroneo AM et al, Effectiveness and Safety of Citicoline in Mild Vascular Cognitive Impairment: The IDEALE Study Clin Interv Aging, 2013, PMCID: PMC3569046.

[840] Wignall ND et al, Citicoline in addictive disorders: a review of the literature, Amer J Drug and Alcohol Abuse, 2014, PMCID: PMC4139283.

[841] Secades JJ, CDP-choline: pharmacological and clinical review, Methods Find Exp Clin Pharmacol. 1995, PMID: 8709678.

[842] Benton D et al, Vitamin supplementation for 1 year improves mood. Neuropsychobiology, 1995, PMID: 7477807.

[843] Carroll D et al, The effects of an oral multivitamin combination with calcium, magnesium and zinc on psychological well-being in healthy young male volunteers: a double-blind placebo-controlled trial, Psychopharmacology, 2000, PMID: 10907676.

[844] Harris E et al, The effect of multivitamin supplementation on mood and stress in healthy older men, Hum Psychopharmacol. 2011, PMID: 22095836.

[845] Hawkins, D. R. "Orthomolecular Psychiatry: Niacin and Megavitamin Therapy." Psychosomatics, 1970, AMERICAN PSYCHIATRIC PUBLISHING, INC.

[846] Boittelle G et al, Results obtained with high doses of multivitamin perfusions as a treatment for chronic alcoholism, Ann Med Psychol, 1958, PMID: 13534105.

[847] Kampman KM et al, Open trials as a method of prioritizing medications for inclusion in controlled trials for cocaine dependence, Addic Behav, 1999, PMID: 10336110.

[848] Davidson JR. Effectiveness of chromium in atypical depression: a placebo-controlled trial. Biol Psychatry 2003, PMID: 12559660.

[849] Docherty JP. A double-blind, placebo-controlled, exploratory trial of chromium picolinate in atypical depression: effect on carbohydrate craving. J Psychiatr Pract 2005, PMID: 16184071.

[850] Linder MC, Biochemistry of Copper, Plenum Press, 1991.

[851] Pfeiffer C, Excess Copper as a Factor in Human Diseases, Jof Orthomolecular Medicine, 1987, http://goo.gl/tQlibJ.

[852] Morgan RF, Effect of copper deficiency on the concentrations of catecholamines and related enzyme activities in the rate brain, J Neurochem, 1977, http://goo.gl/QDoJMr.

[853] Rao TSS et al, Understanding nutrition, depression and mental illnesses, Indian J Psychiatry. 2008, PMCID: PMC2738337.

[854] Hunt J et al, Iron status and depression in premenopausal women: An MMPI study, Behavl Med, 1999, PMID: 10401535.

[855] Bear JL, et al, Maternal Iron Deficiency Anemia Affects Postpartum Emotions and Cognition, J Nutr, 2005, PMID: 15671224.

[856] Chen MH et al, Association between psychiatric disorders and iron deficiency anemia among children and adolescents: a nationwide population-based study, BMC Psychiatry, 2013, PMID: 23735056.

[857] Shaw W, LITHIUM DEFICIENCY: COMMON IN MENTAL ILLNESS AND SOCIAL ILLS, 2015, https://goo.gl/T8vMec.

[858] Greenblatt J, Lose Dose Lithium for the treatment of mood, behavioral, and cognitive disorders, a video, 2015, https://goo.gl/jfgJxV.

[859] Knudsen N et al, Lithium in Drinking Water and Incidence of Suicide: A Nationwide Individual-Level Cohort Study with 22 Years of Follow-Up, Int J Environ Res Public Health. 2017, PMCID: PMC5486313.

[860] Getz H, The Little Lauded Benefits of Lithium. Great Plains Laboratory, http://goo.gl/Q9NBYk.

[861] Fierro A, Natural low dose lithium supplementation in manic-depressive disease., Nutrition Perspect, 1988.

[862] Sun YR et al, Global grey matter volume in adult bipolar patients with and without lithium treatment: A meta-analysis, J Affect Disord. 2018, PMID: 28886501.

[863] Sartori SE, Lithium orotate in the treatment of alcoholism and related conditions, Alcohol. 1986, PMID: 3718672.

[864] Schrauzer GN, Effects of nutritional lithium supplementation on mood. A placebo-controlled study with former drug users, Biol Trace Elem Res, 1994, PMID: 7511924.

[865] Adams JB et al, Analyses of toxic metals and essential minerals in the hair of Arizona children with autism and associated conditions, and their mothers, Biol Trace Elem Res. 2006, PMID: 16845157.

[866] Great Plains Laboratory, Lithium Deficiency: Common in Mental Illness and Social Ills, http://goo.gl/HjJJu7.

[867] Mauer S et al, Standard and trace-dose lithium: A systematic review of dementia prevention and other behavioral benefits, Aust N Z J Psychiatry. 2014, PMID: 24919696, https://goo.gl/b8upE5.

[868] Nat'l Inst of Mental Hlth, Lithium Shows Promise Against Alzheimer's in Mouse Model, Nature 2003, http://goo.gl/JTJPtm.

[869] Gerhard T et al, Lithium treatment and risk for dementia in adults with bipolar disorder: population-based cohort study, Br J Psychiatry. 2015, PMID: 25614530.

[870] Nunes PV et al, Lithium and risk for Alzheimer's disease in elderly patients with bipolar disorder, Br J Psychiatry. 2007, PMID: 17401045.

[871] Greenblatt J, Magnesium: the missing ink in mental health?, 2016, Integrative Medicine for Mental Health, https://goo.gl/epKm3o.

[872] Swaminathan R, Magnesium Metabolism and its Disorders, Clin Biochem Rev. 2003, PMCID: PMC1855626.

[873] Derom ML. Magnesium and depression: a systematic review. Nutr Neurosci 2013, PMID: 23321048.

[874] T. S. Sathyanarayana Rao et al, Understanding nutrition, depression and mental illnesses, Indian Journal of Psychiatry, 2008, PMCID: PMC2738337.

[875] Chouinard G et al, A pilot study of magnesium aspartate hydrochloride (Magnesiocard) as a mood stabilizer for rapid cycling bipolar affective disorder patients. Prog Neuropsychopharm Biol Psych, 1990, PMID: 2309035.

[876] Giannini AJ et al, Magnesium oxide augmentation of verapamil maintenance therapy in mania. Psychiatry Res. 2000, PMID: 10699232.

[877] Heiden A et al. Treatment of severe mania with intravenous magnesium sulphate as a supplementary therapy, Psychiatry Res, 1999, PMID: 10708270.

[878] Weston P, Magnesium as a sedative, Read at the 77th annual meeting of the American Medico-Psychological Association, now the Amer Psychiatric Assoc, 1921.

[879] Memis D, Comparison of sufentanil with sufentanil plus magnesium sulphate for sedation in the intensive care unit using bispectral index, Crit Care. 2003, PMCID: PMC270723.

[880] Durlach J, Clinical aspects of chronic magnesium deficiency, in MS Seeling, Ed Magnesium in Health and Disease. New York, Spectrum Publications, 1980

[881] Romani A, Magnesium homeostasis and alcohol consumption, Magnesium Res 2008, PMID: 19271417.

[882] Altura B et al, Association of alcohol in brain injury, headaches and stroke with brain-tissue and serum levels of ionized magnesium: A review of recent findings and mechanisms of action, Alcoholism, 1999, PMID: 10548155.

[883] Margolin A et al, A preliminary, controlled investigation of magnesium L-aspartate hydrochloride for illicit cocaine and opiate use in methadone-maintained patients, J Addict Dis 2003, PMID: 12703668.

[884] Abbasi B et al, The effect of magnesium supplementation on primary insomnia in elderly: A double-blind placebo-controlled clinical trial, J Res Med Sci. 2012, PMCID: PMC3703169.

[885] Walsh W, Depression, Presentation by William Walsh, Walsh Institute, http://goo.gl/VlYnHK.

[886] Benton D, Selenium intake, mood and other aspects of psychological functioning, Nutr Neurosci. 2002, PMID: 12509066.

[887] Mokhber N. Effect of supplementation with selenium on postpartum depression: a randomized double-blind placebo-controlled trial, PMID: 20528214.

[888] Benton D et al, The impact of selenium supplementation on mood, Biological Psychiatry, 1991, http://goo.gl/J1XVJ8.

370   *References*

[889] Brown J, Role of Selenium and Other Trace Elements in the Geography of Schizophrenia, Schizophrenia Bulletin, 1994, PMID: 8085140, http://goo.gl/USJvsE.

[890] Lai J et al, The efficacy of zinc supplementation in depression: systematic review of randomised controlled trials. J of Affective Disorders 2012, PMID: 21798601.

[891] Nolan K, Copper Toxicity syndrome, J Orthomolecular Psychiatry, 1983.

[892] Popper CW, Single-micronutrient and broad-spectrum micronutrient approaches for treating mood disorders in youth and adults, Child Adolesc Psychiatr Clin N Am. 2014, PMID: 24975626.

[893] Starobrat-Hermelin B, The effect of deficiency of selected bioelements on hyperactivity in children with certain specified mental disorders, Ann Acad Med Stetin, 1998, PMID: 9857546.

[894] Greenblatt J, Understanding the Role of Amino Acids in the Treatment of Mental Health, presentation, for Great Plains Labs, 7/21/2015.

[895] Tsai, Guochuan E, D-Alanine Added to Antipsychotics for the Treatment of Schizophrenia, Biological Psychiatry, 2006, PMID: 16154544.

[896] Smith, Sean M. "The Therapeutic Potential of D-Amino Acid Oxidase (DAAO) Inhibitors." Open Medicinal Chemistry Journal, 2010, Bentham Science Publishers.

[897] Hofmann SG et al, Augmentation of Exposure Therapy With D-Cycloserine for Social Anxiety Disorder, Arch Gen Psychiatry. 2006, PMID: 16520435, http://goo.gl/ieK8BE.

[898] Heresco-Levy U, D-serine efficacy as add-on pharmacotherapy to risperidone and olanzapine for treatment-refractory schizophrenia. Biol Psychiatry 2005, PMID: 15780844.

[899] Sabelli HC et al. Clinical studies on the phenylethylamine hypothesis of affective disorder: urine and blood phenylacetic acid and phenylalanine dietary supplements. J Clin Psychiatry 1986, PMID: 3944066.

[900] Beckmann H et al, DLPhenylalanine in depressed patients: an open study. J Neural Transm 1977, PMID: 335027.

[901] Beckmann H et al, DL-phenylalanine versus imipramine: a double-blind controlled study. Arch Psychiatr Nervenkr 1979, PMID: 387000.

[902] Abdou AM et al, Relaxation and immunity enhancement effects of gamma-aminobutyric acid (GABA) administration in humans, Biofactors, 2006, PMID: 16971751.

[903] Gawryluk J et al, Decreased levels of glutathione, the major brain antioxidant, in post-mortem prefrontal cortex from patients with psychiatric disorders, Int J Neuropsychopharmacol. 2011, PMID: 20633320.

[904] Gysin R et al, Impaired glutathione synthesis in schizophrenia: Convergent genetic and functional evidence, Proc Natl Acad Sci U S A. 2007, PMCID: PMC2034265.

[905] Neeman G et al, Relation of plasma glycine, serine, and homocysteine levels to schizophrenia symptoms and medication type, Am J Psychiatry, 2005, PMID: 16135636.

[906] Strzelecki, Dominik, Changes in positive and negative symptoms, general psychopathology in schizophrenic patients during augmentation of antipsychotics with glycine: a preliminary 10-week open-label study, Psychiatria Polska, 2011, PANSTWOWY ZAKAD WYDAWNICTW LEKARSKICH, PMID: 22335126.

[907] Heresco-Levy, U. "Efficacy of High-Dose Glycine in the Treatment of Enduring Negative Symptoms of Schizophrenia." Archives of General Psychiatry, 1999, PMID: 9892253.

[908] Nia S, Psychiatric signs and symptoms in treatable inborn errors of metabolism, J Neurol. 2014, PMCID: PMC4141145.

[909] Bersani G. l-Acetylcarnitine in dysthymic disorder in elderly patients: A double-blind, multicenter, controlled randomized study vs. fluoxetine. Eur Neuropsychopharmacol 2013, PMID: 23428336.

[910] Chengappa, K. N. Roy, "A Preliminary, Randomized, Double-Blind, Placebo-Controlled Trial of L-Carnosine to Improve Cognition in Schizophrenia." Schizophrenia Research, 2012, PMID: 23099060.

[911] Rogers LL et al, Glutamine in the treatment of alcoholism, Q J Stud Alcohol, 1957, PMID: 13506018.

[912] Zeinoddini, Atefeh, L-Lysine as an Adjunct to Risperidone in Patients with Chronic Schizophrenia: A Double-Blind, Placebo-Controlled, Randomized Trial, Journal of Psychiatric Research, 2014, PMID: 25227564.

[913] Smriga M et al, Oral treatment with L-lysine and L-arginine reduces anxiety and basal cortisol levels in healthy humans, Biomed Res 2007, PMID: 17510493.

[914] Ritsner MS. L-theanine relieves positive, activation, and anxiety symptoms in patients with schizophrenia and schizoaffective disorder: an 8 week, randomized, double-blind, placebo-controlled, 2-center study. J Clin Psychiatry, 2011, PMID: 21208586.

[915] Banderet LE, Treatment with tyrosine, a neurotransmitter precursor, reduces environmental stress in humans, Brain Res Bull. 1989, PMID 2736402.

[916] Kishimoto H et al, The level and diurnal rhythm of plasma tryptophan and tyrosine in manic-depressive patients, Yokohama Medical Bulletin, 1976,

[917] Byerley W, Depression and serotonin metabolism: rationale for neurotransmitter precursor treatment, J clin Psychopharmacol, 1985, PMID: 2410463.

[918] Van Hiele, L-5-Hydroxytryptophan in depression: the first substitution therapy in psychiatry? The treatment of 99 outpatients with therapy-resistant depressions, Heuropsychobiology, 1980, PMID: 6967194.

[919] Jangid P. Comparative study of efficiency of l-5-hydroxytryptophan and fluoxetine in patients presenting with first depressive episode, PMID: 23380314.

[920] Zmilacher K, L-5-hydroxytryphan alone and in combination with a peripheral decarboxylase inhibitor in the treatment of depression. Neuropsychobiology 1988, PMID: 3265988.

[921] US Library of Medicine, Medline Plus 5-HTP, http://goo.gl/bDTwZZ.

[922] Hughes JH et al, Effects of acute tryptophan depletion on cognitive function in euthymic bipolar patients, European Neuropsychopharmacology, 2002, PMID: 11872328.

[923] Van Praag HM et al, Chemoprophylaxis of depression. An attempt to compare lithium with 5-hydroxytryptophan, Acta Psychiatr Scand Suppl, 1981, PMID: 6164250.

[924] Chouinard G et al, A controlled clinical trial of L-trytophan in acute mania, Biological Psych, 1985, PMID: 3886024.

[925] Brewerton T. et al, Lithium carbonate and L-tryptophan in the treatment of bipolar and schizoaffective disorders, Amer J of Psych, 1983, PMID: 6405638.

[926] Schruers K et al, L-5-hydroxytryptophan administration inhibits carbon dioxide-induced panic in panic disorder patients, Psychiatry Res, 2002, PMID: 1255948.

[927] De Luca V et al, Peripheral Amino Acid Levels in Schizophrenia and Antipsychotic Treatment, Psychiatry Investig. 2008, PMCID: PMC2796006.

[928] Levkovitz, Yechiel, "Effect of L-Tryptophan on Memory in Patients with Schizophrenia." The JI of Nervous and Mental Disease, 2003, PMID: 14504565.

[929] Lindsley JG et al, Selectivity in response to L-tryptophan among insomniac subjects: A preliminary reports, Sleep, 1983, PMID: 6353523.

[930] Bowen DJ et al, Tryptophan and high-carbohydrate diets as adjuncts to smoking cessation therapy, J Behav Med, 1991, PMID: 188079.

[931] European College of Neuropsychopharmacology, Amino acid offers potential therapeutic alternative in psychiatric disorders, 2013, http://goo.gl/zt0E8m.

[932] Sarris, Mischoulon D, Schweitzer I. Adjunctive nutraceuticals with standard pharmacotherapies in bipolar disorder: a systematic review of clinical trials. Bipolar Disord. 2011, PMID: 22017215.

[933] Dean O, Giorlando F, Berk M. N-acetylcysteine in psychiatry: current therapeutic evidence and potential mechanisms of action. J Psychiatry Neurosci. 2011, PMCID: PMC3044191.

[934] Berk M et al, N-acetyl cysteine for depressive symptoms in bipolar disorder—a double-blind randomized placebo-controlled trial. Biol Psychiatry. 2008, PMID: 18534556.

[935] LaRowe SD et al, Is cocaine desire reduced by N-acetylcysteine?, Am J Psychiatry, 2007, PMID: 17606664.

[936] Brambilla F et al, Beta-endorphin concentration in peripheral blood mononuclear cells of elderly depressed patients – effects of phosphatidylserine therapy, Neuropsychobiology, 1996, PMID: 8884754.

[937] Maggioni M et al, Effects of phosphatidylserine therapy in geriatric patients with depressive disorders, Acta Psychiatr Scand 1990, PMID: 1693032.

[938] Crook TH et al, Effects of phosphatidylserine in age-associated memory impairment, Neurology, 1991, PMID: 2027477.

[939] Lane, HY et al, Sarcosine or D-Serine Add-on Treatment for Acute Exacerbation of Schizophrenia: A Randomized, Double-Blind, Placebo-Controlled Study, Archives of General Psychiatry, 2005, PMID: 16275807.

[940] Lane HY et al, A Randomized, Double-Blind, Placebo-Controlled Comparison Study of Sarcosine (N-Methylglycine) and D-Serine Add-on Treatment for Schizophrenia, Int'l J of Neuropsychopharmacology, 2010, PMID: 19887019.

[941] Strzelecki D et al, Supplementation of antipsychotic treatment with sarcosine – GlyT1 inhibitor – causes changes of glutamatergic (1)NMR spectroscopy parameters in the left hippocampus in patients with stable schizophrenia, Neurosci Lett. 2015, PMID: 26306650.

[942] Tsai, Guochuan, "Glycine Transporter I Inhibitor, N-Methylglycine (sarcosine), Added to Antipsychotics for the Treatment of Schizophrenia." Biological Psychiatry, 2004, PMID: 15023571.

[943] Latif Z et al, P03-261 - Use of sarcosine to augment treatment of schizophrenia- review of evidence, J of European Psychiatric Association, 2011, http://goo.gl/NhaJuR.

[944] Lane et al, Sarcosine (N-Methylglycine) Treatment for Acute Schizophrenia: A Randomized, Double-Blind Study, BiologPsych, 2008.

[945] Barrett S et al, Acute phenylalanine/tyrosine depletion: A new method to study the role of catecholamines in psychiatric disorders, Primary Psychiatry, 2004.

[946] Scarna A et al, Effects of a branched-chain amino acid drink in mania, British J of Psychiatry, 2003, PMID: 12611783.

[947] Gately D et al, Database Analysis of Adults with Bipolar Disorder Consuming a Micronutrient Formula, Clinical Med: Psychiatry 2009.

[948] Kaplan B et al, Effective mood stabilization with a chelated mineral supplement: an open-label trial in bipolar disorder, J Clin Psychiatry, 2001, PMID: 11780873.

[949] Rucklidge J, Vitamin-mineral treatment of attention-deficit hyperactivity disorder in adults: double-blind randomised placebo-controlled trial, BJPsych, 2014, PMID: 24482441.

[950] Boston PF et al, Cholesterol and mental disorder, BJ Psych, 1996, PMID: 8968624, http://goo.gl/pqMHyi.

[951] Steegmans P et al, Higher Prevalence of Depressive Symptoms in Middle-Aged Men With Low Serum Cholesterol Levels, Psychosom Med. 2000, PMID: 10772398.

[952] Horsten M et al, Depressive symptoms, social support, and lipid profile in healthy middle-aged women, Psychosom Med. 1997, PMID: 9316185.

[953] Kaplan A, Statins, Cholesterol Depletion–and Mood Disorders: What's the Link?, Psychiatric Times, 2010, PMID: 8968624, http://goo.gl/IE88Bp.

[954] Ellison L et al, Low Serum Cholesterol Concentration and Risk of Suicide, Epidemiology, 2001, PMID: 11246576.

[955] Mehrpooya M et al, Evaluating the Effect of Coenzyme Q10 Augmentation on Treatment of Bipolar Depression: A Double-Blind Controlled Clinical Trial, J Clin Psychopharmacol. 2018, PMID: 30106880, https://goo.gl/B87R2P.

[956] Forester B et al, Coenzyme Q10 Effects on Creatine Kinase Activity and Mood in Geriatric Bipolar Depression. J Geriatr Psych Neurol. 2012, PMCID: PMC4651420; Forester BP et al, Antidepressant effects of open label treatment with Coenzyme Q10 in geriatric bipolar depression. J Clin Psychopharmacol. 2015, PMCID: PMC4414830.

[957] Roitman S. Creatine monohydrate in resistant depression: a preliminary study. Bipolar Disord 2007.

[958] Voronkova KV et al, Use of Noben (idebenone) in the treatment of dementia and memory impairments without dementia, Neurosci Behav Physiol. 2009, PMID: 19430983.

[959] Gutzmann H et al, Sustained efficacy and safety of idebenone in the treatment of Alzheimer's disease: update on a 2-year double-blind multicentre study, J Neural Transm Suppl. 1998, PMID: 9850939.

[960] Silvestri R et al, Indole-3-pyruvic acid as a possible hypnotic agent in insomniac subjects, J Int Med Res. 1991, PMID: 1748233.

[961] Hager K et al, Alpha-lipoic acid as a new treatment option for Alzheimer type dementia, Arch Gerontol Geriatr, 2001, PMID: 11395173.

[962] Sarris J, Omega-3 for bipolar disorder: meta-analyses of use in mania and bipolar depression, J Clin Psychiatry, 2012, PMID: 21903025.

[963] Freeman MP, et al, Omega-3 fatty acids: Evidence basis for treatment and future research in psychiatry, J Clin Psychiatry. 2006, PMID: 17194275.

[964] Frangou S et al, Efficacy of ethyl-eicosapentaenoic acid in bipolar depression: Randomised double-blind placebo-controlled study, British Journal of Psychiatry, 2006, PMID: 16388069.

[965] Omega 3 fatty acids in bipolar disorder: a preliminary double-blind, placebo-controlled trial. Arch Gen Psych, 1999, PMID: 10232294.

[966] Su K et al, Association of Use of Omega-3 Polyunsaturated Fatty Acids With Changes in Severity of Anxiety Symptoms A Systematic Review and Meta-analysis, JAMA Network Open, 2018, https://goo.gl/QKM3ay.

[967] Puri BK. Eicosapentaenoic acid in the treatment-resistant depression associated with symptom remission, structural brain changes and reduced neuronal phospholipid turnover. Int J Clin Pract 2001, PMID: 11695079.

[968] Jazayeri et al. Comparison of therapeutic effects of omega-3 fatty acid eicosapentaenoic acid and fluoxetine, separately and in combination, in major depressive disorder. Aust N Z J Psychiatry 2008, PMID: 18247193.

[969] Peet M, Omega-3 polyunsaturated fatty acids in the treatment of schizophrenia, Israel Journal of Psychiatry and related sciences, 2008, PMID: 18587166.

[970] Berger GE et al, Ethyl-eicosapentaenoic acid in first-episode psychosis: a randomized, placebo-controlled trial. J Clin Psychiatry. 2007, PMID: 18162017.

[971] Amminger GP et al, Long-chain omega-3 fatty acids for indicated prevention of psychotic disorders: a randomized, placebo-controlled trial, Archives of General Psychiatry, 2010, PMID: 20124114.

[972] Richardson, AJ, "Laterality Changes Accompanying Symptom Remission in Schizophrenia Following Treatment with Eicosapentaenoic Acid." International Journal of Psychophysiology, 1999, PMID: 10610057.

[973] Buydens-Branchey L, n-3 Polyunsaturated fatty acids decrease anxiety feelings in a population of substance abusers, Journal of Clinical Psychopharmacology, 2006, PMID: 17110827.

[974] Georgetown University Medical Center, Resveratrol appears to restore blood-brain barrier integrity in Alzheimer's disease, 2016, https://goo.gl/EqcxN4.

[975] Xingrong Ma, Resveratrol improves cognition and reduces oxidative stress in rats with vascular dementia, Neural Regen 2013, PMCID: PMC4146064.

[976] National association of mental health planning and advisory council, Evidence-based alternative therapies for mental illness - omega-3 fatty acids and sam-e, http://goo.gl/kijoaG.

[977] Sarris J et al, Major depressive disorder and nutritional medicine: a review of monotherapies and adjuvant treatments, Nutrition Reviews, PMID: 19239627, http://goo.gl/433tDe.

[978] Carpenter DJ. St John's wort and S-adenosyl methionine as "natural" alternatives to conventional antidepressants in the era of the suicidality boxed warning: what is the evidence for clinically relevant benefit? Altern Med Rev. 2011, PMID: 21438644.

[979] Pancheri P, A double-blind, randomized parallel-group, efficacy and safety study of intramuscular S-adenosyl-L-methionine 1,4-butanedisulphonate (SAMe) versus imipramine in patients with major depressive disorder. Int J Neuropsychopharma 2002, PMID: 12466028.

[980] Levkovitz Y. Effects of S-adenosylethionine augmentation of serotonin-reuptake inhibitor antidepressants on cognitive symptoms of major depressive disorder. J Affect Disord 2012, PMID: 21665441.

[981] Anstee Q, S-adenosylmethionine (SAMe) therapy in liver disease: A review of current evidence and clinical utility, J of Hepatology, 2012, PMID: 22659519.

[982] Cibin M et al, S-Adenosylmethionine (SAMe) is effective in reducing ethanol abuse in an outpatient program for alcoholics. Proceedings of the 4th congress of biomedical and social aspects of alcohol and alcoholism.

[983] Pataracchia R, Optimal Dosing for Schizophrenia, Journal Orthomolecular Med V 20/2, 2005, http://goo.gl/gcSXVm.

[984] (a) Greenblatt James, Integrative Psychiatrist http://vimeo.com/49454442; (b) Pataracchia R, Orthomolecular Treatment Response, Journal of Orthomolecular Medicine, Volume 25, Number 1, 2010, http://goo.gl/TSC83x; (c) Prousky J, The Orthomolecular Treatment of Schizophrenia: A primer for clinicians, http://goo.gl/Gj3V26; (d) Hoffer A, Chronic Schizophrenic Patients Treated Ten Years Or More, http://goo.gl/R0UbIQ; Hoffer A, Orthomolecular Treatment for Schizophrenia, Keats Good Health Guide, 1999.

[985] Safe Harbor, Dramatic Recovery from "Catatonic Schizophrenia" Case History: Treatment of Severe "Schizophrenia" without Drugs, https://goo.gl/7DxmPS, copied 9/17/16.

[986] Wang W, Case report of mental disorder induced by niacin deficiency, Shanghai Archives of Psychiatry, 2012, PMCID: PMC4198903.

[987] Gomez-Bernal GJ, Vitamin B12 Deficiency Manifested as Mania: A Case Report, Prim Care Companion J Clin Psychiatry. 2007, PMCID: 1911186.

[988] Gelenberg A, Tyrosine for the treatment of depression, Nutr Health. 1984, PMID: 6443584, https://goo.gl/Vf1YBK.

[989] Hamill S, Pittsburgh researchers may have found 'cure' for some untreatable depression, Pittsburgh Post-Gazette, 2016, http://goo.gl/m3iF27.

[990] Gaby A, Intravenous Nutrient Therapy: the "Myers' Cocktail", (Altern Med Rev 2002, PMID: 12410623, https://goo.gl/jSm5GJ.

[991] O'Connor D et al, Effects of Testosterone on Mood, Aggression, and Sexual Behavior in Young Men: A Double-Blind, Placebo-Controlled, Cross-Over Study, J of Clinical Endocrinology & Metabolism, 2013, PMID: 15181066, http://goo.gl/P2b5vx.

[992] Abdullatif HD, Reversible subclinical hypothyroidism in the presence of adrenal insufficiency. Endocr Pract, 2006, PMID: 17002934.

[993] Golden SH et al, Clinical review: Prevalence and incidence of endocrine and metabolic disorders in the United States: a comprehensive review, J Clin Endocrinol Metab. 2009, PMID: 19494161, http://goo.gl/4HYMFn.

[994] Deshmukh V et al, Prevalence, clinical and biochemical profile of subclinical hypothyroidism in normal population in Mumbai, In J Endo Met 2013, PMC3712376.

[995] Gharib H et al, Subclinical Thyroid Dysfunction: A Joint Statement on Management from the American Association of Clinical Endocrinologists, the American Thyroid Association, and The Endocrine Society, J of Clinical Endocrinology & Metabolism, PMID: 15643019, http://goo.gl/QxEt72.

[996] Levenson J, Psychiatric Issues in Endocrinology, Primary Psychiatry, 2006, http://goo.gl/2630sw.

[997] Canaris GJ, The Colorado thyroid disease study prevalence. Arch Intern Med 2000.

[998] Awad A, The Thyroid and the Mind and Emotions/Thyroid Dysfunction and Mental Disorders, Thyroid foundation of Canada. www.thyroid.ca/e10f.php.

[999] Schizophrenia.com, Hypothyroidism and psychiatric illness, December 15, 2006, http://goo.gl/6ibqeT,

[1000] Awad A, The Thyroid and the Mind and Emotions/Thyroid Dysfunction and Mental Disorders, Thyroid foundation of Canada. www.thyroid.ca/e10f.php.

[1001] Rack SK et al, Hypothyroidism and depression: A therapeutic challenge, Ann Pharmacother, 2000, PMID: 11054982.

[1002] Bahls S, The relation between thyroid function and depression: a Review, Rev Bras Psiquiatr, 2004, PMID: 15057840, http://goo.gl/oUHrUC.

[1003] Holtorf Medical Group, copied 10/29/13. http://goo.gl/O1fQEJ.

[1004] Rev. Bras. Psiquiatr, The relation between thyroid function and depression: a review, SCI ELO, http://goo.gl/hVmDWv.

[1005] Brogan K, The Oft-Ignored Link Between Mental Illness and Hypothyroid Disease, Mercola.com, 2014, http://goo.gl/wgtQVw.

[1006] Cole DP et al, Slower treatment response in bipolar depression predicted by lower pretreatment thyroid function. Am J Psychiatry 2002, PMID: 11772699.

[1007] Radhakrishnan R et al, Thyroid dysfunction in major psychiatric disorders in a hospital based sample, Indian J Med Res. 2013, PMCID: PMC3978977.

[1008] Langlois MC et al, Impact of antipsychotic drug administration on the expression of nuclear receptors in the neocortex and striatum of the rat brain. Neuroscience. 2001, PMID: 11564442.

[1009] Schizophrenia.com, Hypothyroidism and psychiatric illness, Dec 15, 2006, http://goo.gl/lLtR7i, copied 10/29/2013.

[1010] Anglin R, The Neuropsychiatric Profile of Addison's Disease: Revisiting a Forgotten Phenomenon, J of Neuropsych and Clinical Neurosci 2006; PMID: 17135373.

[1011] Anglin RE et al, The neuropsychiatric profile of Addison's disease: revisiting a forgotten phenomenon, J Neuropsychiatry Clin Neurosci. 2006, PMID: 17135373.

[1012] Camilla AM et al, Reduced DNA methylation and psychopathology following endogenous hypercortisolism... Scientific Reports, 2017, PMCID: PMC5353706.

[1013] The difference between Cushing's disease and other forms of Cushing's syndrome, http://goo.gl/M5L9Ic.

[1014] Schmidt PJ. Dehydroepiandrosterone monotherapy in midlife-onset major and minor depression. Arch Gen Psychiatry 2005, PMID: 15699292.

[1015] Wolkowitz OM. Dehydroepiandrosterone (DHEA) treatment of depression. Biol Psychiatry 1997, PMID: 9024954.

[1016] Wolkowitz OM. Double-blind treatment of major depression with dehydroepiandrosterone. Am J Psychiatry 1999, PMID: 10200751.

[1017] Strous RD. Dehydroepiandrosterone augmentation in the management of negative, depressive, and anxiety symptoms in schizophrenia. Arch Gen Psychiatry 2003, PMID: 12578430.

[1018] Friess E et al, DHEA administration increases rapid eye movement sleep and EEG power in the sigma frequency range, Amer J of Physiol, 1995, PMID: 7840167.

[1019] Wolkowitz OM et al, Dehydroepiandrosterone (NPI-34133) treatment of Alzheimer's disease: a randomized, double-blind, placebo-controlled, parallel group study, APA, 1999,

[1020] Marx CE et al, Pregnenolone as a novel therapeutic candidate in schizophrenia: emerging preclinical and clinical evidence, Neuroscience. 2011, PMID: 21756978.

[1021] Ritsner, Michael S, Pregnenolone Treatment Reduces Severity of Negative Symptoms in Recent-Onset Schizophrenia: An 8-Week, Double-Blind, Randomized Add-on Two-Center Trial. Psychiatry and Clinical Neurosciences, 2014, PMID: 24548129.

[1022] Marx CE, et al, Proof-of-concept trial with the neurosteroid pregnenolone targeting cognitive and negative symptoms in schizophrenia. Neuropsychopharmacology 2009, PMCID: PMC3427920.

[1023] Sripada R et al, Allopregnanolone Elevations Following Pregnenolone Administration are Associated with Enhanced Activation of Emotion Regulation Neurocircuits, Biol Psychiatry. 2013, PMCID: PMC3648625.

[1024] Ossewaarde L et al, Neural mechanisms underlying changes in stress-sensitivity across the menstrual cycle, Psychoneuroendocrinology, 2010, PMID: 19758762.

[1025] Osuji IJ et al, Pregnenolone for cognition and. mood in dual diagnosis patients. Psych Res 2010, PMID: 20493557.

[1026] Michael L et al, Brain Oxytocin as a Main Regulator of Prosocial Behaviour - Link to Psychopathology, Autism - A Neurodevelopmental Journey from Genes to Behaviour, 2011, http://goo.gl/1kKgtE.

[1027] Nagasawa M et al, Dog's gaze at its owner increases owner's urinary oxytocin during social interaction, Hormones and Behavior, 2009, PMID: 19124024, https://goo.gl/cJsdwa.

[1028] Bakharev, V. D., "[Psychotropic properties of oxytocin]." Problemy Endokrinologii, 1967: 6718333.

[1029] Gordon I e al, Oxytocin enhances brain function in children with autism, PNAS, 2013, PMID: 24297883.

[1030] Van Cappellen P et al, Effects of oxytocin administration on spirituality and emotional responses to meditation, Soc Cogn Affect Neurosci. 2016, PMID: 27317929.

[1031] Ishak WW et al, Oxytocin role in enhancing well-being: a literature review, J of Affective Disorders, 2011, PMID: 20584551.

[1032] Prange, A. J. "Behavioral and Endocrine Responses of Schizophrenic Patients to TRH (protirelin)." Archives of General Psychiatry 36, no. 10 (September 1979), PMID: 112944.

[1033] Govorin, NV, Use of thymic peptide thymalin in the complex treatment of therapy-resistant schizophrenia, Zhurnal Nevropatologii I Psikhiatrii Imeni S.S. Korsakova (Moscow, Russia: 1952), 1990, PMID: 2163147.

[1034] Velasco PJ, Psychiatric Aspects of Parathyroid Disease, Psychosomatics, 1999, PMID: 10581976.

[1035] Brezezinski A et al, Effects of exogenous melatonin on sleep: A meta-analysis, Sleep Med Review, 2005, PMID: 15649737.

[1036] Anderson G et al, Melatonin: an overlooked factor in schizophrenia and in the inhibition of anti-psychotic side effects. Metab Brain Dis, 2012, PMID: 22527998.

[1037] Monti JM, Sleep disturbance in schizophrenia. Int Rev Psychiatry. 2005, PMID: 16194796.

[1038] Dolberg OT. Melatonin for the treatment of sleep disturbances in major depression. Am J Psychiatry 1998.

[1039] Sarfaty MA. A randomized double-blind placebo-controlled trial of treatment as usual plus exogenous slow-release melatonin (6mg) or placebo for sleep disturbance and depressed mood. Int Clin Psychopharm, 2010, PMID: 20195158.

[1040] Zhdanova IV, Melatonin treatment attenuates symptoms of acute nicotine withdrawal in humans, Pharmacol Biochem Behav 2000, PMID: 11113492.

[1041] Garfinkel D et al, Facilitation of benzodiazepine discontinuation by melatonin: a new clinical approach. Arch Intern Med 1999, PMID: 10665894.

[1042] University of Maryland Medical Center, Melatonin, 2016, copied 1/19/17, https://goo.gl/Chahvp.

[1043] Thompson, Rest easy: MIT study confirms melatonin's value as sleep aid, MIT News, 2005, https://goo.gl/gDnnZx.

[1044] Pfeiffer C, Nutrition and Mental Illness An Orthomolecular Approach to Balancing Body Chemistry, Healing Arts Press, 1987.

[1045] Salzer H, Relative Hypoglycemia as a Cause of Neuropsychiatric Illness, J Nat Med Assoc, 1966, PMCID: PMC2611193.

[1046] Levitt J, Conquering Anxiety, Depression and Fatigue Without Drugs - the Role of Hypoglycemia, http://goo.gl/1YLQXt.

[1047] Ding Y et al, Neuropsychiatric profiles of patients with insulinomas, Eur Neurol. 2010, PMID: 20029216.

[1048] WebMd, http://diabetes.webmd.com/diabetes-hypoglycemia, copied on 10/29/2013.

[1049] Hypoglycemia Support Foundation, http://hypoglycemia.org/hypoglycemia-diet/, copied 10/29/2013.

[1050] Molteni R et al, A high-fat, refined sugar diet reduces hippocampal brain-derived neurotrophic factor, neuronal plasticity, and learning, Neuroscience. 2002, PMID: 12088740.

[1051] Krabbe KS et al, Brain-derived neurotrophic factor (BDNF) and type 2 diabetes, Diabetologia. 2007 Feb; Epub 2006 Dec 7, PMID: 17151862.

[1052] Holcomb S, DiSalvo D, The Brain in Your Kitchen: A Collection of Essays on How What We Buy, Eat, and Experience Affects Our Brains, Quoted from Forbes.Com on March 8, 2012.

[1053] Weiner M et al, Cardiovascular Morbidity and Mortality in Bipolar Disorder, Ann Clin Psychiatry. 2011, PMCID: PMC3190964.

[1054] Pete M, Eicosapentaenoic acid in the treatment of schizophrenia and depression: rationale and preliminary double-blind clinical trial results, Prostaglandins Leukot Essent Fatty Acids. 2003, PMID: 14623502.

[1055] National Alliance on Mental Illness, NAMI Hearts and Minds, http://goo.gl/FJmS1b, copied 10/29/13.

[1056] Skovlund CW et al, Association of Hormonal Contraception With Depression, JAMA Psychiatry. 2016, PMID: 27680324.

[1057] Rasgon N et al, Depression in women with polycystic ovary syndrome: clinical and biochemical correlates, J Affect Disord. 2003, PMID: 12738050.

[1058] Cochrane, Estrogen for schizophrenia, 2005, copied 12/16/16, https://goo.gl/08WIso.

[1059] Ghafari, Emel, Combination of Estrogen and Antipsychotics in the Treatment of Women with Chronic Schizophrenia: A Double-Blind, Randomized, Placebo-Controlled Clinical Trial, Clinical Schizo & Related Psychoses,2013, PMID: 23302446.

[1060] Gregoire AJ et al, Transdermal oestrogen for treatment of severe postnatal depression, Int J Gynaecol Obstet, 1996, PMID: 8598756.

[1061] Barak Y et al, Breast cancer in women suffering from serious mental illness, Schiz Res, 2008, PMID: 18455368.

[1062] Barron ML et al, Associations between Psychiatric Disorders and Menstrual Cycle Characteristics, Arch Psychiatr Nurs. 2008, PMCID: PMC2588420.

[1063] Rasgon N et al, Menstrual cycle related mood changes in women with bipolar disorder. Bipolar Disorders, 2003, PMID: 12656938.

[1064] Harlow BL et al, Depression and its influence on reproductive endocrine and menstrual cycle markers associated with perimenopause: the Harvard Study of Moods and Cycles. Archives of General Psychiatry, 2003, PMID: 12511170.

[1065] Ko, Young-Hoon, Short-Term Testosterone Augmentation in Male Schizophrenics: A Randomized, Double-Blind, Placebo-Controlled Trial, J of Clinical Psychopharmacology, 2008, PMID: 18626263.

[1066] Pope HG Jr. Testosterone gel supplementation for men with refractory depression: a randomized, placebo-controlled trial. Am J Psych 2003, PMID: 12505808.

[1067] Levenson, JL. Psychiatric issues in endocrinology. Primary Psychiatry 2006.

[1068] Hendrick V et al, Psychoneuroendocrinology of mood disorders. The hypothalamic-pituitary-thyroid axis. Psychitric Clin N Am 1998, PMID: 9670226.

[1069] Bahtiyar G et al, Novel endocrine disrupter effects of classic and atypical antipsychotic agents and divalproex: induction of adrenal hyperandrogenism, reversible with metformin or rosiglitazone, Endocr Pract. 2007, PMID: 17954415.

[1070] Pike MC et al, Estrogens, progestogens, normal breast cell proliferation and breast cancer risk, Epidemiolgic Reviews, 1993, PMID: 8405201.

[1071] Formica M, Anxiety Disorder or Hyperthyroidism?, Psychology Today, Dec 2011, https://goo.gl/ohAFQI.

[1072] Department of Psychiatry and Behavioral Science, Course of Specialized Clinical Science, Tokai University School of Medicine, Could subclinical hypothyroidism cause periodic catatonia with delusional misidentification syndrome? Psychiatry and Clinical Neurosciences, 2010, http://goo.gl/JbNH76.

[1073] Hertz P et al, CUSHING'S SYNDROME AND ITS MANAGEMENT, Amer J of Psychiatry, 1955, PMID: 13238637.

[1074] Brogan K, "Is It Her Hormones? A Case of Psychiatry Missing the Mark", Mad in America, 2016, http://goo.gl/r1Qry.

[1075] Rettenbacher M et al, Improvement of Psychosis During Treatment With Estrogen and Progesterone in a Patient with Hypoestrogenemia, J Clin Psychiatry, 2004, PMID: 15003086, http://goo.gl/r9WNjY.

[1076] Safe Harbor, Recovery from "Schizophrenia", http://goo.gl/O76Fmx.

[1077] Newbold H et al, Ecologic Mental Illness Produced by Allergies: Ecologic Mental Illness, Orthomolec Psych, 1973.

[1078] Bürk K, et al. Neurological symptoms in patients with biopsy proven celiac disease. Mov Disord 2009, PMID: 19845007.

[1079] Jackson J et al, Neurologic and Psychiatric Manifestations of Celiac Disease and Gluten Sensitivity, Psychiatric Quarterly, March 2012, PMCID: PMC3641836.

[1080] Hadjivassiliou M et al. Clinical, radiological, neurophysiological, and neuropathological characteristics of gluten ataxia. Lancet. 1998, PMID: 9843103.

[1081] Mayo Clinic., Celiac disease is a disease for the masses, Note: Mayo Clinic gastroenterologist Joseph A. Murray, M.D., thinks "…celiac testing may become routine for everyone… we have to screen people rather than just waiting for the disease to become apparent…", http://goo.gl/D5rph8, copied 10/30/2013.

[1082] Neumann J, Celiac disease showing up in many forms and at all ages, Reuters, 2014, http://goo.gl/637SsC.

[1083] Dickerson F, Markers of gluten sensitivity and celiac disease in bipolar disorder, Bipolar Disorders, 2011, PMID: 21320252.

[1084] Ciacci C, Depressive symptoms in adult coeliac disease, Scandanavian Journal of gastroenterology, 1998, PMID: 9548616.

[1085] Kalaydjian AE et al, The gluten connection: The association between schizophrenia and celiac disease. Acta Psychiatrica Scandinavica, 2006, PMID: 16423158.

[1086] Eaton W et al, Coeliac disease and schizophrenia: population based case control study with linkage of Danish national registers. BMJ 2004, PMID: 14976100.

[1087] Dohan C, Genetic Hypothesis of Idiopathic Schizophrenia: Its Exorphin Connection, Schizophrenia Bulletin, 1988, PMID: 2851166.

[1088] Dohan FC. Prevalence of celiac disease and gluten sensitivity in the United States clinical antipsychotic trials of intervention effectiveness study population, Schizo Bulletin, 2011, PMCID: PMC3004201.

[1089] Dohan FC. Relapsed schizophrenics: more rapid improvement on a milk-and cereal free diet. Br J Psychiatry 1969, PMID: 5820122.

[1090] Dohan, F. C."Relapsed Schizophrenics: Earlier Discharge from the Hospital after Cereal-Free, Milk-Free Diet." American Jof Psychiatry, 1973 PMID: 4739849.

[1091] Dohan FC, Wheat Consumption and Hospital Admissions for Schizophrenia During World War II, Amer Journ of Clinical Nutrition, 1966, PMID: 5900428.

[1092] Storms LH et al, Effects of gluten on schizophrenics, Arch Gen Psychiatry, 1982, PMID: 7065842.

[1093] Cade R et al, Autism and schizophrenia: intestinal disorders, Nutritional Neuroscience 2000.

[1094] Wilt T, Lactose Intolerance and Health, Agency for Healthcare Research and Quality, Pub 10-E004, 2010, http://goo.gl/IABd3G.

[1095] Severance EG et al, Subunit and whole molecule specificity of the anti-bovine casein immune response in recent onset psychosis and schizophrenia, Schizophr Res. 2010, PMID: 20071146.

[1096] Ledochowski et al, Lactose Malabsorption is Associated with Early Signs of Mental Depression in Females, Digestive Diseases and Sciences, Vol 43, No 11, Nov 1998, PMID: 9824144.

[1097] Bell IR, et al. Depression and allergies: survey of a nonclinical population. Psychother Psychosom, PMID: 1866437.

[1098] Johnson K, Allergy statistics and facts, 2012, WebMD, http://goo.gl/JZpgf8.

[1099] Postolache TT et al, Changes in severity of allergy and anxiety symptoms are positively correlated in patients with recurrent mood disorders who are exposed to seasonal peaks of aeroallergens. Int J Child Health Hum Dev 2008, PMID: 19430577.

[1100] Pelsser L, A randomised controlled trial into the effects of food on ADHD, Eur Child Adoles Psych 2008, PMID: 18431534, http://goo.gl/Xw4wxZ.

[1101] Dohan FC et al, Is schizophrenia rare if grain is rare? Biological Psychiatry, 1984, PMID: 6609726.

[1102] Amir S et al, The role of endorphins in stress: evidence and speculations, Neurosci Biobehav Rev. 1980, PMID: 6250104.

[1103] University of Wisconsin School of Medicine, Integrative Approaches to Anxiety, http://goo.gl/GNkTqn. .

[1104] De Santis A et al, Schizophrenic symptoms and SPECT abnormalities in a coeliac patient: regression after a gluten-free diet, J Intern Med. 1997, PMID: 9408073.

[1105] Bernardo J, Aluminum Toxicity, Medscape, 2015, http://goo.gl/ykuwUw.

[1106] Martyn, CN et al, Geographical relation between Alzheimer's disease and aluminum in drinking water. Lancet, 1989, PMID: 2562879.

[1107] Rahman A et al, Zinc, Manganese, Calcium, Copper, and Cadmium Level in Scalp Hair Samples of Schizophrenic Patients, Biol Trace Elem Res, 2009, PMID: 18810332, http://goo.gl/qWWsSb.

[1108] Amer Acad Of Neurology, On-The-Job Lead Exposure Could Increase Alzheimer's Risk, ScienceDaily 2000, http://goo.gl/vwJ0Xl.

[1109] Brain Research 1998 July;27(2):168-76.

[1110] Wojcik DP, Mercury toxicity presenting as chronic fatigue, memory impairment and depression: diagnosis, treatment, susceptibility, and outcomes in a New Zealand general practice setting, 1994-06, PMID: 16891999.

[1111] Rajanna B et al, Influence of mercury on uptake of dopamine and norepinephrine by rat brain synaptosomes Toxicol Let, 1985.

[1112] Genuis SJ, Fielding a current idea: exploring the public health impact of electromagnetic radiation, Public Health. 2008, PMID: 17572456, http://goo.gl/BUB07U.

[1113] Poole C et al, Depressive symptoms and headaches in relation to proximity of residence to an alternating-current transmission line right-of-way. Am J Epidemiol 1993, PMID: 8452140.

[1114] Silke T et al, Exposure to radio-frequency electromagnetic fields and behavioural problems in Bavarian children…, Eur J Epidemiol, 2010, PMID: 19960235.

[1115] Havas M et al, Dirty electricity and electrical hypersensitivity: five case studies. World Health Organization workshop on Electrical Hypersensitivity. Prague, Czech Republic; 2004, http://goo.gl/hk2P4m.

[1116] Beard J, Pesticide Exposure and Depression among Male Private Pesticide Applicators in the Agricultural Health Study, Env Health Perspect, 2014, PMC4154212.

[1117] Wagner-Schuman M et al, Association of pyrethroid pesticide exposure with attention-deficit/hyperactivity disorder in a nationally representative sample of U.S. children, Environ Health 2015, PMCID: PMC4458051.

[1118] Bienkowski B, Pesticide use by farmers linked to high rates of depression suicides, Env Hlth News, 2014, http://goo.gl/wRP5St.

[1119] Aschengrau A et al, Occurrence of mental illness following prenatal and early childhood exposure to tetrachloroethylene (PCE)-contaminated drinking water: a retrospective cohort study, Environmental Health 2012, PMCID: PMC3292942.

[1120] Grasso P, Neurophysiological and psychological disorders and occupational exposure to organic solvents, Food Chem Toxicol. 1984, PMID: 6541621.

[1121] Walker M, The Chelation Way, New York: Avery, 1989.

[1122] Flora S, Chelation in Metal Intoxication, Int J Environ Res Public Health, Jul 2010, PMCID: PMC2922724.

[1123] Atwood KC IV et al, Why the NIH Trial to Assess Chelation Therapy (TACT) should be abandoned, Medscape Journal of Medicine, 2008, PMCID 2438277

[1124] Benros M et al, Autoimmune Diseases and Severe Infections as Risk Factors for Mood Disorders, JAMA Psychiatry. 2013, PMID: 23760347.

[1125] Yolken R, Viruses and schizophrenia: a focus on herpes simplex virus, Herpes. 2004, PMID: 15319094.

[1126] Giacometti a et al, Epidemiologic features of intestinal parasitic infections in Italian mental institutions, Eur J Epidemiol. 1997, PMID: 9384271.

[1127] Johns Hopkins Medicine, Algae in Your Throat? Scientists Discover Algae Virus in Humans, 2014, http://goo.gl/GszzVZ.

[1128] Schaller J et al, Do Bartonella Infections Cause Agitation, Panic Disorder, and Treatment-Resistant Depression?, MedGenMed. 2007, PMCID: PMC2100128.

[1129] Hatalski CG, Borna disease, Emerg Infect Dis. 1997, PMID: 9204293.

[1130] Irving G et al, Psychological factors associated with recurrent vaginal candidiasis: a preliminary study, Sex Transm Infect. 1998, PMCID: PMC175814.

[1131] Severance EG et al, Candida albicans exposures, sex specificity and cognitive deficits in schizophrenia and bipolar disorder. npj Schizophrenia, 2016, https://goo.gl/Xd4sla.

[1132] Samonis G et al, Prospective study of the impact of broad spectrum antibiotics on the yeast flora of the human gut. Eur J Clin Microbiol Infect Dis 1994, PMID: 7813500.

[1133] Krone CA, Does gastrointestinal Candida albicans prevent ubiquinone absorption?, Med Hypotheses. 2001, PMID: 11735312.

[1134] Rucklidge J, Could Yeast Infections Impair Recovery From Mental Illness? A Case Study Using Micronutrients and Olive Leaf Extract for the Treatment of ADHD and Depression, ADVANCES, 2013, PMID: 23784606, http://goo.gl/mz2Otd.

[1135] William Shaw, Increased urinary excretion of a 3-(3-hydroxyphenyl)-3-hydroxypropionic acid (HPHPA), an abnormal phenylalanine metabolite of Clostridia spp. in the gastrointestinal tract, in urine samples from patients with autism and schizophrenia, Nutr Neurosci. 2010, PMID: 20423563, http://goo.gl/U7i6S9.

[1136] Manor I et al, Recurrence pattern of serum creatine phosphokinase levels in repeated acute psychosis, Biol Psychiatry. 1998, PMID: 9513739.

[1137] Walsh M, Clostridia, 3-{3-hydroxy-phenyl}-3-hydroxypropionic acid (HPHPA) & Psychosis, from Great Plains Laboratory web site under Digestive Disorders & Dysbiosis, copied 6/15/15, http://goo.gl/gCVS6v.

[1138] Wright M, Neuropsychiatric Illness in Systemic Lupus Erythematosus: Insights From a Patient With Erotomania and Geschwind's Syndrome, Am J Psychiatry 2010, PMID: 20439397.

[1139] Lupus Foundation of America, Can lupus cause depression?, 2013, http://goo.gl/jaiDyD.

[1140] Lupus Foundation of America, 15 Questions - Depression and Lupus, http://goo.gl/7WW0ne.

[1141] Center for Disease Control, Infectious Diseases and Mental Illness: Is There a Link?, Mar 1998, http://goo.gl/G6bhdL.

[1142] Fallon BA et al, Lyme disease: a neuropsychiatric illness, Am J Psychiatry. 1994, PMID: 7943444.

[1143] Hájek T, Higher Prevalence of Antibodies to Borrelia Burgdorferi in Psychiatric Patients Than in Healthy Subjects, Am J Psychiatry 2002, PMID: 11823274, http://goo.gl/7Jlmcn.

[1144] Horowitz R, Antibiotics Found Effective in Schizophrenia, Psychology Today, 2014, https://goo.gl/7SjVs0.

[1145] Horowitz R, Horowitz Lyme - MSIDS Questionnaire, http://goo.gl/zjSvtU.

[1146] Benke T, Lyme encephalopathy: long-term neuropsychological deficits years after acute neuroborreliosis, Acta Neurol Scand. 1995, PMID: 7639064.

[1147] Grisolia JS et al, CNS Cysticercosis, Archives of Neurology, 1982, PMID: 7115142.

[1148] Forlenza OV et al, Psychiatric manifestations of neurocysticercosis: a study of 38 patients from a neurology clinic in Brazil, Neurol Neurosurg Psych, 1997, PMC1074146.

[1149] Walker DH, Rickettsia, Medical Miocrobiology 4th edition, 1996, http://goo.gl/vmxZJE.

[1150] Swedo S, as quoted in From Throat to Mind: Strep Today, Anxiety Later?, Scie Amer, 2010, http://goo.gl/PkJEJY.

[1151] Westly E, From Throat to Mind: Strep Today, Anxiety Later?, Scientific Amer, 2010, http://goo.gl/ZiWRLu.

[1152] Sutterland AL et al, Beyond the association. Toxoplasma gondiiin schizophrenia, bipolar disorder, and addiction: systematic review and meta-analysis, Acta Psych Scand, 2015, http://goo.gl/jJChkx.

[1153] Penn News, Epidemiological Study by Penn Vet Professor Investigates Parasite-Schizophrenia Connection, 2014, http://goo.gl/HBxHcJ.

[1154] Sugden K et al, Is Toxoplasma Gondii Infection Related to Brain and Behavior Impairments in Humans? Evidence from a Population-Representative Birth Cohort, 2016, PMID: 26886853, http://goo.gl/FsbLqf.

[1155] Chaudhry, et al., Preventing clinical deterioration in first episode psychosis: potential role of minocycline in neuroprotection (abstract). Biol Psychiatry 2009.

[1156] Levkovitz Y et al, A double-blind, randomized study of minocycline for the treatment of negative and cognitive symptoms in early-phase schizophrenia. J Clin Psychiatry, 2010, PMID: 19895780.

[1157] Levine J et al, Possible antidepressant effect of minocycline (letter). Am J Psychiatry 1996, PMID: 8599421.

[1158] Hedaya R, Functional Medicine for Depressive Disorder: Advances in the Treatment Paradigm, presentation, 2016.

[1159] Fallon BA et al, Psychiatric manifestations of Lyme borreliosis, The J of Clinical Psychiatry, 1993, PMID: 8335653.

[1160] Bhatia B et al, Neurocysticercosis Presenting as Schizophrenia: A Case Report, Indian J of Psychiatry, 1994, PMCID: PMC2972502.

[1161] Walker S, A Dose of Sanity: Mind Medicine and Misdiagnosis, 1997, http://goo.gl/EmcxOr.

[1162] University of Buffalo, What happens when the brain is artificially stimulated? Science Daily, 2016, https://goo.gl/Vi9NzW.

[1163] Wolfson P et al, An investigation into the efficacy of Scutellaria lateriflora in healthy volunteers, Altern Ther Health Med, 2003, PMID: 12652886.

[1164] Hou Z et al, Effect of Anthocyanin-Rich Extract from Black Rice (Oryza sativa L. Japonica) on Chronically Alcohol-Induced Liver Damage in Rats, J Agric Food Chem. 2010, PMID: 20143824.

[1165] Joseph JA et al, Reversals of age-related declines in neuronal signal transduction, cognitive, and motor behavioral deficits with blueberry, spinach, or strawberry dietary supplementation, J Neurosci. 1999, PMID: 10479711.

[1166] Sayyah M. A preliminary randomized double blind clinical trial on the efficacy of aqueous extract of Echium amoenum in the treatment of mild to moderate major depression. Prog Neuropsychopharmacol Biol Psychiatry. 2006, PMID: 16309809.

[1167] Sayyah M et al, Efficacy of aqueous extract of Echium amoenum in treatment of obsessive–compulsive disorder. Prog Neuropsychopharmacol Biol Psychiatry, 2009, PMID: 19737592.

[1168] Sayyah M, A double-blind, placebo-controlled study of the aqueous extract of Echium amoenum for patients with Generalized Anxiety Disorder. Iran J Pharm Res 2012, PMID: 24250495.

[1169] Hanus M et al, Clinical Trial on Fixed Combination of Hawthorn, California Poppy, and Magnesium for Anxiety Disorders Found Safe and Effective, Curr Med Res Opin. 2004.

[1170] Leweke FM, Cannabidiol enhances anandamide signaling and alleviates psychotic symptoms of schizophrenia, Translational Psych, 2012, PMCID: PMC3316151.

[1171] Campos AC et al, Multiple mechanisms involved in the large-spectrum therapeutic potential of cannabidiol in psychiatric disorders, Philos Trans R Soc Lond B Biol Sci. 2012, PMCID: PMC3481531.

[1172] Zuardi A et al, Action of cannabidiol on the anxiety and other effects produced by delta 9-THC in normal subjects. Psychopharmacology, 1982, PMID: 6285406.

[1173] Bergamaschi M, Safety and side effects of cannabidiol, a Cannabis sativa constituent, Curr Drug Saf. 2011 Sep, PMID: 22129319.

[1174] Amsterdam J, Chamomile (Matricaria recutita) May Have Antidepressant Activity in Anxious Depressed Humans - An Exploratory Study, Altern Ther Health Med. 2012, PMCID: PMC3600408.

[1175] Amsterdam J et al, A randomized, double-blind, placebo-controlled trial of oral Matricaria recutita (chamomile) extract therapy for generalized anxiety disorder, 2009, J. Clin. Psychopharmacol, PMCID: PMC3600416.

[1176] Chang HM et al, Pharmacology and Applications of Chinese Materia Medica vol 1. Singapore: World ScientiInc., 1986.

[1177] Kumar S, Anti-anxiety Activity Studies on Homoeopathic Formulations of Turnera aphrodisiaca Ward, Evid Based Compl Alt Med. 2005, PMCID: PMC1062162.

[1178] Haller J, The effect of Echinacea preparations in three laboratory tests of anxiety: comparison with chlordiazepoxide, Phytother Res. 2010, PMID: 21031616.

[1179] Hermann N et al, Galantamine Treatment of Problematic Behavior in Alzheimer Disease: Post-hoc Analysis of Pooled Data from Three Large Trials, Am J Geriatr Psychiatry, 2005, PMID: 15956273.

[1180] Herrera-Arellano A. Therapeutic effectiveness of Galphimia glauca vs. lorazepam in generalized anxiety disorder. A controlled 15-week clinical trial, Planta Med 2012, PMID: 22828921.

[1181] Fugh-Berman A, Cott JM. Dietary supplements and natural products as psychotherapeutic agents. Psychosom Med. 1999, PMID: 10511018.

[1182] Marasco A et al, Double-blind study of a multivitamin complex supplemented with ginseng extract, Drugs Under Experimental and Clinical Research, 1996, PMID: 9034759.

[1183] Chen EY, HT1001, a proprietary North American ginseng extract, improves working memory in schizophrenia: a double-blind, placebo-controlled study. Phyther Res 2012, PMID: 22213250.

[1184] Chatterjee M, Evaluation of the antipsychotic potential of Panax quinquefolium in ketamine induced experimental psychosis model in mice. Neurochem Res 2012, PMID: 22189635.

[1185] Li N et al, Protective effects of ginsenoside Rg2 against glutamate-induced neurotoxicity in PC12 cells, J Ethnopharmacol, 2007, PMID: 17257792.

[1186] Spollen J et al, Psychiatric side effects of herbal medicinals, Journal of Pharmacy Practice 1999, http://goo.gl/rSoxRm.

[1187] National Center for Complementary and Alternative Medicine, Asian Ginseng, 2012, http://goo.gl/5uAdES.

[1188] Schiller H et al, Sedating effects of Humulus lupulus L extracts, Phytomedicine 2006, PMID: 16860977.

[1189] Volz HP, Kava-kava extract WS 1490 versus placebo in anxiety disorders--a randomized placebo-controlled 25-week outpatient trial, Pharmacopsychiatry, 1997, PMID: 9065962.

[1190] Schmidt M, Is kava hepatoxic, Deutsch Apotheker-Zeitung, Witung, 2002.

[1191] Akhondzadeh S et al, Comparison of Lavandula angustifolia Mill. Tincture and imipramine in the treatment of mild to moderate depression: a double-blind, randomized trial, Prog Neuropsychopharmacol Biol Psychiatry 2003, PMID: 12551734.

[1192] Lee IS et al, Effects of lavender aromatherapy on insomnia and depression in women college students, Taehan Knho Hakhoe Chi, 2006, PMID: 16520572.

[1193] Kennedy DO et al, Modulation of mood and cognitive performance following acute administration of single doses of Melissa officinalis (lemon balm) with human CNS nicotine and muscarinic receptor-binding properties, Neuropsychopharmacology, 2003, PMID: 12888775.

[1194] Sayyah M. Comparison of Silybum marianum (L.) Gaertn with fluoxetine in the treatment of obsessive-compulsive disorder. Prog Neuropsychopharmacol Biol Psychiatry 2010, PMID: 20035818.

[1195] National Center for Complementary and Alternative Medicine, Milk Thistle, 2012, http://goo.gl/bhnOUQ.

[1196] Salin-Pascual RJ. Antidepressant effect of transdermal nicotine patches in nonsmoking patients with major depression. J Clin Psych 1996, PMID: 9746444.

[1197] Hindmarch I et al, Efficacy and tolerance of vinpocetine in ambulant patients suffering from mild to moderate organic psychosyndromes, Int Clin Psychopharmacol, 1991, PMID: 2071888.

[1198] Moreno FA. Safety, tolerability, and efficacy of psilocybin in 9 patients with obsessive-compulsive disorder. J Clin Psych 2006, PMID: 17196053.

[1199] BYSTRITSKY A, A Pilot Study of Rhodiola rosea (Rhodax®) for Generalized Anxiety Disorder (GAD), J Alt and Comp Med, 2008, PMID: 18307390.

[1200] Cao LL et al, The effect of salidroside on cell damage induced by glutamate and intracellular free calcium in PC 12 cells, J Asian Natural Prod Res, 2006, PMID: 16753799.

[1201] Darbinyan V. Clinical trial of Rhodiola rosea L. extractSHR-5 in the treatment of mild to moderate depression. Nord J Psychiatry 2007, PMID: 17990195.

[1202] Linde K, Hypericum St John's wort for depression--an overview and meta-analysis of randomised clinical trials, BMJ 1996, http://goo.gl/HQK4q5.

[1203] Shelton RC, Effectiveness of St John's wort in major depression: a randomized controlled trial, JAMA 2001, PMID: 11308434.

[1204] Hypericum Depression Trial Study Group: Effect of Hypericum perforatum (St. John's Wort) in major depressive disorder: a randomized controlled trial, JAMA 2002, PMID: 11939866.

[1205] Szedgedi A et al, Acute treatment of moderate to severe depression with hypericum exteract WS5570 (St. John's Wort): Randomized controlled double blind non-inferiority trial versus paroxetine, BMJ, 2005.

[1206] Nierenberg AA, Burt T, Matthews J, Weiss AP. Mania associated with St. John's wort. Biol Psychiatry. 1999, PMCID: PMC2993537.

[1207] Taylor LH. An open-label trial of St. John's Wort (Hypericum pertoratum) in obsessive-compulsive disorder. J Clin Psych 2000, PMID: 10982200.

[1208] Kobak KA et al, St. John's Wort versus placebo in obsessive-compulsive disorder: Results from a double-blind study, Int Clinic Psychopharm, 2005, PMID: 16192837.

[1209] Perfumi M et al, Effects of Hypericum perforatum extraction on alcohol intake in Marchigian Sardinian alcohol-preferring rats. Alcohol 1999, PMID: 10528811.

[1210] Coskun I et al, Attenuation of ethanol withdrawal syndrome by extract of Hypericum perforatum in Wistar rats. Fund Clin Pharm 2006, PMID: 16968419.

[1211] NIH Office of Dietary Supplements, Dietary Supplements: What You Need to Know, 2011, http://goo.gl/IV2AyQ.

[1212] Bent S et al, Valerian for Sleep: A Systematic Review and Meta-Analysis. The American Journal of Medicine. 2006, PMCID: PMC4394901.

[1213] Krystal AD et al, The use of valerian in neuropsychiatry, CNS Spectr. 2001, PMID: 15334039.

[1214] Blumenthal M. German Federal Institute for Drugs and Medical Devices. Commission E. The Complete German Commission E monographs: therapeutic guide to herbal medicines. Austin, Tex: American Botanical Council, 1998.

[1215] Bauer B, Insomnia, I read that the herbal supplement valerian can help you fall asleep if you have insomnia. Is valerian safe, and does it actually work?, Mayo Clinic, http://goo.gl/PLP6w8.

[1216] Du S-L et al, Protective effects of saponins derived from Aralia Elata (Miq.) seem. on alcoholic liver disease in rats, J of Jilin Univ. of Med, 2005.

[1217] Coppola M, Potential Action of Betel Alkaloids on Positive and Negative Symptoms of Schizophrenia: A Review. Nordic J of Psych 66, 2012, PMID: 21859398.

[1218] Sullivan R J, Effects of Chewing Betel Nut (Areca Catechu) on the Symptoms of People with Schizophrenia in Palau, Micronesia. The British Journal of Psychiatry: The Journal of Mental Science, 2000, PMID: 11026959.

[1219] Koushik A et. al, Clinical evaluation of medhya rasayana compound in cases of non depressive anxiety neurosis. Ancient Sci of Life, 1982, PMCID: PMC3336698.

[1220] Bradwejn J, et al, A double-blind placebo controlled study on the effects of gotu kola (centella asiatica) on acoustic startle response in healthy subjects, Journal of Clinical Psychopharmacology, 2000, PMID: 11106141.

[1221] Jana U. A clinical study on the management of generalized anxiety disorder with Centella asiatica. Nepal Med Coll J 2010, PMID: 20677602.

[1222] Butler L et al, Chinese Herbal Medicine and Depression: The Research Evidence, Evid Based Complement Alternat Med. 2013, PMCID: PMC3582075.

[1223] Wang Y. Meta-analysis of the clinical effectiveness of traditional Chinese medicine formula Chaihu-Shugan-San in depression. J Ethnopharma 2012, PMID: 21933701.

[1224] Yi ZH. Clinical observation on treatment of major depressive disorder by paroxetine combined with chaihu xiaoyao mixture, Zhongguo Zhong Xi Yi Jie He Za Zhi, 2010, PMID: 21302485.

[1225] Terasawa K, Choto-san in the treatment of vascular dementia: a double-blind, placebo-controlled study, Phytomedicine, 1997, PMID: 23195240.

[1226] Zhang Y et al, Chinese Herbal Formula Xiao Yao San for Treatment of Depression: A Systematic Review of Randomized Controlled Trials, Evid Based Complement Alternat Med. 2012, PMCID: PMC3159992.

[1227] Li LT et al, The beneficial effects of the herbal medicine Free and Easy Wanderer Plus (FEWP) and fluoxetine on post-stroke depression. J Altern Complement Med. 2008, PMID: 18721085.

[1228] Zhang LD. Traditional Chinese medicine typing of affective disorders and treatment. Am J Chin Med 1994, PMID: 7872244.

[1229] Meng XZ et al, A Chinese Herbal Formula to Improve General Psychological Status in Posttraumatic Stress Disorder: A Randomized Placebo-Controlled Trial on Sichuan Earthquake Survivors, Evid Based Complement Alternat Med. 2012, PMCID: PMC3199055.

[1230] Woelk H et al, Ginkgo bilboa special extract EGb 761 in generalized anxiety disorder and adjustment disorder with anxious mood: a randomized, double-blind placebo-controlled trial, J Psych Res, 2007, PMID: 16808927.

[1231] Brondino N et al, A Systematic Review and Meta-Analysis of Ginkgo biloba in Neuropsychiatric Disorders: From Ancient Tradition to Modern-Day Medicine, Evidence-Based CAM, 2013, PMID: 23781271, http://goo.gl/zxy5xd.

[1232] Hemmeter U et al, Polysomnographic effects of adjuvant ginkgo biloba therapy in patients with major depression medicated with trimipramine, Pharacopsychiatry, 2001, PMID: 11302564.

[1233] Hopfenmuller W, Evidence for a therapeutic effect of Ginkgo biloba special extract: meta-analysis of 11 clinical studies in patients with cerebrovascular insufficiency in old age, Arzneimittelforschung, 1994, PMID: 7986236.

[1234] Le Bars PL, et al, A placebo-controlled, double-blind, randomized trial of an extract of Ginkgo biloba for dementia. JAMA, 1997, PMID: 9343463.

[1235] **Note**: Recommendation made by Mental Health America (http://goo.gl/fTQlAo). See Drugs RD, 2003, http://goo.gl/7GIRHm.

[1236] Zhang Z et al, Huperzine A as Add-on Therapy in Patients with Treatment-Resistant Schizophrenia: An Open-Labeled Trial, Schizo Res, 2007, PMID: 17383858.

[1237] Li J, Huperzine A for Alzheimer's disease (Review), Cochrane Collaboration, 2009, http://goo.gl/zEOGBE.

[1238] McGregor N, Pueraria lobata (Kudzu root) hangover remedies and acetaldehyde-associated neoplasm risk, Alcohol, 2007, PMID: 17980785, http://goo.gl/Ykt8nW.

[1239] Lukas SE et al, An extract of the Chinese herbal root kudzu reduces alcohol drinking by heavy drinkers in a naturalistic setting, Alcohol Clin Exp Res 2005, PMID: 15897719.

[1240] Shebek J, Rindone JP. A pilot study exploring the effect of kudzu root on the drinking habits of patients with chronic alcoholism. J Alt Comp Med 2000, PMID: 10706235.

[1241] Akhondzadeh S et al, Passionflower in the treatment of generalized anxiety: a pilot double-blind randomized controlled trial with oxazepam. J Clin Pharm Ther, 2001, PMID: 11679026.

[1242] Movafegh A et al, Preoperative oral Passiflora incarnata reduces anxiety in ambulatory surgery patients: a double-blind, placebo-controlled study. Anesth Analg, 2008, PMID: 18499602.

[1243] Bourin M et al, A combination of plant extracts n the treatment of outpatients with adjustment disorder with anxious mood: controlled study versus placebo. Fundam Clin Pharmacol 1997.

[1244] Fiebich BL. Pharmacological studies in an herbal drug combination of St. John's Wort and passion flower: in vitro and vivo of synergy between Hypericum and Passiflora in antidepressant pharmacological models. Fitoterapia 2011, PMID: 21185920.

[1245] Akhondzadeh S et al, Passionflower in the treatment of opiates withdrawal: a double-blind randomized controlled trial, J Clin Pharm Ther, 2001, PMID: 11679027.

[1246] Dwyer AV et al, Herbal medicines, other than St John's wort, in the treatment of depression: a systematic review. Altern Med Rev. 2011, PMID: 21438645.

[1247] Moshiri E. Crocus sativus L. (petal) in the treatment of mild-to-moderate depression: a double-blind, randomized and placebo-controlled trial. Phytomedicine, 2006, PMID: 16979327.

[1248] Panossian A. Pharmacology of Schisandria Chinensis Bail: An overview of Russian research and uses in medicine. Journal of Ethhopharmacology, 2008.

[1249] Aizawa R, Effects of Yoku-kan-san-ka-chimpi-hange on the sleep of normal healthy adult subjects, Psychiatry Clin Neurosci. 2002, PMID: 12047606.

[1250] Fan-Chin Kung, New possibility of traditional Chinese and Japanese medicine as treatment for behavioral and psychiatric symptoms in dementia, Clin Interv Aging. 2012, http://goo.gl/9kA54G.

[1251] Miyaoka T et al, Efficacy and Safety of Yokukansan in Treatment-Resistant Schizophrenia: A Randomized, Double-Blind, Placebo-Controlled Trial (a Positive and Negative Syndrome Scale, Five-Factor Analysis), Psychopharma, 2014, PMID: 24923986.

[1252] Miyaoka I et al, Yokukansan (TJ-54) for Treatment of Very Late Onset Schizophrenia-like Psychosis: An Open-Label Study, Phytomedicine: Int'l J Phytotherapy and Phytopharmacology, 2013, PMID: 23453830.

[1253] Miyaoka T et al, Yi-Gan San as Adjunctive Therapy for Treatment-Resistant Schizophrenia: An Open-Label Study, Clinical Neuropharma 2009, PMID: 19471183.

[1254] Li YJ. Effect of Danzhi Xiaoyao Powder on neuro-immuno-endocrine system in patients with depression. Zhongguo Zhong Xi Yi Jie He Za Zhi 2007, PMID: 17432674.

[1255] Yeung WF. A meta-analysis of the efficacy and safety of traditional Chinese medicine formula Ganmai Dazao decoction for depression. J Ethnopharmacol 2014, PMID: 24632021.

[1256] Shen ZM. Comparative observation on efficacy of jieyu pill and maprotiline in treating depression. Zhongguo Zhong Xi Yi Jie He Za Zhi 2004, PMID: 15199625.

[1257] Ushiroyama T. Efficacy of kampo medicine xiong-gui-tiao-xue-yin (kyuki-chouketsuin), a traditional herbal medicine, in the treatment of maternity blues syndrome in postpartum period. Am J Chin Med 2005.

[1258] WebMD, Use Caution With Ayurvedic Products, http://goo.gl/9YI8H5.

[1259] Singh RH, Singh L, Studies on the anti-anxiety effect of the Medhya Rasayana drug Brahmi (Bacopa monniera Wet.), Journ Res Ayurveda and Siddha, 1980.

[1260] Stough C et al, The chronic effects of an extract of Bacopa monniera (Brahmi) on cognitive function in healthy human subjects. Psychopharm, 2001, PMID: 11498727.

[1261] Calabrese C et al, Effects of a standardized Bacopa monnieri extract on cognitive performance, anxiety, and depression in the elderly: a randomized, double-blind, placebo-controlled trial, J Altern Complement Med, 2008, PMID: 18611150.

[1262] Sarkar S et al, Add-on effect of Brahmi in the management of schizophrenia, J Ayurveda Integr Med, 2012, PMCID: PMC3545244.

[1263] Cochrane Database of Systematic Reviews, 2007, http://goo.gl/6P8hef.

[1264] Sanmukhani J. Efficacy and safety of curcumin in major depressive disorder: A randomized controlled trial. Phytother Res 2013, PMID: 23832433.

[1265] Fiala M et al, Innate immunity and transcription of MGAT-III and Toll-like receptors in Alzheimer's disease patients are improved by bisdemethoxycurcumin, Proc Natl Acad Sci USA, 2007, PMCID: PMC1937555.

[1266] Shah L et al, A comparative study of Geriforte in anxiety neurosis and mixed anxiety-depressive disorders, Probe, 1993, http://goo.gl/fdZhsI.

[1267] Sharma KP, A Placebo-Controlled Trial on the Efficacy of Mentat in Managing Depressive Disorders, Probe, 1993, http://goo.gl/qr2Orl.

[1268] Das S, BR-16 in Schizophrenia, J. Comm. Psychiatry, 1989, http://goo.gl/xWkjh3.
[1269] Trivedi BT, A clinical trial on Mentat, Probe, 1999, http://goo.gl/VDOkBh.
[1270] Kumari R et al, Rauvolfia serpentina L. Benth. ex Kurz.: Phytochemical, Pharmacological and Therapeutic Aspects, Int. J. Pharm. Sci. Rev, 2013, http://goo.gl/QBI4WQ.
[1271] Lopez-Munoz F et al, Historical approach to reserpine discovery and its introduction in psychiatry, Actas Esp Psiquiatr, 2004, PMID: 15529229.
[1272] Christison GW et al, When symptoms persist: choosing among alternative somatic treatments for schizophrenia, Schizophr Bull. 1991, PMID: 1679252, http://goo.gl/XdtNNY.
[1273] Bacher NM et al, Lithium plus reserpine in refractory manic patients,Am J Psych, 1979, PMID: 443466.
[1274] Bertlant JL, Neuroleptics and reserpine in refractory psychosis, J Clin Psychopharmacol, 1986, PMID: 2872238.
[1275] Chengappa KN et al, Randomized Placebo-Controlled Adjunctive Study of an Extract of Withania Somnifera for Cognitive Dysfunction in Bipolar Disorder, J of Clinical Psychiatry, 2013, PMID: 24330893.
[1276] Pratte MA et al, An Alternative Treatment for Anxiety: A Systematic Review of Human Trial Results Reported for the Ayurvedic Herb Ashwagandha (Withania somnifera), J Altern Complement Med. 2014, PMCID: PMC4270108.
[1277] Chandre R. Clinical evaluation of Kushmanda Ghrita in the management of depressive illness. Ayu 2011, PMCID: PMC3296346.
[1278] Costa-Campos L. Antipsychotic-like profile of alstonine. Pharmacology Biochemistry and Behavior, 1998, PMID: 9610935.
[1279] Sotoing Taïwe G, Antipsychotic and Sedative Effects of the Leaf Extract of Crassocephalum Bauchiense (Hutch.) Milne-Redh (Asteraceae) in Rodents. J of Ethnopharmacology, 2012, PMID: 22750453.
[1280] Omogbiya IA. Jobelyn® pretreatment ameliorates symptoms of psychosis in experimental models. J Basic Clin Physiol Pharmacol 2013, PMID: 23412872.
[1281] Wooten V, Effectiveness of yohimbine in treating narcolepsy, Southern Medical Journal, 1994.
[1282] Dominguez RA, Valerian as a hypnotic for Hispanic patients, Cultur Divers Ethnic Minor Psychol. 2000, http://goo.gl/k5K64m.
[1283] Zuardi A et al, Antipsychotic effect of cannabidiol. J. Clin. Psychiatry, 1995, PMID: 7559378.
[1284] Boerner RJ, Case study: Kava is effective in the treatment of anxiety disorder, simple phobia and specific social phobia. - GreenMedInfo Summary, Phytother Res. 2001, http://goo.gl/9U8VgH.
[1285] Lam RW et al, Efficacy of bright light treatment, fluoxetine, and the combination in patients with nonseasonal major depressive disorder: a randomized clinical trial, JAMA Psychiatry, 2016 PMID: 26580307.
[1286] Terman M et al, Light therapy. In: Kryger MH, Roth T, Dement WC, eds. Principles and Practice of Sleep Medicine. 5th ed. St Louis: Elsevier/Saunders; 2010.
[1287] Golen RN, The efficacy of light therapy in the treatment of mood disorders: a review and meta-analysis of the evidence, Am J Psychiatry, 2005, PMID: 15800134.
[1288] Oren DA, Bright Light Therapy for Schizoaffective Disorder, Amer Jof Psychiatry, 2001, PMID: 11729035.
[1289] Medical News today, Panic attacks associated with fear of bright daylight, 2014, http://goo.gl/7DrUCw.
[1290] Barbini B et al, Dark therapy for mania: a pilot study, Bipolar Disord. 2005, PMID: 15654938.
[1291] Phelps J, Dark therapy for bipolar disorder using amber lenses for blue light blockade, Med Hypotheses. 2008, PMID: 17637502.
[1292] Wirz-Justice A, The Implications of Chronobiology for Psychiatry, 2014, Psych Times,http://goo.gl/XLf2Av.
[1293] Evans James, Handbook of Neurofeedback: Dynamics and Clinical Applications, Binghamtom, NY, Haworth Press, 2006.
[1294] Shealy N et al, A comparison of depths of relaxation produced by various techniques and neurotransmitters produced by brainwave entrainment. A study done for Comprehensive Health Care, Shealy and Forest Institute of Professional Psychology, 1989.
[1295] Morrow BK et al, The effect of audio-visual entrainment on seasonal affective disorder in a northern latitude, J of Neurotherapy, 1999, http://goo.gl/E4l3xg.
[1296] Lopez HH et al, Evidence based complementary interventions for insomnia, Hawaii Medical Journal, 2002.
[1297] Yutaka Kaneko, Geriatrics Gerontology Intl., Efficacy of white noise therapy for dementia patients with schizophrenia, 2013, PMID: 23819634.
[1298] Bloch, Boaz, "The Effects of Music Relaxation on Sleep Quality and Emotional Measures in People Living with Schizophrenia." Journal of Music Therapy, 2010.
[1299] Hongratanaworakit T. Relaxing effect of rose oil on humans. Nat Prod Commun 2009, PMID: 19370942.
[1300] Holmes C et al, Lavender oil as treatment for agitated behavior in severe dementia: a placebo controlled study. Int J Geriatr Psychiatry 2002.
[1301] Holmes Clive, Aromatherapy in dementia, Advances in Psychiatric Treatment, 2004, http://goo.gl/XLf2Av.
[1302] Harmon RB, Hydrotherapy in state mental hospitals in the mid-twentieth century, 2009, PMID: 19591022.
[1303] Giannini AJ. Treatment of acute mania with ambient air anionization: variants of climatic heat stress and serotonin syndrome. Psychol Rep 2007, PMID: 17451018.
[1304] Terman M, Controlled trial of naturalistic dawn simulation and negative air ionization for seasonal affective disorder, Am J Psychiatry, 2006, PMID: 17151164.
[1305] Terman M et al, A controlled trial oftimed bright light and negative air ionization for treatment of winter depression, Arch Gen Psychiatry, 1998, PMID: 9783557.
[1306] Terman M et al, Treatment of seasonal affective disorder with a high-output negative ionizer, J Altern Complement Med, 1995, PMID: 9395604.
[1307] Collinge W, Promoting reintegration of National Guard veterans and their partners using a self-directed program of integrative therapies: a pilot study, Mil Med. 2012 Dec, PMCID: PMC3645256.
[1308] Richards D et al, Use of complementary and alternative therapies to promote sleep in critically ill patients, Crit Care Nurs Clin North Am, 2003, PMID: 12943139.
[1309] Kaneko Y et al, Two cases of intractable auditory hallucination successfully treated with sound therapy, Int'l Tinnitus J, 2010, PMID: 21609910, http://goo.gl/xam4Ej.
[1310] Wirz-Justice A et al, Case Report A Rapid-Cycling Bipolar Patient Treated with Long Nights, Bedrest, and Light, Biol Psych, 1999, https://goo.gl/7v4hiF.
[1311] Reti I, ELECTROCONVULSIVE THERAPY TODAY, Johns Hopkins Medicine, p22, http://goo.gl/12RrSw.
[1312] University of Michigan Dept. of Psychiatry, Electroconvulsive Therapy Program How Does ECT Work?, copied 9/23/15, http://goo.gl/QQDTYs.
[1313] APA, The Practice of Electroconvulsive Therapy: Recommendations for Treatment, Training, and Privileging (A Task Force Report of the APA), American Psych Pub, 2008, http://goo.gl/a12Ewb.
[1314] Abrams R (Professor of Psychiatry, The Chicago Medical School), Electroconvulsive Therapy, Oxford University Press, Jun 27, 2002, http://goo.gl/uHsDo9.
[1315] Prudic J et al, Effectiveness of electroconvulsive therapy in community settings, Biol. Psychiatry, 2004, PMID: 14744473, http://goo.gl/u414EB.
[1316] Ross, The sham ECT literature: Implications for consent to ECT, Ethical Human Psychol & Psych, 2006, PMID: 16856307, http://goo.gl/CwGOk3.
[1317] Read J, The effectiveness of electroconvulsive therapy: A literature review, Epidem e Psich Soc, 2010, PMID: 21322506, http://goo.gl/TzDfJ6.
[1318] Read J et al, 'Is electroconvulsive therapy for depression more effective than placebo? A systematic review of studies since 2009.', Ethical Human Psychology and Psychiatry, In Press, 2017, https://goo.gl/KmxeZG.
[1319] Johnstone EC et al, The Northwick Park electroconvulsive therapy trial. Lancet 1980, PMID: 6109147, http://goo.gl/NHapAX.
[1320] Rose D et al, Patients' perspectives on electroconvulsive therapy: systematic review, BMJ. 2003, PMCID: PMC162130.
[1321] Bauer M, Review: electroconvulsive therapy may be an effective short term treatment for people with depression, Evid Based Ment Health. 2003, PMID: 12893794, http://goo.gl/cOVHYb.
[1322] Sackeim H et al, Effects of Stimulus Intensity and Electrode Placement on the Efficacy and Cognitive Effects of Electroconvulsive Therapy, 1993, PMID: 8441428.
[1323] Sackeim H et al, The Cognitive Effects of Electroconvulsive Therapy in Community Settings, Neuropsychopharmacology, 2007, PMID: 16936712, http://goo.gl/DYiMn2.
[1324] Barnes, R Information about ECT (Electro-convulsive therapy), Royal College of Psychiatrists, 2015, http://goo.gl/ZS5oWK, copied 3/10/16.
[1325] Tor PC et al, A systematic review and meta-analysis of brief versus ultrabrief right unilateral electroconvulsive therapy for depression, J Clin Psychiatry. 2015, PMID: 26213985.
[1326] Buchanan R, The 2009 Schizophrenia PORT Psychopharmacological Treatment Recommendations and Summary Statements, Schiz Bulletin, 2010, http://goo.gl/pcS8gO.
[1327] Tharyan P et al, Electroconvulsive therapy for schizophrenia, Cochrane Collaboration, 2005, http://goo.gl/E4kgVG.
[1328] Wall Street Journal, Using Electricity, Magnets for Mental Illness, Jan. 11 2011, http://goo.gl/ENzXUi.
[1329] Lowry F, FDA Panel Wants Electroconvulsive Therapy to Retain High-Risk Class III Status, Medscape, 2011, http://goo.gl/kN57Ad.
[1330] Wilson D, F.D.A. Panel Is Split on Electroshock Risks, The New York Times, 2011, http://goo.gl/NG8hxz.
[1331] FDA Neurological Devices Panel, FDA Executive Summary of the Meeting to Discuss the Classification of Electroconvulsive Therapy Devices (ECT), 2011, http://goo.gl/Y7fHvW.
[1332] Reti I, Electroconvulsive Therapy Today, Johns Hopkins Medicine, copied 9/12/15, http://goo.gl/YlgbPO.
[1333] National Institute for Health and Care Excellence, Guidance on the use of electroconvulsive therapy, 2009, https://goo.gl/UW1Y28.
[1334] DeWilde KE, The promise of ketamine for treatment-resistant depression: current evidence and future directions, Ann N Y Acad Sci. 2015, PMID: 25649308.
[1335] Moore J, The 57th Maudsley Debate: Interview with Professor John Read and Doctor Sue Cunliffe, Mad in America, 2018, https://goo.gl/6xUGGz.
[1336] Persaud R, t: Ruth's experience: Dr Raj Persaud in conversation with Ruth, about her experience of ECT and its effect on her depression, RC Psych podcast, http://goo.gl/QjGWnP.
[1337] Maddock M, Electroshock Causes More Harm Than Good, 2014, Mad in America, http://goo.gl/WA5IKI.
[1338] Rodriguez-Martin JL, Transcranial magnetic stimulation (TMS) for depression, Cochrane Collaborative, 2002, http://goo.gl/Ea9sBY.

[1339] Klein E, Kreinin I, Chistyakov A, et al. Therapeutic efficacy of right prefrontal slow repetitive transcranial magnetic stimulation in major depression: a double-blind controlled study. Arch Gen Psychiatry, 1999, PMID: 10197825.

[1340] Yesavage J et al, Effect of repetitive transcranial magnetic stimulation on treatment-resistant major depression in US veterans: A randomized clinical trial. JAMA Psychiatry, JAMA Psychiatry. 2018, PMID: 29955803.

[1341] Dougall N et al, Transcranial magnetic stimulation (TMS) for the treatment of schizophrenia, Cochrane Collaboration, 2015, http://goo.gl/34zSX8.

[1342] Jin Y, Therapeutic effects of individualized alpha frequency transcranial magnetic stimulation (alphaTMS) on the negative symptoms of schizophrenia, Schizophr Bull. 2006, PMID: 16254067.

[1343] Freitas C et al, Meta-analysis of the effects of repetitive transcranial magnetic stimulation (rTMS) on negative and positive symptoms in schizophrenia, Schizophr Res. 2009, PMCID: 2748189.

[1344] Wassermann E et al, Transcranial Magnetic Brain Stimulation: Therapeutic Promises and Scientific Gaps, Pharmacol Ther, 2013, PMCID: 3241868.

[1345] Lefaucheur, JP et al., Evidence-based guidelines on the therapeutic use of repetitive transcranial magnetic stimulation (rTMS), Clinical Neurophysiology, 2014, PMID: 25034472.

[1346] European College of Neuropsychopharmacology (ECNP), media release, 2017, https://goo.gl/S7LokM.

[1347] Saba G et al, Repetitive transcranial magnetic stimulation as an add-on therapy in the treatment of mania: a case series of eight patients, Psychiatry Res, 2004, PMID: 15488963.

[1348] Grisaru N et al, Transcranial magnetic stimulation in mania: A controlled study. Am J Psychiatry. 1998, PMID: 9812128.

[1349] Eichhammer P et al, Highfrequency repetitive transcranial magnetic stimulation decreases cigarette smoking. J Clin Psychiatry 2003, PMID: 12927012.

[1350] Camprodon JA et al, One session of high frequency repetitive transcranial magnetic stimulation (rTMS) to the right prefrontal cortex transiently reduces cocaine craving. Drug Alcohol Depend 2007, PMID: 16971058.

[1351] B Basil et al, Is There Evidence for Effectiveness of Transcranial Magnetic Stimulation in the Treatment of Psychiatric Disorders?, Psychiatry. 2005, PMC2993526.

[1352] Demitrack M, Med Gadget, The Promise of TMS: Interview with Neuronetics, 2012, http://goo.gl/WOJOwl.

[1353] Demitrack M, A multisite, longitudinal, naturalistic observational study of transcranial magnetic stimulation (TMS) for major deoression in clinical practice, 2013 preliminary abstract, http://goo.gl/8p2Zxb.

[1354] Loo CK, et al. Double-blind controlled investigation of bilateral prefrontal transcranial magnetic stimulation for the treatment of resistant major depression. Psychol Med. 2003, PMID: 12537034.

[1355] Mayo Clinic, as reported in CNN.Com Health Library, Vagus nerve stimulation: A new depression treatment option.

[1356] Univ. of Michigan Department of Psychology, Vagus Nerve Stimulation, www.psych.med.umich.edu/vns.

[1357] Corcoran et al, Vagus nerve stimulation in chronic treatment-resistant depression Preliminary findings of an open-label study, The British Journal of Psychiatry,2006, PMID: 16946367, http://goo.gl/dvgPfq.

[1358] Conway C, as reviewed in Brain and Behavior Research Foundation, May 2013, Brain Imaging Shows How Vagus Nerve Stimulation Improves Symptoms of Depression, http://goo.gl/VnxNaQ.

[1359] University of Michigan Department of Psychology, Vagus Nerve Stimulation, www.psych.med.umich.edu/vns.

[1360] Hein E et al, Auricular transcutaneous electrical nerve stimulation in depressed patients: a randomized controlled pilot study, J Neural Transm, 2013, PMID: 23117749.

[1361] FDA Briefing document, SUMMARY OF SAFETY AND EFFECTIVENESS DATA, http://goo.gl/gK2aMY.

[1362] Mayo Clinic, as reported in CNN.Com Health Library, URL.

[1363] Gershon M, The Second Brain, 1998 Harper Collins as quoted in Scientific American, Think Twice: How the Gut's "Second Brain" Influences Mood and Well-Being,2/24/2010, http://goo.gl/z8wbjh.

[1364] Keltner D, Born to Be Good: The Science of a Meaningful Life (W. W. Norton, 2009), as extracted from Scientific American Interview, http://goo.gl/1oe0G0.

[1365] Science Daily, Unique Type Of MRI Scan Shows Promise In Treating Bipolar Disorder, 2004, http://goo.gl/cYnj9G.

[1366] Rohan M, Low-field magnetic stimulation in bipolar depression using an MRI-based stimulator, Am J Psychiatry. 2004 , http://goo.gl/sDtqqe.

[1367] Pelka RB et al, Impulse magnetic-field therapy for insomnia: a double blind, placebo-controlled study, Advances in Therapy, 2001, PMID: 11571822.

[1368] Johns Hopkins Psychiatry and Behavioral Sciences, Transcranial Direct Current Stimulation, copied 10/13/2016, https://goo.gl/W5kGGq.

[1369] Philip N et al, Low-Intensity Transcranial Current Stimulation in Psychiatry, Am J Psychiatry 2017, https://goo.gl/gDCqoU.

[1370] Arul-Anandam AP et al, Induction of hypomanic episode with transcranial direct current stimulation. J ECT. 2010, PMID: 19483641.

[1371] Brunoni AR et al, Transcranial direct current stimulation (tDCS) in unipolar vs. bipolar depressive disorder, Prog Neuropsychopharm Biol Psych. 2011, PMID: 20854868.

[1372] Brunelin J et al, Examining transcranial direct-current stimulation (tDCS) as a treatment for hallucinations in schizophrenia, Am J Psych, 2012, PMID: 22581236.

[1373] Palm U et al, Prefrontal Transcranial Direct Current Stimulation for Treatment of Schizophrenia With Predominant Negative Symptoms: A Double-Blind, Sham-Controlled Proof-of-Concept Study, Schizophrenia Bulletin, http://goo.gl/OojU9z.

[1374] Orlov ND et al, Stimulating thought: a functional MRI study of transcranial direct current stimulation in schizophrenia, Brain, 2017, https://goo.gl/wdoUkC.

[1375] Meng Z, Transcranial direct current stimulation of the frontal-parietal-temporal area attenuates smoking behavior, J Psychiatr Res. 2014, PMID: 24731752.

[1376] den Uyl TE, Transcranial direct current stimulation, implicit alcohol associations and craving, Biol Psychol. 2015, PMID: 25541515.

[1377] da Silva MC, Behavioral effects of transcranial direct current stimulation (tDCS) induced dorsolateral prefrontal cortex plasticity in alcohol dependence, J Physiol Paris. 2013, PMID: 23891741.

[1378] Boggio PS, Modulation of risk-taking in marijuana users by transcranial direct current stimulation (tDCS) of the dorsolateral prefrontal cortex (DLPFC), Drug and Alcohol Dependence, 2010. PMID: 20729009.

[1379] Agarwal Sri M, Transcranial Direct Current Stimulation in Schizophrenia, Clin Psychopharmacol Neurosci. 2013, PMCID: 3897759.

[1380] Kavirajan HC et al, Alternating current cranial electrotherapy stimulation in the treatment of depression, Cochrane, 2014, https://goo.gl/svw87W.

[1381] Zaghi S et al, Noninvasive brain stimulation with low-intensity electrical currents: putative mechanisms of action for direct and alternating current stimulation, Neuroscientist. 2010, PMID: 20040569, https://goo.gl/SfGBFV.

[1382] Klimke A et al, Case Report: Successful Treatment of Therapy-Resistant OCD with Application of Transcranial Alternating Current Stimulation (tACS), Brain Stimulation, 2016, PMID: 27068232, http://goo.gl/oFxfpJ.

[1383] Pasche B et al, Effects of low energy emission therapy in chronic psychophysiological insomnia, Sleep, 1996, PMID: 8776791.

[1384] Gottlief PD, Successful treatment of post-traumatic stress disorder and chronic pain with paraspinal square wave stimulation, Alternatie Therapies in Health and Medicine, 2004, PMID: 14727505.

[1385] Sokal K et al, Earthing the human body influences physiologic processes, J Altern Complement Med. 2011, PMCID: PMC3154031.

[1386] Chevalier G, The effects of grounding the human body on mood, Psychological Reports: Mental & Physical Health, 2015, https://goo.gl/C0dgHZ.

[1387] Oschman J et al, The effects of grounding (earthing) on inflammation, the immune response, wound healing, and prevention and treatment of chronic inflammatory and autoimmune diseases, J Inflamm Res. 2015, PMCID: PMC4378297.

[1388] Ghaly M et al, The biologic effects of grounding the human body during sleep as measured by cortisol levels and subjective reporting of sleep, pain, and stress, J Altern Complement Med. 2004, PMID: 15650465.

[1389] Chevalier G et al, Earthing: Health Implications of Reconnecting the Human Body to the Earth's Surface Electrons, J Environ Pub Hlth. 2012, PMCID: PMC3265077.

[1390] Heroux M et al, Questionable science and reproducibility in electrical brain stimulation research, Plos One, 2017, PMCID: PMC5405934.

[1391] Rakesh G et al. Monotherapy with tDCS for Schizophrenia: a case report. Brain Stimul. 2013, PMID: 2343387.

[1392] Katsnelson A, Hopeful Currents, Psychology Today, 2015, https://goo.gl/wJipL2.

[1393] Anderson K, Psychiatric Medications Kill More Americans than Heroin, Pro Talk, 2016, https://goo.gl/K41rU4.

[1394] Sharfstein SS, Big Pharma and American Psychiatry: The Good, the Bad, and the Ugly, Psych News 2005, http://goo.gl/IzjQSW.

[1395] Hollins S, Prescribed drugs associated with dependence and withdrawal - building a consensus for action, British Med Assoc Rpt, 2015, http://goo.gl/HejuUD.

[1396] Raghavan R, Psychotropic Medication Use in a National Probability Sample of Children in the Child Welfare System, J of Child and Adolescent Psychopharmacology, 2005, PMID: 15741791.

[1397] R. Raghavan et al. Interstate Variation in Psychotropic Medication Use Among a National Sample of Children in the Child Welfare System, Child Maltreatment, 1998, http://goo.gl/DntPQS.

[1398] L. Leslie et al, Investigating Geographic Variation in Use of Psychotropic Medications Among Youth in Child Welfare, Child Abuse & Neglect, 1998, PMID: 21620160.

[1399] Walsh W et al, Psychotropic Medication Use Among Children in the Child Welfare System, Carsey Institute, 2012, http://goo.gl/rMQ80y.

[1400] Smith BL, Inappropriate prescribing, America Psychological Association, 2012, http://goo.gl/U9OY5e.

[1401] BCBS of Illinois, National Initiative Examines Antipsychotic Drug Use in the Elderly, Open Letter, August 2014, http://goo.gl/HmU3YL.

[1402] Mientka M, Antipsychotic Medications Overprescribed For Everything, From Hyper Children To Nursing Home Residents, Med Daily, 2013, http://goo.gl/aCXHQn.

[1403] James Scully (MD, APA Medical Director and CEO), excerpt from a video of him speaking to the APA's participation in the *Choosing Wisely®* campaign, 2013, http://goo.gl/TrEZdx, copied 2015.

[1404] Lunsky Y et al, Antipsychotic Use With and Without Comorbid Psychiatric Diagnosis Among Adults with Intellectual and Developmental Disabilities, 2017, Canadian J Psych, PMID: 28830241.

[1405] Pharmaceutical Journ, Most GPs are over-prescribing antidepressants, 2004, http://goo.gl/LIHNr2.

[1406] Smith B, Inappropriate prescribing, American Psychological Association, 2012, http://goo.gl/6d2PUY.

[1407] Fournier JC et al, Antidepressant drug effects and depression severity: a patient-level meta-analysis. JAMA. 2010, PMID: 20051569.

[1408] Smith, B, Inappropriate prescribing. Monitor on Psychology, 2012.

[1409] Lane C, Why DSM-5 Concerns European Psychiatrists, Psychology Today, 2013, https://goo.gl/vezKNs.

[1410] Gøtzsche P, Why Few Patients Benefit from Psychiatric Medication, Mad in America Education, copied 1/27/17, https://goo.gl/Rn3Xvi.

[1411] Brauser D, Caffeine Withdrawal Recommended for Inclusion in DSM-5, Medscape, 2011, http://goo.gl/Ko3B7z.

[1412] Insel T, Transforming Diagnosis, National Institute of Mental Health, 2013, https://goo.gl/WOhw5A.

[1413] Encyclopedia of Mental Disorders, Generalized anxiety disorder, 2015, http://goo.gl/pJZRjH.

[1414] Buchanan R et al, The 2009 Schizophrenia PORT Psychopharmacological Treatment Recommendations and Summary Statements, Schiz Bul, 2010, PMC2800144.

[1415] NIH, Medications for patients with first episode psychosis may not meet guidelines, 2014, http://goo.gl/LiKBO3.

[1416] Davis JM, Chen N. Dose response and dose equivalence of antipsychotics. J Clin Psychopharmacol 2004, PMID: 15206667.

[1417] Hiroto I, Polypharmacy and excessive dosing: psychiatrists' perceptions of antipsychotic drug prescription, BJ Psych, 2005, PMID: 16135861, http://goo.gl/A5pL9W.

[1418] Harrington, M et al, The results of a multi-centre audit of the prescribing of antipsychotic drugs for in-patients in the UK. Psych Bulletin, 2002, http://goo.gl/H0JybN.

[1419] Ostrow L et al, Discontinuing psychiatric medications: A survey of long-term users. Psychiatric Services, 2017, https://goo.gl/4hm487.

[1420] Qato DM et al, Prevalence of Prescription Medications With Depression as a Potential Adverse Effect Among Adults in the United States, JAMA. 2018, PMID: 29896627.

[1421] Health Quality Ontario, Looking for balance – antipsychotic medication use in Ontario long-term care homes, http://goo.gl/xNTEhV.

[1422] Frances A, A Debate Between Allen Frances and Robert Whitaker, 2014, http://goo.gl/raAxyd.

[1423] American Psychiatric Association. Position statement. Patient Access to Treatments Prescribed by Their Physicians. 2007, http://goo.gl/CN347f.

[1424] Radley DC et al, Off-label prescribing among office-based physicians. Arch Intern Med. 2006, PMID: 16682577, https://goo.gl/swRvVr.

[1425] Eguale T et al, Association of Off-label Drug Use and Adverse Drug Events in an Adult Population, JAMA, 2016, PMID: 26523731.

[1426] Haw, C et al, A survey of the off-label use of mood stabilizers in a large psychiatric hospital. J of Psychopharmacology, 2005, PMID: 15982996.

[1427] Hodgson R et al, Off-label prescribing by psychiatrists. Psychiatric Bulletin, 2006, http://goo.gl/Fjrt8a.

[1428] Mojtabai R et al, Proportion Of Antidepressants Prescribed Without A Psychiatric Diagnosis Is Growing, Health Affairs, 2011, PMID: 21821561, https://goo.gl/mbXzFb.

[1429] US Department of Veterans Affairs, PTSD: National Center for PTSD, copied 10/2/2016, https://goo.gl/ESwJDA.

[1430] Krystal J et al, Adjunctive Risperidone Treatment for Antidepressant-Resistant Symptoms of Chronic Military Service–Related PTSD, JAMA 2011, PMID: 21813427, http://goo.gl/q8hF3S.

[1431] French D et al, How Well do Psychotropic Medications Match Mental Health Diagnoses? A National View of Potential Off-Label Prescribing in VHA Nursing Homes, Oxford University Press, 2007, PMID: 17158114, http://goo.gl/43nFaO.

[1432] Weiss, E et al,Off-label use of antipsychotic drugs. J of ClinicPsychopharmacology, 2000, PMID: 11106144.

[1433] Chen DT et al, U.S. physician knowledge of the FDA-approved indications and evidence base for commonly prescribed drugs: results of a national survey, Pharmacoepidemiology and Drug Safety, 2009, PMID: 19697444.

[1434] Kukreja S et al, Polypharmacy In Psychiatry: A Review, Mens Sana Monogr. 2013, PMCID: PMC3653237; Medical Directors Council and State Medicaid Directors. Alexandria, Virginia: 2001. National Association of State Mental Health Program Directors; Technical Report on Psychotropic Polypharmacy.

[1435] Kreyenbuhl J, Long-Term Antipsychotic Polypharmacy in the VA Health System: Patient Characteristics and Treatment Patterns, Psych Sycs 2007, PMC3673552.

[1436] Kingsbury S, Psychopharmacology: Rational and Irrational Polypharmacy, Psychiatric Times, Aug 2001, PMID: 11474046, http://goo.gl/PFE3Rk.

[1437] Kingsbury S, Psychiatric Polypharmacy: The Good, the Bad, and the Ugly, Psychiatric Times, 1007, http://goo.gl/KlIsId.

[1438] Akici A, Rational pharmacotherapy and pharmacovigilance, Curr Drug Saf. 2007, PMID: 18690951.

[1439] Preskorn SH et al, Polypharmacy: when is it rational? J Psychiatr Pract, 2007, 17414685.

[1440] Kukreja S et al, Polypharmacy In Psychiatry: A Review, Mens Sana Monogr. 2013, PMCID: PMC3653237.

[1441] Hunt L et al, The Changing Face of Chronic Illness Management in Primary Care: A Qualitative Study of Underlying Infl uences and Unintended Outcomes, ANNALS OF FAMILY MEDICINE, 20120, http://goo.gl/mZ7uw1.

[1442] Lapham's Quarterly Journal, Charts & Graph's, graphic concept from "The Pfizer Circle of Hell", Fall 2009, http://goo.gl/OD2gOi, copied 3/16/2016.

[1443] American Society for Consultant Pharamacists, The Prescribing Cascade, https://goo.gl/P5z4uJ, copied 3/21/2016.

[1444] Frye MA et al, The increasing use of polypharmacy for refractory mood disorders: 22 years of study, J Clin Psychiatry, 2000, http://goo.gl/VRvRdW.

[1445] Patrick V et al, Antipsychotic polypharmacy: is there evidence for its use? J Psychiatr Pract 2005, PMID: 16041235.

[1446] Waddington JL, Mortality in schizophrenia. Antipsychotic polypharmacy and absence of adjunctive anticholinergics over the course of a 10-year prospective study, Br J Psychiatry 1998, PMID: 9926037.

[1447] Joukamaa M et al, Schizophrenia, neuroleptic medication and mortality. Br J Psychiatry, 2006, PMID: 16449697.

[1448] Ito H et al, Polypharmacy and excessive dosing: psychiatrists' perceptions of antipsychotic drug prescription. Br J Psychiatry. 2005, PMID: 16135861.

[1449] Correll CU et al, Does antipsychotic polypharmacy increase the risk for metabolic syndrome?, Schizophr Res. 2007, PMCID: PMC2718048.

[1450] Paton C et al, Patterns of antipsychotic and anticholinergic prescribing for hospital inpatients. J Psychopharmacol. 2003, PMID: 12870571.

[1451] Correll CU et al, Efficacy of 42 pharmacologic cotreatment strategies added to antipsychotic monotherapy in schizophrenia: Systematic overview and quality appraisal of the meta-analytic evidence, 2017, JAMA Psychiatry, PMID: 28514486.

[1452] Kukreja S et al, Polypharmacy In Psychiatry: A Review, Mens Sana Monogr. 2013, PMCID: PMC3653237.

[1453] Mojtabai R et al, National Trends in Psychotropic Medication Polypharmacy in Office-Based Psychiatry, Arch Gen Psych. 2010, PMID: 20048220, http://goo.gl/1jlYk0.

[1454] American Psychiatric Association, Five Things Physicians and Patients Should Question, Choosing Wisely, 2015, http://goo.gl/t3blZ8.

[1455] Thompson W et al, Deprescribing: What Is It and What Does the Evidence Tell Us?, Can J Hosp Pharm. 2013, PMCID: PMC3694945.

[1456] Plakiotis C et al, Deprescribing psychotropic medications in aged care facilities: the potential role of family members, Adv Exp Med Biol. 2015, PMID: 25416108.

[1457] Durkin M, When less is more: De-prescribing medications, ACP Hospitalist, 2016, https://goo.gl/mwCnKc.

[1458] Hideaki T, Interventions to reduce antipsychotic polypharmacy: A systematic review, Elsevier Schizophrenia Research, http://goo.gl/WAIY4h.

[1459] Protection & Advocacy, Inc, Psychiatric Polypharmacy: A Word of Caution, 2004, http://goo.gl/HI0UEa.

[1460] Gurevich M, Medication-free Alternatives for Long-term Maintenance of Bipolar Disorder: A Case Series, Glob Adv Health Med. 2015, PMCID: 4424923.

[1461] SAMHSA, Working Definition of Recovery, https://goo.gl/H8wStv.

[1462] Improving the Quality of Health Care for Mental and Substance-Use Conditions: Quality Chasm Series, National Academies Press, 2006, https://goo.gl/TJsbNM.

[1463] Sarris J et al, Herbal Medicine in Depression, Anxiety and Insomnia: A Review of Psychopharmacology and Clinical Evidence, U of Mel, http://goo.gl/HW6w71. .

[1464] Agency for Healthcare Research and Quality, Design and Implementation of N-of-1 Trials: A User's Guide, 2014, http://goo.gl/fKaYlI.

[1465] UYEMURA B, Should You Consider Alternative Treatments for Anxiety Disorders?, PsychCentral, 2011, http://goo.gl/atTwYt.

[1466] Holmes SE et al, Elevated Translocator Protein in Anterior Cingulate in Major Depression and a Role for Inflammation in Suicidal Thinking: A Positron Emission Tomography Study, Biological Psych, 2017, https://goo.gl/QvmHMV.

[1467] Schwartz J et al, Ketamine for treatment-resistant depression: recent developments and clinical applications, Evid Based Ment Health. 2016, PMID: 27053196.

[1468] Hu XH et al, Incidence and duration of side effects and those rated as bothersome with selective serotonin reuptake inhibitor treatment for depression: patient report versus physician estimate. J Clin Psych. 2004, PMID: 15291685.

[1469] Kelly K et al, Toward achieving optimal response: understanding and managing antidepressant side effects, Dialogues Clin Neurosci, 2008, PMC3181894.

[1470] Khan, A et al, Antidepressants versus placebo in major depression: an overview. World Psychiatry, 2015, PMCID: PMC4592645.

[1471] Ghaemi SN, Seasonal Affective Disorder (SAD): Facts and Misconceptions, Medscape, 2016, https://goo.gl/4htV34.

[1472] Firth J et al, The effects of vitamin and mineral supplementation on symptoms of schizophrenia: a systematic review and meta-analysis, Psychol Med. 2017, PMID: 28202095.

[1473] Read J et al, Childhood trauma, psychosis and schizophrenia: a literature review with theoretical and clinical implications, Acta Psychiatr Scand 2005, PMID: 16223421.

[1474] Read et al, Negative childhood experiences and mental health: theoretical, clinical and primary prevention implications, Brit J Psych, 2012, PMID: 22297585; Bailey T et al, Childhood Trauma Is Associated With Severity of Hallucinations and Delusions in Psychotic Disorders: A Systematic Review and Meta-Analysis, Schizophrenia bulletin, 2018, PMID: 29301025.

[1475] Shevlin et al, Cumulative Traumas and Psychosis: an Analysis of the National Comorbidity Survey and the British Psychiatric Morbidity Survey, Schizophr Bull. 2008, PMCID: PMC2632373.

[1476] Garety P, The future of psychological therapies for psychosis, 2003, World Psychiatry, PMCID: PMC1525111.

[1477] Husa AP et al, Lifetime antipsychotic medication and cognitive performance in schizophrenia at age 43 years in a general population birth cohort, Psychiatry Res. 2016, PMID: 27888683.

[1478] Harding CM, The Vermont longitudinal study of persons with severe mental illness, II: Long-term outcome of subjects who retrospectively met DSM-III criteria for schizophrenia, Am J Psychiatry. 1987, PMID: 3591992.

[1479] Morgan C et al, Reappraising the Long-term Course and Outcome of Psychotic Disorders The ÆSOP-10 Study, Psychol Med. 2014, PMCID: PMC4134320.

[1480] Wils RS et al, Antipsychotic medication and remission of psychotic symptoms 10 years after a first-episode psychosis, 2016, Schiz Res, https://goo.gl/iNTdkW.

[1481] Murray G et al, The clinical significance of creativity in bipolar disorder, Clin Psychol Rev, 2012, PMCID: PMC3409641.

[1482] Palmier-Claus JE et al, Relationship between childhood adversity and bipolar affective disorder: systematic review and meta-analysis, BJPsych, 2016, https://goo.gl/tuOQLl.

[1483] Johns Hopkins Medicine, Beef Jerky and Other Processed Meats Associated with Manic Episodes, copied on 7/26/18 from https://goo.gl/iC8GSH.

[1484] DiazGranados N et al, Rapid Resolution of Suicidal Ideation after a Single Infusion of an NMDA Antagonist in Patients with Treatment-Resistant Major Depressive Disorder, J Clin Psychiatry. 2010, PMCID: PMC3012738.

[1485] Sachs GS et al, Effectiveness of Adjunctive Antidepressant Treatment for Bipolar Depression, N Engl J Med. 2007, PMID: 17392295.

[1486] Etain B et al, Childhood Trauma Is Associated With Severe Clinical Characteristics of Bipolar Disorders, J Clin Psych, 2013, PMID: 24229750.

[1487] **Note: Bipolar Drug Benefits, Risks, and Limitations.** [1] See www.OnwardMentalHealth.com/definitions. [2] Weinstock LM et al, Medication burden in bipolar disorder: a chart review of patients at psychiatric hospital admission. Psychiatry Res. 2014, PMCID: PMC3968952. [3] Gazalle FK et al, Polypharmacy and suicide attempts in bipolar disorder, Rev Bras Psiquiat, 2007, PMID: 17435926, https://goo.gl/4nC2S1. [4] Alda M et al, Is Monotherapy as Good as Polypharmacy in Long-Term Treatment of Bipolar Disorder?, Can J Psychiatry. 2009, PMID: 19961659, https://goo.gl/ZqpHbq. [5] Glick I, Undiagnosed Bipolar Disorder: New Syndromes and New Treatments, Prim Care Companion J Clin Psychiatry. 2004, PMCID: PMC427610. [6] Duckworth K, The Sensible Use of Psychiatric Medications, NAMI Advocate, Winter 2013, https://goo.gl/GMluSU. [7] Judd LL et al, The long-term natural history of the weekly symptomatic status of bipolar I disorder. Arch Gen Psychiatry. 2002, PMID: 12044195. Judd LL et al. Long-term symptomatic status of bipolar I vs. bipolar II disorders. Int J Neuropsychopharmacol. 2003, PMID: 12890306. [37]. This statement is equivalent to saying that bipolar drugs have overall ARRs in the 15%-25% range. [38] Dell'Osso B et al, Bridging the gap between education and appropriate use of benzodiazepines in psychiatric clinical practice, Neuropsychiatr Dis Treat. 2015, PMCID: PMC4525786. Cascade EF et al, Antidepressants in Bipolar Disorder, Psychiatry (Edgmont). 2007, PMCID: PMC2922360. [39] Hitti M, WebMD, Epilepsy Drugs Get Suicide Risk Warning, https://goo.gl/WK8FqE. Bielefeldt AØ et al, Precursors to suicidality and violence on antidepressants: systematic review of trials in adult healthy volunteersJ R Soc Med. 2016, PMC5066537. [40] Duckworth K, Prescribed Benzodiazepines and Suicide Risk: A Review of the Literature, Prim Care Companion CNS Disord. 2017, PMID: 28257172. [41] Koranyi EK et al, Physical illnesses underlying psychiatric symptoms, Psycho Psychosom. 1992, PMID: 1488499, http://goo.gl/V9Wi23. [42] Brown R et al, How to Use Herbs, Nutrients and Yoga in Mental Health Care, WW Norton & Co, 2009, http://goo.gl/cWlG0g. [43] Duckworth K, The Sensible Use of Psychiatric Medications, NAMI Advocate Magazine, Winter 2013, https://goo.gl/GMluSU.

[1488] Cipriani A, Lithium in the prevention of suicide in mood disorders: updated systematic review and meta-analysis, BMJ. 2013, PMID: 23814104.

[1489] Carman JS et al, Calcium: Bivalent cation in the bivalent psychoses, Biol Psychiatry, 1979, PMID: 476221.

[1490] Attenburrow MJ et al, Chromium treatment decreases the sensitivity of 5-HT2A receptors, Psychopharmacology, 2002, PMID: 11823896.

[1491] Mebane AH, L-Glutamine and mania, Am J Psychiatry, 1984, PMID: 6486273.

[1492] Carney MWP et al, The switch mechanism in affective illness and oral S-adenosylmethionine (SAM), Br J Psychiatry, 1987.

[1493] Kaustubh GJ et al, Mania and Psychosis Associated with St. John's Wort and Ginseng, Psychiatry (Edgmont). 2005, PMCID: 2993537.

[1494] Vazquez I et al, Herbal products and serious side effects: a case of ginseng-induced manic episode, Acta Psychiatr Scand, 2002, PMID: 12086230.

[1495] Jamison K, An Unquiet Mind, Vintage Books, 1995.

[1496] **Note:** Levinson H, "Phobia Free" is perhaps the best introduction to inner ear/anxiety issues. Also, Nagaratnam N, The vestibular dysfunction and anxiety disorder interface: a descriptive study with special reference to the elderly, Arch Gerontol Geriatr, 2005.

[1497] Scarmeas N et al, Mediterranean diet and risk for Alzheimer's disease, Ann Neurol 2006, PMCID: PMC3024594.

[1498] Larson EB et al, Exercise is associated with reduced risk for incident dementia among persons 65 years of age and older, Annals of Int Med 2006, PMID: 16418406.

[1499] Brechin et al, Alternatives to antipsychotic medication: Psychological approaches in managing psychological and behavioural distress in people with dementia, 2013, British Psychological Society, https://goo.gl/HU5W7v.

[1500] Beasley JD et al, Follow-up cohort of alcoholic patients through 12 months of comprehensive biobehavioral treatment, J Subst Abuse 1991, PMID: 1660078.

[1501] Guenther RM, Role of nutritional therapy in alcoholism treatment, Int J Biosoc Res, 1983, http://goo.gl/9AZep9.

[1502] Patkarr AA et al, Transdermal selegiline, Drugs Today (Barc) 2007.

[1503] Knibb RC et al, Psychological characteristics of people with perceived food intolerance in a community sample, J Psychosom Res, 1999.

[1504] Slade M, Mental illness and well-being: the central importance of positive psychology and recovery approaches, BMC Hlth Svcs Research, 2010, http://goo.gl/fOIbG3. Mr. Slade referenced: Keyes CLM, Lopez SJ: Toward a Science of Mental health. Handbook of Positive Psychology, .2002.

[1505] Yogananda P, Where there is Light, Self-Realization Fellowship, 1988.

[1506] Insel, TR, Translating scientific opportunity into public health impact: A strategic plan for research on mental illness. Archives of

[1507] Sprooten E et al, Addressing reverse inference in psychiatric neuroimaging: Meta-analyses of task-related brain activation in common mental disorders, Hum Brain Mapp. 2017, PMID: 28067006.

[1508] De Hert M et al, Physical illness in patients with severe mental disorders. I. Prevalence, impact of medications and disparities in health care, World Psychiatry. 2011, http://goo.gl/awbVFo.

[1509] Walsh W, Evaluation & treatment of over- and under-methylation in the psychiatric population, Walsh Research Institute, 2015, https://goo.gl/aO3nbp.

[1510] Bains AS, Abnormal calcium level in a psychiatric presentation? Rule out parathyroid disease, Current Psychiatry 2015, http://goo.gl/JRWg.

[1511] Moyer M, It's Not Dementia, It's Your Heart Medication: Cholesterol Drugs and Memory, Scientific American, 2010, https://goo.gl/AQbgJV.

[1512] Pan LA et al, Neurometabolic Disorders: Potentially Treatable Abnormalities in Patients With Treatment-Refractory Depression and Suicidal Behavior, Am J Psych, online pub, http://goo.gl/B79g2A.

[1513] FDA, FDA permits marketing of mobile medical application for substance use disorder, 2017, FDA News Release, https://goo.gl/fpdZHZ.

[1514] SAMHSA National Registry of Evidence-based Programs and Practices, Matrix Model, http://goo.gl/QqGTDW.

[1515] Rawson RA et al, An intensive outpatient approach for cocaine abuse treatment: The Matrix model. J of Substance Abuse Treatment, 1995, PMID: 7623389.

[1516] Matrix Institute of Addictions, Matrix model success rates, copied from http://goo.gl/fIoILh on 9/5/15.

[1517] Rawson RA et al, A multi-site comparison of psychosocial approaches for the treatment of methamphetamine dependence, Addiction. 2004, PMID: 15139869.

[1518] Cook J, Copeland ME et al, Initial Outcomes of a Mental Illness Self-Management Program Based on Wellness Recovery Action Planning, PSYCHIATRIC SERVICES 2009, PMID: 19176420.

[1519] Ziqiang L, Effectiveness of illness self-management programmes for adults with schizophrenia and other psychotic disorders: a systematic review, http://goo.gl/y3wkYs.

[1520] Jungfer, H et al, Reduction of Seclusion on a Hospital-Wide Level: Successful Implementation of a Less Restrictive Policy. J Psych Res, 2014, PMID: 24726637.

[1521] Stovall J, Is assertive community treatment ethical care?, Harv Rev Psychiatry, 2009, PMID: 11287409.

[1522] Watts J, Phenomenological account of users' experiences of ACT, Bioethics 2002, http://goo.gl/kSLo8l.

[1523] Scott JE, Assertive community treatment and case management for schizophrenia. Schizophr Bull 1995, PMID: 8749892.

[1524] Kisely S et al, Compulsory community and involuntary outpatient treatment for people with severe mental disorders, Cochrane DB Sys Rev. 2011, PMC4164937.

[1525] Rand Corp Health Division, Does Involuntary Outpatient Treatment Work?, 2000, http://goo.gl/AVoipW.

[1526] Burns T et al, Community treatment orders for patients with psychosis (OCTET): a randomised controlled trial, Lancet, 2013, https://goo.gl/5kM3U.

[1527] Coldwell C et al, The Effectiveness of Assertive Community Treatment for Homeless Populations With Severe Mental Illness: A Meta-Analysis, Am J Psychiatry. 2007, PMID: 17329462.

[1528] Brodsky M, Residential Treatment – When to Consider It, What to Look For, Social Work Today, 2012, http://goo.gl/of5czf.

[1529] NAMI, Dual Diagnosis and Integrated Treatment of Mental Illness and Substance Abuse Disorder, https://goo.gl/WEhd9e.

380 *References*

[1530] Hopper,K, Deviance and dwelling space: Notes on the resettlement of homeless persons with alcohol and drug problems. Cont Drug Problems, 1989.
[1531] Hellerstein,D. J. & Meehan,B. (1987). Outpatient group therapy for schizophrenic substance abusers. Amer Journal of Psych, PMID: 3661769.
[1532] Martino S, Dual Diagnosis Motivational Interviewing: a modification of Motivational Interviewing for substance-abusing patients with psychotic disorders, J Subs Abuse Treat. 2002, PMCID: PMC3865805.
[1533] Bien TH, Miller WR, Boroughs JM. Motivational interviewing with alcohol outpatients. Behavioural and Cognitive Psychotherapy. 1993.
[1534] Kemper K, CAM Therapies to Promote Healthy Moods. Pediatric clinics of North Amer 2007, PMCID: PMC2329575.
[1535] Krall EA et al, Smoking and bone loss among postmenopausal women, J Bone Miner Res, 1991, PMID: 1858519.
[1536] Kuhnert BR et al, The effect of maternal smoking on the relationship between maternal and fetal zinc status and infant birth weight, J Am Coll Nutr, 1988, PMID: 3209781.
[1537] Hall SM et al, Weight gain prevention and smoking cessation: Cautionary findings, Am J Public Health, 1992, PMCID: PMC1694191.
[1538] Stead LF et al, Can nicotine replacement therapy (NRT) help people quit smoking?, Cochrane Group, PMID: 23152200.
[1539] Fucito LM, Addressing the evidence for FDA nicotine replacement therapy label changes: a policy statement of the Association for the Treatment of Tobacco use and Dependence and the Society for Research on Nicotine and Tobacco, Nicotine Tob Res. 2014, PMID: 24919399.
[1540] Stead LF et al, Group behaviour therapy programmes for smoking cessation, Cochrane Database Syst Rev 2005, PMID: 15846610.
[1541] Spiegel D et al, Predictors of smoking abstinence following a single-session restructuring intervention with self-hypnosis, Am J Psych, 1993, PMID: 8317582.
[1542] Elkins G et al, Intesnsive hypnotherapy for smoking cessation: a prospective study, Int J Clin Exp Hypn, 2006, PMID: 16766441.
[1543] Davis JM et al, A pilot study on mindfulness based stress reduction for smokers, BMC Complement Altern Med, 2007, PMCID: PMC1794538.
[1544] Wynd CA, Personal power imagery and relaxation techniques used in smoking cessation programs, Am J Health Promot, 1992, PMID: 10148676.
[1545] Wynd CA, Guided health imagery for smoking cessation and long-term abstinence, J Nurs Scholarsh, 2005, PMID: 16235865.
[1546] He D et al, Effects of acupuncture on smoking cessation or reduction for motivated smokers, Prev Med, 1997, PMID: 9085389.
[1547] Christakis N et al, Quitting in Droves: Collective Dynamics of Smoking Behavior in a Large Social Network, NEJM, 2008, PMCID: PMC2822344.
[1548] USA Today, Veteran stress cases up sharply, 10/22/2007, http://goo.gl/IALbtb.
[1549] Seal KH, Bringing the war back home: mental health disorders among 103,788 US veterans returning from Iraq and Afghanistan seen at Department of Veterans Affairs facilities, Arch Intern Med. 2007, PMID: 17353495.
[1550] Jeff Hargarten et al, Veteran Suicides Twice as High as Civilian Rates, News21, 2013. Retrieved: 12/25/14.
[1551] Mission Reconnect (www.MissionReconnect.com). Kahn JR, Post-9/11 Veterans and Their Partners Improve Mental Health Outcomes with a Self-directed Mobile and Web-based Wellness Training Program: A Randomized Controlled Trial, J Med Internet Res. 2016, PMC5059485.
[1552] Veterans Stress Project, VA Therapists offering Energy Psychology, http://goo.gl/m8yV3j.
[1553] Yount RA et al, Service dog training program for treatment of posttraumatic stress in service members, US Army Med Dep J. 2012, PMID: 22388685.
[1554] Joan Esnayra, quoted from ABC News, Dog Helps Man Manage PTSD Symptoms, 2011, http://goo.gl/vwVqzy.
[1555] Mawanda F et al, PTSD, Psychotropic Medication Use, and the Risk of Dementia Among US Veterans: A Retrospective Cohort Study, J Am Geriatric Soc, 2017, https://goo.gl/1psWYU.
[1556] **Note**: The Diagnostic and Statistical Manual of Mental Disorders, Fifth Edition (DSM-5) is the American Psychiatric Association's widely criticized classification and diagnostic tool.. A research specialist calls it "astonishingly arbitrary" (Caplan P, http://goo.gl/1UJZxA). There is little scientific underpinning and the pharmaceutical industry has had significant influence on content (psychiatric diagnoses are created by an APA committee, 69 percent of whom have financial ties to Big Pharma, https://goo.gl/inmdpv). This criticism resulted in an open letter of protest from the American Psychological Association signed by 13,000 people. Additionally, the Director of the NIMH indicates that the DSM-5 has a "weakness [in] its lack of validity... It is critical to realize that we cannot succeed if we use DSM categories as the 'gold standard'." (Insel T, Director's Blog: Transforming Diagnosis, April 29, 2013).
[1557] Simson SD, Is the randomized clinical trial the gold standard of research?, J Androl. 2001, http://goo.gl/cN6zoq.

CPSIA information can be obtained
at www.ICGtesting.com
Printed in the USA
LVHW031729090519
617265LV00014B/1180